Concise Medical Textbo

Ophthalmology

Concise Medical Textbooks

Antimicrobial Chemotherapy / Greenwood

Biochemistry / Ottaway & Apps

Cardiology / Julian

Community Health, Preventive Medicine and Social Services / Meredith Davies

Dermatology / Pegum & Harvey Baker

Embryology / Craigmyle & Presley

Gastroenterology / Bouchier

Geriatrics / Hamdy

Introduction to General Practice / Drury & Hull

Medical Microbiology / Thomas

Obstetrics and Gynaecology / Taylor & Brush

Ophthalmology / Wybar & Kerr Muir

Paediatrics / Apley

Pathology / Tighe & Davies

Pharmacology / Penn

Psychiatry / Trethowan & Sims

Renal Medicine / Gabriel

Respiratory Medicine / Flenley

Rheumatology / Grennan

Sociology as Applied to Medicine / Patrick & Scambler

Ophthalmology

Kenneth Wybar

MD, ChM, FRCS

Former Ophthalmic Surgeon, The Hospital for Sick Children, Great Ormond Street, and the Royal Marsden Hospital. Surgeon, Moorfields Eye Hospital. Lecturer in Ophthalmology, University of London. Civilian Consultant in Ophthalmology, The Royal Navy

Malcolm Kerr Muir

MRCP, FRCS, DTM&H

Lecturer in Clinical Ophthalmology, Moorfields Eye Hospital, London. Honorary Lecturer, School of Tropical Medicine, Liverpool

Third Edition

Baillière Tindall

London   Philadelphia   Toronto
Mexico City   Rio de Janeiro   Sydney   Tokyo   Hong Kong

Baillière Tindall 1 St Anne's Road
W.B. Saunders Eastbourne, East Sussex BN21 3UN, England

West Washington Square
Philadelphia, PA 19105, USA

1 Goldthorne Avenue
Toronto, Ontario M8Z 5T9, Canada

Apartado 26370— Cedro 512
Mexico 4, DF Mexico

Rua Evaristo da Veiga 55, 20° andar
Rio de Janeiro – RJ, Brazil

ABP Australia Ltd, 44–50 Waterloo Road
North Ryde, NSW 2113, Australia

Ichibancho Central Building, 22–1 Ichibancho
Chiyoda-ku, Tokyo 102, Japan

10/fl, Inter-Continental Plaza, 94 Granville Road
Tsim Sha Tsui East, Kowloon, Hong Kong

First published 1966
Second edition 1974
Third edition 1984

Typeset by MML
Printed in Great Britain at the Alden Press, Oxford

British Library Cataloguing in Publication Data

Wybar, K.
    Ophthalmology.—3rd ed.—(concise
    medical textbooks)
    1. Eye — Diseases and defects
    I. Title   II. Kerr Muir, M.
    617.7   RE46

ISBN 0-7020-1005-7

Contents

Preface

In the Preface to the first edition of this series of Concise Medical Textbooks dealing with Ophthalmology in April, 1966, I indicated that the purpose of the book was to provide a factual, and yet concise account of the essential features of the practice of ophthalmology at that time with regard to the medical student who is without any previous experience of the subject, to the general practitioner who is concerned with the recognition and day-to-day management of the more common ophthalmic disorders, and to the specialist in some other branch of medicine or surgery who is aware of the impact of the recognition of an ocular disorder in an adequate assessment of certain forms of systemic disease.

In the Preface to the second edition of this series in March, 1974, I indicated that the scope of the book had been increased because of the interest which had been shown by the postgraduate student working for the Diploma or Fellowship examination of the Royal College of Surgeons, and even by the established ophthalmic surgeon who wanted a comprehensive and yet concise evaluation of a particular topic. Several alterations and additions were made to the original text in 1974, but recently it become apparent that the ever-increasing knowledge of many ophthalmic disorders—the role of the immune and autoimmune influences in certain surface and intraocular conditions, the role of lensectomy and vitrectomy, the role of laser therapy in retinal disease, etc.—demanded a considerable rewriting of the original text.

I am delighted, therefore, that Mr Malcolm Kerr Muir agreed to join me in producing this third edition, and I have every confidence that it will be received with enthusiasm in a similar way to the previous two editions.

KENNETH WYBAR

Acknowledgements

We are most grateful to Dr P. Hansell, Director of the Medical Illustration Department of the Institute of Ophthalmology, and to Mr T. Tarrant of that department who so skilfully prepared the original illustrations and diagrams from rough sketches. Many of these have been used in previous editions and other publications, and we should like to thank the following publishers for permission to use them again: H.K. Lewis & Co. Ltd for Figs 50–57 from Lyle and Wybar's *Practical Orthoptics in the Treatment of Squint*; The National Society of Children's Nurseries for Fig. 58 from *The Eyes in the Early Years of Life* (1963); The Ophthalmological Society of the United Kingdom for Figs 76–81 and 84–92 from *The Functional Anatomy of the Afferent Visual Pathways* (1962); and Mr R. Hill and Mrs J. Howe for Fig. 93.

We should also like to thank Mr Tarrant for having supplied the drawings for Figs 16, 17, 21, 22, 30, 32, 36, 37, 38, 39, 40, 41, 42, 43, 44, 45, 46, 47, 48, 66, 68, 72 and 75; Sir Stephen Miller and *The Practitioner* for Figs 71 and 74; Marie Restori for Fig. 69; Dr Glyn Lloyd for Fig. 70; and Kulwant Sehmi for Figs 31, 33 and 35. Fig. 1 from *Ophthalmic Nursing* by Vera H. Darling and Margaret R. Thorpe and Figs 7, 9, 10 and 49 from May & Worth's *Manual of Diseases of the Eye* by Mr Keith Lyle and Mr A.G. Cross are reproduced with permission of the publishers, Baillière Tindall. The manuscript was patiently prepared by Miss C. Smyth, to whom we are greatly indebted.

KENNETH WYBAR

February 1984 MALCOLM KERR MUIR

1

Basic Methods of Examination

A distinctive feature of the art and science of ophthalmology is the comparative ease with which many parts of the eye may be examined in detail using relatively simple techniques. It follows that the ophthalmologist is frequently able to come to precise conclusions on the state of health or disease of the various parts of the eye during a purely routine examination, and for this reason it is essential to adopt systematic methods of examination at all times. Indeed it is likely that more errors in diagnosis are made as a result of an inadequate method of examination leading to a failure to detect the true nature of the lesion rather than as a result of ignorance of its exact significance.

Most of the special methods of examination which are applied to the different parts of the eye are described in the separate chapters dealing with the diseases of these structures, but there are various more general methods of examination which are considered here.

General assessment of the patient

Before proceeding to an examination of the eyes, it is important to make an assessment of the patient as a whole, including the general physique, the state of well-being, the facial expression and complexion, the position of the head, and the gait.

Methods of illumination

Diffuse illumination

This is a diffuse and even type of illumination which is achieved using daylight from a conveniently situated window or artificial light from an electric light source, and it provides a general view of the patient and of the eye, thus obviating the danger of overlooking some fairly obvious defect by concentrating too rapidly on the more localized methods of illumination.

Focal illumination

This is a concentrated and usually bright type of illumination which is directed to particular parts of the eye so that they are revealed with

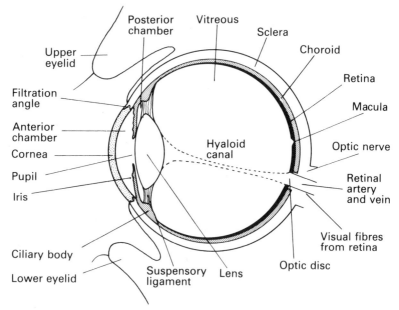

Fig. 1.   The normal eye in horizontal section.

great clarity against the relatively dark background of the other structures. It is achieved by the use of a projection lamp which incorporates a condensing lens within its own case, for example the 'pen' torch or the ophthalmoscope which is held by the examiner so that a focused beam of light is directed to a certain part of the eye.

The examination of the eye by focal illumination is enhanced by the use of some form of magnification. For many years emphasis was placed on the use of the uniocular loupe. However, this particular method of eye examination has largely fallen into abeyance as the result of the ready availability of the slit-lamp microscope which provides a much more precise examination.

The slit-lamp microscope. The slit-lamp microscope is an essential instrument in the critical examination of the fine structural details of both the anterior and posterior segments of the eye (Fig. 1). It is also available in a portable and hand-held form, the latter being particularly useful for field and survey work.

The beam of light from the slit lamp is maintained accurately in focus on different parts of the eye by means of a movable mechanical arm which houses the projection lamp, and the light may be varied in intensity and in shape (circular, vertical slit or horizontal slit beams). Such a beam is usually narrow so that it passes through the optical media of the eye (the cornea, anterior chamber, lens and anterior part of the vitreous) without much diffusion, and a section of these structures is readily seen. The microscope is capable of being adjusted to provide varying magnifications and is maintained accurately in different positions by its attachment to a second movable mechanical arm. It is customary in modern slit-lamp microscopes for the light source and the microscope arms to be mounted together so that each is maintained in focus on different parts of the eye by movement of a single controlling lever, thus leaving one hand free to control the eyelids of the patient. During this examination the patient's head is fixed in a steady position by a chin rest which is attached to the table supporting the microscope and projection lamp, and the patient and examiner sit on stools at opposite ends of the table.

There are extra attachments available for use with the slit lamp, providing facilities for a detailed examination of the region of the filtration angle (gonioscopy) and for precise measurements of the intraocular pressure (applanation tonometry), corneal thickness (pachometry) and anterior chamber depth.

The fundus may be examined by artificially creating a flat anterior surface to the cornea with the use of a strong concave lens ($-55\,\mathrm{D}$) held near the cornea or a specially designed contact lens incorporating three mirrors at differing angles to allow a binocular view of all regions of the retina.

The optical system of the slit lamp can also be used as the vehicle for accurate delivery of photocoagulation burns from a laser source to the trabecular meshwork, iris and retina.

Ophthalmoscopic examination

Direct ophthalmoscopy

Light from the projection lamp of the ophthalmoscope is reflected into the eye of the patient by an angled mirror, and the light which emerges from the eye is viewed by the observer through a small hole in the centre of the mirror. An inverted image (which appears to the observer as an erect one) of the illuminated part of the eye, in particular the fundus (retina, choroid and optic nerve), is formed. The image is focused by a system of lenses mounted on a movable circular disc in the head of the ophthalmoscope, which compensate for any errors in the refraction of different parts of the fundi. If a green filter is also mounted in the circular disc, then the details of blood vessels and the nerve fibre layer will be enhanced. The ophthalmoscope provides a magnified view of the fundus, usually of about $\times 15$. It is held close to the eye of the patient and to the eye of the observer during this examination. The observer's right eye should be used in examination of the patient's right eye with the ophthalmoscope held in the right hand. The process is reversed for the patient's left eye, which is viewed by the observer's left eye with the instrument held in the left hand. It is usual to steady the patient's head using the other hand placed on the patient's forehead, which also permits the retraction of the upper lid by the thumb if there is any tendency for the patient to close the lid.

The ophthalmoscope may also be used to detect defects in the media of the eye (the cornea, anterior chamber, lens and vitreous), and in fact this should precede the more detailed assessment of the fundus. The ophthalmoscope is held some distance from the patient's eye so that the fundus appears to the observer simply as a red reflex without any details of its structure, but defects of the media are revealed as dark areas against the normal bright red background of the fundus, particularly if a fairly high convex (+) lens is used in the head of the ophthalmoscope. Sometimes it is difficult to determine the exact situation of any defect detected by this method, but this is facilitated by making use of the phenomenon of parallax so that the direction of apparent movement of an opacity in relation to a fixed point, such as the iris, is observed on movement of the patient's eye; when the eye moves upwards an opacity in front of the pupil will appear to move up but an opacity behind the pupil will appear to move down. Sometimes, of course, a defective red reflex on direct ophthalmoscopy may be the result of some fairly gross disease of the vitreous, retina or choroid.

Indirect ophthalmoscopy

If the retina is brightly illuminated, the emergent rays may be converged by a strong (+ 20 D) convex lens to produce a real inverted image of about 5 × magnification which lies between the lens and the observer. Although the technique requires considerable practice, it has the advantage of a wider field of view, which is binocular, and an ability to penetrate, to some extent, opacities in the media. With the source of light attached to a head-band, one hand is free to hold the lens while the other may be used to manipulate a scleral indenter, which permits a detailed examination of the peripheral retina.

2

Visual Acuity

The visual acuity of each eye separately is recorded in two ways: the distant visual acuity and the near visual acuity. This distinction is sometimes of great importance, such as in congenital idiopathic nystagmus, when the near vision is usually good despite a relatively poor level of distant acuity, and in some forms of cataract where distant or near vision is disproportionately affected.

Distant visual acuity

This measures the form sense of the eye, which is made up of two components: first, the resolving power of the eye to discriminate between two separate but adjacent stimuli (the smallest measurement of which is the *minimum separable*), and secondly, the ability of the visual cortex to appreciate the nature of a stimulus by a perceptual process (the smallest measurement of which is the *minimum cognisable*). In general the miminum separable under conditions of normal illumination is about one minute (1') and this represents the angle which the object subtends at the nodal point of the eye (Fig. 2). This is used as a basis for the construction of square-shaped serif letters or the figures of Snellen's test types (Fig. 3); the strokes which compose them and the intervals between them subtend this angle, although each letter or figure as a whole subtends 5' at the nodal point, which may be regarded as an average measurement of the minimum cognisable.

Letters or figures of different sizes are constructed which subtend this angle of 5' at the nodal point when they are placed at 60, 36, 24, 18, 12, 9, 6 and 5 m, respectively, from the eye, and they are then placed on a card with a gradual reduction in size from above down so that the largest letter or figure is placed at the top of the card and the smallest letters or figures are placed as a line at the foot of the card. The distant visual acuity of each eye is recorded as an expression of the line of letters which can be discerned at a particular distance (usually 6 m) from the eye; if, for example, only the top letter is read, the acuity is recorded as 6/60, where 6 equals the distance of the chart from the eye in metres and 60 equals the distance at which the letter subtends 5' at the nodal point of the eye. It follows, therefore, that a normal level of vision is 6/6, although under conditions of good illumination a level of 6/5 is usual. If the patient is unable to read the top letter at 6 m, he is

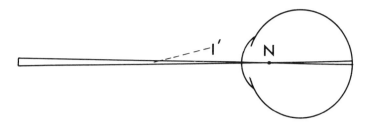

Fig. 2. The minimum separable—an angle of 1' at the nodal point of the eye (N).

Fig. 3. Construction of a Snellen's serif test type letter.

asked to approach the chart until he is able to read it; if this distance is, for example, 3 m the vision is recorded as 3/60. It should be appreciated that, although this method of recording vision is suggestive of a 'fraction' with a numerator (the distance from the chart) and a denominator (the line of letters which is read), it is incorrect to regard it as such and, for example, a vision of 6/12 should not be considered as 'half or 50% vision'.

If the vision is less than 2/60, a test is made of the ability to count figures (CF) at different distances (2m, 1m, 0.5m) or, failing that, the ability to appreciate hand movements (HM), or to perceive light (PL). When this is absent, the eye is blind (no PL).

In testing the vision of the young child who is unable to read or of the illiterate or foreign patient, a suitable method to use is the *E test*. This is carried out conveniently using a cube which has different-sized letter Es on each side; the cube is held by the examiner to show the different Es in different orientations at different distances from the eye, and the child mimics the position of the E throughout the test with a cut-out E which he holds in his hand. It is also possible to use a Snellen's type chart with the letter Es of different sizes arranged in lines in different orientations. A further test for the young child is the *Sheridan-Gardiner test*, based on Stycar charts which are composed of nine standard Snellen's letters without serifs — H L C T O X A V U. The child is given a card containing the Snellen letters and points to the correct letter when the examiner presents isolated letters to him of varying sizes and at different distances; a co-operative three-year-old child is able to carry out this test, but it may be necessary initially to carry out the test with both eyes open because the child may resent a patch on one eye.

It should be noted that it is easier to identify an isolated letter than letters arranged in a line. It follows that the simple methods of testing visual acuity may not be comparable strictly with the conventional methods, and this is illustrated particularly when there is some degree of amblyopia (p.230), so that an amblyopic eye after treatment may achieve a level of 6/9 by a simple test but subsequently only 6/12 by a conventional test. However, in the slightly older child, it is possible to perform the Sheridan-Gardiner test using letters arranged as in the Snellen's test type, and this provides a more accurate measurement.

Near visual acuity

This is a measure of the ability to read words composed of letters of different sizes at the normal reading distance of 33 cm. Jaeger's types represent a random series of different sizes of printers' types—the smallest being J 1 and the largest J 20, but the modern N types are more exact because they are based on the 'point' measurement of the height of a body of letters used in printing (one point $= \frac{1}{72}$ in); the letters are of ten different sizes—N5 (which equals five points), N6, N8, N10, N12, N14, N18, N24, N36 and N60. A modification of the Sheridan-Gardiner test using 'reduced' Snellen types may be used for assessing the near visual acuity in the young. A near visual acuity of N5 is equivalent to 6/12.

The refraction of the eye

In estimating the distant and near visual acuities, account must be taken of the spectacle requirement in order to obtain the corrected visual acuity as distinct from the unaided (uncorrected) visual acuity. This determination demands an assessment of the refraction of the eye, which is dependent on two main factors: first, the influence of the refracting structures of the eye, that is, the cornea and the lens, and second, the axial length of the eyeball.

The influence of the refracting structures

Refraction takes place when rays of light travelling in one medium, for example air, fall obliquely on the surface of another medium, for example the cornea, the lens or glass, which has a different optical density from the first medium; the rays of light passing into the second medium become bent or refracted so that they travel in a direction different from their original direction. This change occurs because the rays of light move more rapidly in a medium of low density, for example air, than in a medium of high density, for example glass, and it is illustrated by the deviation of the light rays as they pass through a prism (Fig. 4). It follows that a convex-shaped lens, which may be considered as two prisms joined base to base, causes a convergence of

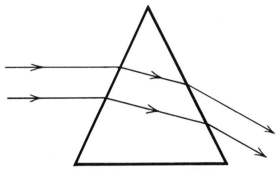

Fig. 4. Refraction of light rays through a prism.

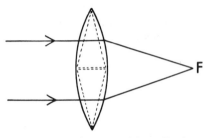

Fig. 5. Convergence of parallel light rays to a point of focus (F) after passing through a convex spherical lens.

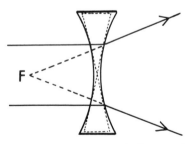

Fig. 6. Divergence of parallel light rays, apparently from a point of focus (F), after passing through a concave spherical lens.

parallel light rays (Fig. 5), whereas a concave-shaped lens, which may be considered as two prisms joined apex to apex, causes a divergence of parallel light rays (Fig. 6). The power of a convex or concave spherical lens is determined by its focal length, which is a measure of the distance from the lens to the point of focus (F) of parallel rays after passing through the lens (Figs. 5 and 6). A lens with a focal length of 1 m is termed a 1 dioptre (1 D) lens, one with a focal length of 0.5 m a 2 dioptre (2 D) lens, and one with a focal length of 2m a 0.50 dioptre

(0.50 D) lens, etc., so that the dioptric power of a lens is inversely proportional to its focal length. Convex and concave spherical lenses are distinguished from one another by the prefix plus (+) for convex lenses and minus (−) for concave lenses in front of the dioptric power. The structures concerned in the refraction of the eye are the cornea and the lens.

The cornea. The influence of the cornea on refraction is exerted almost entirely by its anterior surface, which is a curved convex surface producing convergence of parallel light rays entering the eye. This surface has a high refracting value, and contributes significantly to the final refraction of the eye, because the corneal substance has a much greater optical density than the medium, i.e. the air, with which it is in contact. The posterior corneal surface contributes little because of the negligible difference in the optical densities of the opposing media (the cornea and the aqueous).

The lens. The anterior and posterior surfaces of the lens are curved convex surfaces so that they cause increased convergence of light rays passing through the lens, although this effect is limited to some extent by the absence of any marked differences between the density of the lens and the densities of the surrounding media (the aqueous and the vitreous). Its effect is enhanced, however, by the fact that there is usually a slight increase in the optical density of the central part of the lens, the nucleus, as compared with the peripheral part of the lens, the cortex. It follows that a relative increase in the density of the nuclear portion increases the refracting value of the lens, and a relative increase in the density of the cortical portion decreases the dioptric value of the lens, but these differences are seldom of great significance in the normal lens.

In addition, the influence of the lens is not a static one, because its refractive value may be altered by the act of *accommodation.* An increased effectivity of the lens during accommodation for near sight (*positive accommodation*) is produced by a contraction of the ciliary muscle (the longitudinal fibres, oblique fibres and iridic fibres acting as a whole), which is innerverted by the parasympathetic part of the third cranial nerve, so that there is a forward movement and thickening of the ciliary body with a consequent relaxation of the zonule, or suspensory ligament, which attaches the capsule of the lens to the ciliary body. At one time it was considered that the relaxation of the zonule allowed the lens to assume a more spherical form with an increase in the curvatures of its anterior and posterior surfaces, an increase in its anteroposterior diameter, and a decrease in its transverse diameter (theory of Helmholtz), but it is more likely that the increased curvatures are confined mainly to the regions of the anterior and

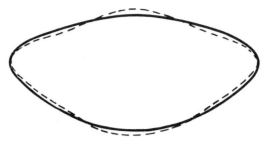

Fig. 7. Alterations in the curvature of the lens from a resting state (solid line) to a fully accommodative state (broken line).

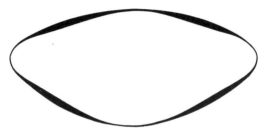

Fig. 8. Variations in the thickness of the lens capsule.

posterior poles and that there is even a slight flattening of the more peripheral parts of these surfaces during accommodation (theory of Fincham) (Fig. 7), perhaps because the capsule of the lens is thicker in its more peripheral parts than in its more central parts (Fig. 8). A decreased effectivity of the lens during accommodation for distance (*negative accommodation*) is achieved by a reversal of this process, although there is some evidence that this may involve the activity of the sympathetic nervous system, and it is certainly not a mere passive relaxation of the ciliary muscle.

The influence of the axial length of the eye

The axial length of the eyeball also determines the final refraction of the eye; this is discussed below.

Types of refraction

The terms used to denote the different types of refraction are emmetropia and ametropia, which includes hypermetropia, myopia, astigmatism, anisometropia and aniseikonia.

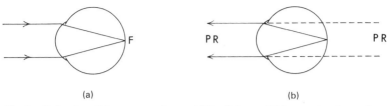

(a)   (b)

Fig. 9. Refraction of the emmetropic eye. (a) Parallel rays of light entering the eye form
a focus (F) on the retina. (b) Rays of light emerging from the eye are parallel and meet at
a far point (punctum remotum, PR) at infinity in front of or behind the eye.

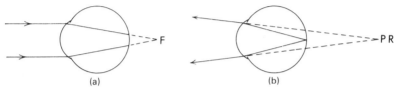

(a)   (b)

Fig. 10. Refraction of the hypermetropic eye. (a) Parallel rays of light entering the eye,
if continued, form a focus (F) behind the retina. (b) Rays of light emerging from the eye
are divergent and appear to arise from a far point (punctum remotum, PR) behind the
eye.

Emmetropia

The emmetropic eye has a normal type of refraction so that parallel rays
of light entering the eye come to focus on the retina (Fig. 9). It follows
that rays of light emerging from the eye are parallel and may be
considered to converge to, or to diverge from, the far point (or *punctum
remotum, PR*) which lies at infinity. Emmetropia is produced by a
perfect correlation of the axial length of the eyeball and the dioptric
power of the refracting media (curvature and index components).

Ametropia

The ametropic eye has an abnormal type of refraction so that parallel
rays of light entering the eye do not come to focus on the retina. There
are several different forms of ametropia.

Hypermetropia. The hypermetropic eye is one in which parallel rays of
light entering the eye would come to focus (if they could be prolonged)
at a point behind the retina (Fig. 10). It follows that rays of light
emerging from the eye are divergent and appear to diverge from the far
point (or punctum remotum, PR) which lies behind the eye.
Hypermetropia is determined by one or more of the following factors:

    1. An axial failure, i.e. an axial length which is shorter than normal.
    2. A curvature failure, i.e. an insufficient degree of corneal or, more
rarely, lenticular curvature.

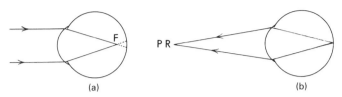

Fig. 11. Refraction of the myopic eye. (a) Parallel rays of light form a focus (F) in front of the retina. (b) Rays of light emerging from the eye are convergent and meet at a far point (punctum remotum, PR) in front of the eye.

3. An index failure, i.e. a decreased density of the lens as a whole or, more particularly, a relative decrease in density of the nuclear portion.

The hypermetropic eye is usually smaller than normal. This affects the anterior segment so that the anterior chamber tends to be somewhat shallow, a factor which may contribute to the development of closed-angle glaucoma (p.310). It also affects the posterior segment, and the optic disc appears ophthalmoscopically to be unduly small; sometimes the disc margins may look blurred so that there is a false impression of papilloedema. Confusion is avoided by careful examination, since there is no true swelling of the tissues or the disc margins and no peripapillary retinal vein dilatation. Uncorrected hypermetropia may cause eyestrain because of the difficulty in maintaining accommodation in the interests of clear vision, and in young children it may precipitate the development of certain forms of convergent squint.

Myopia. The myopic eye is the eye in which parallel rays of light entering the eye come to a focus at a point in front of the retina (Fig. 11). It follows that rays of light emerging from the myopic eye are convergent and converge to the far point (or punctum remotum, PR), which lies in front of the eye. Myopia is determined by one or more of the following factors:

1. An axial failure, i.e. an axial length which is longer than normal.
2. A curvature failure, i.e. an excessive degree of corneal or, more rarely, lenticular curvature.
3. An index failure, i.e. an increased density of the lens as a whole or, more particularly, a relative increase in the density of the nuclear portion.

The myopic eye is usually larger than normal. This affects the anterior segment so that the anterior chamber tends to be deeper than normal, a factor which determines the rarity of closed-angle glaucoma in axial myopia. It also affects the posterior segment, particularly in the region of the optic disc, with the gradual development of a concentric area of choroidal atrophy, the *myopic crescent,* usually along the temporal

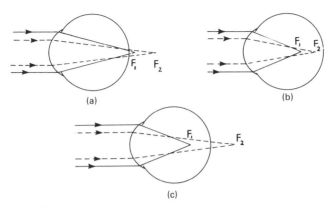

Fig. 12. Refraction of the astigmatic eye: (a) hypermetropic astigmatism; (b) myopic astigmatism; and (c) mixed astigmatism. Note in each diagram the rays of light in the vertical plane (solid lines) are refracted more than those in the horizontal plane (broken lines).

border of the disc but sometimes along some other border of the disc or even around the whole disc (*peripapillary atrophy*). Choroidal atrophy is also liable to occur in the submacular area with the development of degenerative changes in the overlying retina, sometimes in association with haemorrhage from friable new vessels from the choroidal circulation following rupture of the elastic lamina (Bruch's membrane) which separates the retina from the choroid. In extreme cases a thinning of the posterior part of the sclera (including the optic disc) causes a bulging of this part of the eye backwards (*posterior staphyloma*).

In general, the occurrence of a small degree of hypermetropia or myopia is simply the result of a slight failure in correlation between the corneal refracting power and the axial length of the eyeball, but the larger degrees are produced by more elaborate failures, although an abnormality of the axial length is usually the main determining one.

Astigmatism. In the purely emmetropic, hypermetropic or myopic eye, the refracting effect of the eye on parallel rays of light is identical in all meridians, but in the astigmatic eye the refracting effect is different according to the meridian in which these rays traverse the eye. In almost all astigmatic eyes, the meridian of greatest refraction lies at right angles to the meridian of least refraction, and it is often found that one of these meridians lies in or near the vertical plane of the eyeball, with the other meridian lying in or near the horizontal plane of the eyeball. Astigmatism may be associated with hypermetropia (*hypermetropic astigmatism*) (Fig. 12a), with myopia (*myopic astigmatism*) (Fig. 12b) or with hypermetropia and myopia (*mixed astigmatism*) (Fig. 12c).

Anisometropia. This is a condition in which there is an unequal degree of ametropia between the two eyes. It may be of different types: one eye may be emmetropic and the other eye hypermetropic or myopic; both eyes may be hypermetropic or myopic but to unequal degrees; or one eye may be hypermetropic and the other myopic (sometimes called *antimetropia*). It must be appreciated, of course, that small degrees of anisometropia are common and of little significance, but there is evidence that anisometropia is liable to lead to the development of a small-angle esotropia (*microtropia*) when it is present in early childhood (p. 232).

Aniseikonia. This is a condition in which the size of the retinal images in the two eyes is unequal. It may be produced in different ways: (a) as a result of a significant degree of anisometropia—each 0.25 D of difference in refraction causes a 0.5% size difference in the retinal images; (b) as a result of wearing correcting lenses in the wrong positions relative to the eyes; or (c) more rarely, as a result of some abnormality in the density of the retinal mosaic. It is usual for the visual cortex to compensate for certain degrees of aniseikonia— up to 5%—by a perceptual process.

The determination of refraction

The refraction of the eye is determined by two main methods: objectively by the method of retinoscopy and subjectively by the effect of correcting lenses. These methods are discussed only briefly since detailed information about the prescription of glasses is beyond the scope of this book.

Objective test—retinoscopy

When rays of light from an electric self-illuminating retinoscope are projected into the eye, they form an area of illumination on the retina. If the retinoscope is then tilted, this area of illumination moves in the same direction as the tilting of the retinoscope—to the right, to the left, upwards or downwards— and this movement of the illuminated area is independent of the type of refraction of the eye—emmetropia, hypermetropia or myopia. However, the observer who is watching for such a movement through a small hole in the centre of the retinoscope is unaware of the real movement of the light on the retina because he obtains only an impression that the light originates from the punctum remotum, discussed above, which lies at infinity in emmetropia (Fig. 9), behind the eye in hypermetropia (Fig. 10), and in front of the eye in myopia (Fig. 11). It follows, therefore, that the illuminated area appears to move in the same direction as the movement of the

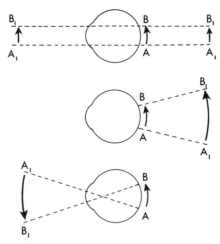

Fig. 13. In retinoscopy the apparent movement of the illuminated retinal areas which is appreciated by the observer as coming from the punctum remotum (i.e. movement from A_1 to B_1) is in the same direction as the real movement of the illuminated retinal areas (i.e. movement from A to B) in emmetropia (top) and in hypermetropia (middle), but in the opposite direction in myopia (bottom).

retinoscope in emmetropia and hypermetropia, and in the opposite direction in myopia (Fig. 13).

In emmetropia, if a convex lens of low power is placed in front of the eye, an artificial myopia is induced because parallel rays of light entering the eye come to a focus just in front of the retina; there is then a reversal of the apparent movement of the illuminated retinal area on moving the retinoscope. Similarly, in hypermetropia a reversal is obtained by placing a sufficiently powerful convex lens in front of the eye to overcorrect the hypermetropic error. In myopia a reversal of the opposite type is obtained by placing a concave lens of sufficient power in front of the eye to overcorrect the myopia. Therefore the measurement of the strength of convex or concave lens which is just sufficient to produce a reversal of the apparent movement of the illuminated retinal areas is a measure of the error of refraction of the eye. In theory this measurement should be recorded by the observer at an infinite distance from the eye, but in practice the observer is placed 1 m from the eye; this introduces an error of 1 dioptre (1 D), so that this must be deducted from the final measurement. Thus, the emmetropic eye is one in which a 1 D convex lens causes a reversal of the apparent movement of the illuminated retinal areas when the observer is 1m from the eye. An astigmatic error is also assessed using retinoscopy by measuring separately the refractive error present in the meridian of greatest refraction and in the meridian of least refraction.

It is sometimes necessary, particularly in children, to carry out retinoscopy after the use of a cycloplegic drug, which temporarily

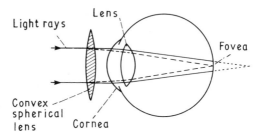

Fig. 14.   Correction of hypermetropia by a convex spherical lens.

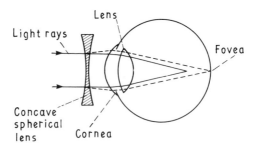

Fig. 15.   Correction of myopia by a concave spherical lens.

paralyses the accommodation of the eye, in order to permit an estimation of the correct amount of hypermetropic error (accommodation during retinoscopy artificially decreases this measurement); such a drug also dilates the pupil (mydriasis) which facilitates the examination of the fundus. In children, atropine 1% ointment once daily for three days prior to retinoscopy provides a complete cycloplegic effect, but cyclopentolate (Mydrilate) 1% or tropicamide (Mydriacyl) 1% drops are used widely in preference to atropine because they produce an adequate level of cycloplegia in 30 minutes and, unlike atropine, the cycloplegic effect is short-lived.

Subjective test—correction of ametropia

The results of the objective method of retinoscopy are verified by a subjective test which determines the best level of distant vision obtained in each eye as measured by the Snellen's test types at 6 m following the use of appropriate correcting lenses. These lenses are convex in hypermetropia (Fig. 14) (although hypermetropia may also be corrected by a simple act of accommodation, but the effectiveness of this correction depends on the amount of accommodation available and on the degree of hypermetropia present), concave in myopia (Fig. 15), and cylindrical convex or concave lenses (which have no refracting effects on rays of light which pass through them in the direction of their axes, but have the same effect as spherical lenses of equivalent dioptric power on rays of light which pass through them at 90° to their axes) in astigmatism; spherical lenses (convex or concave) are used in addition to the cylindrical lenses when there is also a significant hypermetropic or myopic refractive error.

It is important also to determine the level of the near visual acuity of each eye after the correction of the refractive error. In the emmetropic eye there is sufficient accommodation to maintain a clear image of small print (N5) at the normal reading range (33 cm) until about the age of 45 years (except in some eastern countries, for example in India, when this age is usually reduced to about 38 to 40 years). Thereafter, however, the continued reduction in the available accommodation, due to diminished ability of the lens to change its shape in response to a stimulus for accommodation or perhaps due to a diminished ability of the ciliary muscle to produce this change, causes blurring of small print. This is termed *presbyopia*, and a convex spherical lens is then necessary for close reading; in emmetropia the appropriate convex lenses are used alone, but in hypermetropia, myopia or astigmatism they are used in addition to the normal correcting lenses for distant vision. In the early stages of presbyopia it is usually sufficient to prescribe + 0.50 D lenses, but this prescription is increased by + 0.25 D or + 0.50 D every few years up to + 2.50 D (or even + 2.75 D or + 3.00 D) by the age of about 60 years. It should be noted, of course, that in uncorrected hypermetropia, the onset of presbyopia will be earlier than in emmetropia because of the amount of accommodation which is expended in correcting the distant visual acuity, and that, conversely, in myopia the onset of presbyopia will be delayed; indeed in certain degrees of myopia there may be no need for the use of convex lenses for reading because the convex (+) lenses for near vision in presbyopia would merely neutralize the concave (−) lenses required for the myopia.

Correction of ametropia—other methods

Contact lenses

In the search for an ideal contact lens, i.e. one which corrects the refractive error without damaging the cornea and yet can be worn for several hours continuously, a variety of lens types are now in use, each with its own advantages.

A hard plastic material (polymethylmethacrylate), which does not transmit oxygen, is used for corneal lenses which ride on the anterior corneal surface on a cushion of tears through which oxygen freely diffuses. These have excellent optical properties and can correct up to 2.50 D of astigmatism, but may cause central corneal epithelial damage from prolonged continuous use, producing intense pain and photophobia due to apical epithelial hypoxia. Usually no permanent damage results. Moulded sclero-corneal (haptic) lenses, with suitable perforations for oxygen transfer, are made of the same material and are used in eyes with very abnormal corneal contours (keratoconus) or with associated lid abnormalities.

Contact lenses made from several other materials are now available and make up the group known as soft contact lenses. Those made from homogeneous poly-2-hydroxyethylmethacrylate are hydrophilic and allow the passage of oxygen and metabolites to a degree that is dependent on the water content of the lenses. Readily acceptable in terms of comfort, these lenses are limited in their correction of corneal astigmatism (because the lens moulds to the corneal curvature) and require careful cleaning and storage.

The potential for prolonged wearing of such hydrogel lenses using the higher water content material for two to three months has allowed the earlier correction of paediatric aphakia, so reducing the development of stimulus-deprivation amblyopia. A further application of contact lenses is the significant reduction of the aniseikonia which is a feature of uniocular aphakia, and permits a return to normal binocular vision (bifoveal fixation); this is in contrast to the use of a spectacle lens, which fails to correct the aniseikonia.

Another compound, cellulose acetate butyrate, has the advantage of oxygen transmissibility and some rigidity, thereby improving the optics and facilitating handling. Silicone rubber lenses, also in the soft lens category, have excellent oxygen transmission, are strong and are not so susceptible to infection, but being hydrophobic, they need to be surface-treated to allow adequate wetting in order to be tolerated by the eye.

Apart from the correction of refractive errors, contact lenses have therapeutic and cosmetic applications. Therapeutic or bandage lenses can be used in the management of, for instance, recurrent corneal abrasions, permitting re-epithelialization without mechanical trauma of blinking, after corneal perforation, or in the presence of lid anomalies, for example, misdirected lashes which may abrade the cornea. They also have a major use in relieving the pain of bullous keratopathy and the discomfort of the dry-eye syndromes (Riley-Day syndrome and Sjogren's syndrome).

Specially designed shielded lenses which limit the passage of light into the eye may be of value in albinism or aniridia (Chapter 6), while other lenses have purely cosmetic purposes. For example, a lens with a black centre may be used to mask the presence of an opaque cataractous lens in a blind eye, or a lens incorporating a painted eye may be worn over a useless microphthalmic eye or over a shrunken blind eye.

Intraocular lenses

Following cataract extraction it is possible to correct the resulting refractive error (hypermetropia) by spectacles, contact lenses or by the insertion of an acrylic lens within the eye; this is positioned in the anterior chamber, on the surface of the iris where it is held in place by clips, or in the position of the normal lens (i.e. in the posterior chamber), lying within the posterior lens capsule. The more physiological position of the posterior chamber lens has distinct optical advantages, particularly in minimizing the aniseikonia of uniocular aphakia, in improving the field of vision and in eliminating the handling difficulties of spectacles and contact lenses in those with conditions such as rheumatoid arthritis.

Intracorneal lenses

A hydrogel lens inlay may be used within the cornea, but this is seldom carried out purely for refractive errors; it is reserved largely for pathological conditions of the cornea which make the response to other methods of treatment poor (e.g. bullous keratopathy, p.46). Sometimes, however, a donor cornea or a hydrogel lens may be inserted within the corneal stroma after being cryolathed or ground to the appropriate refractive power.

Keratomileusis

An attempt may be made to alter the refraction of the eye by changing the shape of the cornea. This involves removing a disc of the cornea through part of its thickness and, after freezing the tissue, the contours of the corneal disc are altered to counteract the refractive error of the eye. Therefore when the disc is replaced (as in a lamellar keratoplasty), the refractive error of the eye is nearer normal; this operation is termed keratomileusis.

Radial keratotomy

Up to 3 D of myopia can be corrected by a recently introduced operation which is designed to induce flattening of the apical anterior corneal curvature, thereby reducing its refractive power. Leaving the axial area free, 8 to 16 radial incisions, to at least three-quarters corneal depth, are made to the limbus. The exact mechanism of the change in curvature and the permanency of the induced change are not known. Indeed, some patients experience daily fluctuation of acuity due to changes in refraction, while others have glare-induced photophobia as a result of the corneal scars scattering the light.

Colour vision

The colour sense of the eye is its ability to distinguish different colours and, like the form sense, it is mediated essentially by the cones (see Chapter 7). White light consists of impulses of different wavelengths so that it forms a spectrum with the following colours—red, orange, yellow, green, blue-green, blue and violet—from the longest (700 nm) to the shortest (380 nm) wavelengths, respectively. The true nature of colour appreciation in the retina is ill understood, but one of the most acceptable theories (the Young-Helmholtz theory) assumes the existence in the retina of three separate colour-perceiving elements and colour-transmitting mechanisms which are concerned with the three fundamental colours—red, green and blue. All colours are produced by varying degrees of stimulation of these elements and mechanisms, and a white colour is produced by an equal stimulation of all three. In this way the person with normal colour appreciation has all three colour factors present and is termed a *trichromat* (hence its description as the *trichromatic* theory).

In support of the trichromatic theory, there is histological evidence of three types of cones in flat retinal preparations. There is also electrophysiological evidence of three different cone mechanisms, as three groups of modulators which are considered to subserve the function of hue discrimination are known to exist in addition to dominators which are considered to subserve the function of luminosity discrimination. It is suggested also that the laminar system of the lateral geniculate body (see Chapter 16) is further evidence in support of the trichromatic theory, although this is largely a hypothesis. There are, however, certain objections to the theory and it is natural that other theories should have been put forward. Some of these propose a four-colour system, with the addition of the colour yellow to the three other colours (red, green and blue); this is based on psychological rather than physiological (or physical) considerations. It is certainly important to recognize the psychological implications which are inherent in colour discrimination whereby a child is trained to appreciate the colours of different objects by name, although it is likely that such appreciation is widely variable.

There are three different states of abnormal colour appreciation which are of congenital origin.

The trichromat. The trichromat shows an anomaly (not an absence) of one factor. This may be of three types: a *protanomalous trichromat* when the red factor is weak, a *deuteranomalous trichromat* when the green factor is weak, and a *tritanomalous trichromat* when the blue factor is weak. These anomalous trichromats are colour deficient rather than colour blind.

These forms of colour deficiency (dyschromatopsia) occur much more frequently in males than in females (8% as compared with 0.4% in Western countries), and they show a well-marked hereditary pattern with a sex-linked recessive trait. Their recognition is of importance because of the use of colours in so many aspects of life; for example, in the teaching of junior mathematics at school, in the labelling of electronic circuits and in traffic lights.

The dichromat. This person shows an absence (not an anomaly) of one factor and this may be of three types: a *protanope* when the red factor is absent, a *deuteranope* when the green factor is absent, and a *tritanope* when the blue factor is absent.

The monochromat. The monochromat shows an absence of colour appreciation so that there is a total colour blindness (*monochromatism*). This is of two types: *cone monochromatism (cone dysfunction syndrome)* is a rare condition in which there is a disturbance of cone function (with a progressive loss of form and colour vision) but with no disturbance of rod function (so that peripheral vision is not lost). There are no ophthalmoscopic changes and the scotopic electroretinogram (ERG) is normal, but the photopic ERG is abnormal. In the second type, *rod monochromatism*, the visual function of the eye is grossly abnormal with poor visual acuity, nystagmus and a marked intolerance of bright light and, typically, an abnormal ERG.

It should be noted that the anomalous trichromat is much more common than the dichromat, and that in each group disturbance of the green factor is more common than disturbance of the red factor, and disturbance of the blue factor is very rare. The monochromat, particularly the cone monochromat, is extremely rare.

Because 80 to 90% of optic nerve fibres are derived from the region of the macula and therefore subserve cones, disorders of the optic nerve, such as retrobulbar neuritis (p.153), toxic amblyopia (p.135 and 155) and compression, including lesions of the chiasm (p.326), may lead to a change in colour appreciation.

Tests for colour discrimination

The lantern test

There are two main types of lantern: the Edridge-Green lantern, which has a single aperture, and the Board of Trade lantern, which has two apertures. The significance of this difference is related to the phenomenon of *induction*. The physiological changes which occur in the retina as the result of a stimulus are not limited to the time of the actual stimulus because of *successive contrast* or *temporal induction* (the occurrence of positive and negative after-images after the primary stimulus), and are not limited to the area of the retina stimulated by the actual stimulus because of *simultaneous contrast* or *spatial induction* (the occurrence of modifications in the retina adjoining the stimulated area). The single aperture is suitable for assessing successive contrast, but the double aperture is necessary for assessing simultaneous contrast.

The Ishihara or Stilling Test

These tests are concerned with the identification of numbers on each of several plates which are formed of a series of large spots (mostly red or green) against a background of large spots of other colours.

More refined methods of clinical examination of colour vision, especially suitable for children, are the City University system of colour matching, and the Hardy-Rand-Rittler pseudoisochromatic plates, which incorporate geometrical figures rather than numbers. These tests are more subtle than lantern tests and are of value in identifying the anomalous trichromats (of the protanomalous or deuteranomalous types) who are often able to perform the lantern tests successfully.

Adaptation

The effect of a visual stimulus is not uniform because it depends on the state of adapatation of the retina at the time of the stimulus. In a state of light adaptation the vision is mediated largely by the cones, which are concerned with the appreciation of form and colour *(photopic vision)*; in a state of dark adaptation the vision is mediated largely by the rods, which are concerned essentially with the appreciation of light and movement *(scotopic vision)* (Fig. 16). This clear-cut distinction between the photopic and scotopic phases of vision is the basis of the classical duplicity theory. On passing from light into dark, the process of dark adaptation takes place: the retina increases markedly in sensitivity—rapidly during the first ten minutes and then slowly up to a maximum of about 40 minutes. Thus in dim illumination a stimulus which would be invisible under conditions of light adaptation can be perceived. However, because the process of dark adaptation is essentially a function of the rods, it does not occur uniformly throughout the retina; it occurs maximally in the peripheral parts but only minimally in the central part, so that in dim illumination the fovea and parafovea become virtually functionless. Conversely, on passing from dark into light the process of light adaptation occurs. This is a fairly rapid process, so that within a few seconds there is a marked decrease in the sensitivity of the retina; this is demonstrated by the quick acceptance of the light stimulus, despite a momentary intense dazzle.

Night blindness

This is a state in which the vision is usually fairly normal under

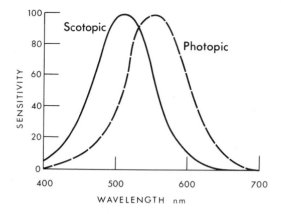

Fig. 16. Retinal sensitivity under different light conditions.

conditions of good illumination, but very defective under conditions of dim illumination. Characteristically, it occurs in a tapetoretinal degeneration of the retinitis pigmentosa type (p.143) and also in the retinal degeneration which occurs in association with keratomalacia as the result of a severe vitamin A deficiency (p.63).

Day blindness

This is not a satisfactory term, but is applied to a state in which there is a central scotoma (e.g. due to toxic amblyopia or macular degeneration) so that the eye appears to function more efficiently in dim illumination.

Depth perception

During the bifoveal fixation of an object, two slightly dissimilar images are formed on the retinae since each eye views the object from a very slightly different angle. The ability to fuse these two images to give a perception of depth is known as stereopsis, and is the highest form of binocular vision. However, it is evident that perception of depth can also be achieved using only one eye (uniocular vision) by the appreciation of various clues: the apparent sizes of different objects (the smaller the apparent size, the farther away is the object), the apparent colours of different objects (the less distinct the colour value, the farther away is the object) and the overlapping of contours of different objects (a near object may partly obliterate a distant object).

3

The Conjunctiva

Structure and function

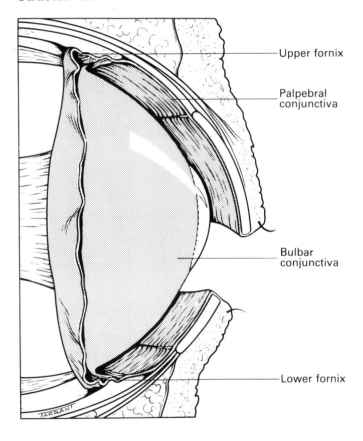

Fig. 17. The extent of the normal conjunctiva (stippled area).

The conjunctiva is a mucous membrane which lines the undersurface of each eyelid (*palpebral conjunctiva*) and covers the surface of the eyeball (*bulbar conjunctiva*) (Fig. 17). The palpebral and bulbar conjunctivae are separated by a potential space (the *conjunctival sac*) which is closed above by the *superior fornix* (where the palpebral conjunctiva is reflected to form the bulbar conjunctiva), below by the *inferior fornix*, medially at the *medial canthus* (where there is a junction of the medial ends of the upper and lower lids), and laterally at the *lateral canthus*. The conjunctival sac is open externally between the upper and lower lid margins (*palpebral fissure*). The bulbar conjunctiva ends at the corneal margin (*limbus*), although its epithelium is continuous with the corneal epithelium. The bulbar conjunctiva is separated from the underlying Tenon's capsule by a space (the subconjunctival space) and this capsule is separated from the underlying sclera by another space (the episcleral space) which contains the episcleral tissues.

The conjunctiva is richly supplied by arteries and veins, but under normal conditions most of these vessels are contracted so that they are scarcely visible. Two other structures lie in the conjunctival sac:

1. The *plica semilunaris*, which is a crescent-shaped fold of conjunctiva arising from the region of the medial canthus immediately lateral to the caruncle, with a free border directed towards the cornea. It corresponds to the third eyelid of certain animals (the nictitating membrane).

2. The *caruncle*, which is a small red fleshy body lying on the medial side of the plica at the medial canthus. It represents a part of the margin of the lower lid which becomes isolated during early development.

The conjunctiva forms a protective coat over the underlying sclera and provides moisture to the eye by means of two types of glands:

1. *Mucous glands.* Mucus is secreted by goblet cells which are widespread in the conjunctival epithelium.

2. *Serous glands.* Lacrimal fluid is secreted by accessory lacrimal glands which are present in various parts of the conjunctiva, although the chief source of tears is from the main lacrimal gland (see Chapter 12).

Injuries

Haemorrhage

Any direct injury of the conjunctiva may cause subconjunctival haemorrhage. This is often widespread owing to the free nature of the subconjunctival space, although the haemorrhage lessens posteriorly and seldom spreads as far as the tissues of the orbit. This is in contrast to a haemorrhage which reaches the subconjunctival space from the orbit (e.g. after a fracture of orbit), which is intense posteriorly and does not have a limiting edge.

Subconjunctival haemorrhages may occur quite spontaneously in normal healthy people because of the exposed situation of the relatively fragile conjunctival vessels, although they are more likely in arteriosclerotic persons, particularly after bouts of coughing. The haemorrhage usually persists for a week or so. It remains red during this time because of free oxygenation of the blood through the thin conjunctival covering.

Lacerations

Any direct injury of the conjunctiva is liable to lacerate it. Such injuries heal readily, but when extensive they should be sutured with collagen.

Foreign bodies

Foreign bodies, such as particles of dirt, cigarette ash, steel from a grinding machine or husks of bird seed, commonly enter the conjunctival sac from the atmosphere. They are readily seen on the bulbar conjunctiva by opening the lids and on the palpebral conjunctiva of the lower lid or in the inferior fornix by pulling down the lower lid, but their identification on the palpebral conjunctiva of the upper lid requires eversion of the lid. This is achieved with the patient looking down and relaxing his lids by keeping them open, pulling the upper lid margin upwards with the forefinger and thumb of one hand whilst pressing on the upper border of the tarsal plate with the forefinger of the other hand or with a glass rod. When it is necessary to expose the full extent of the superior fornix, the fold of conjunctiva which projects from the everted lid is also everted (double eversion of the upper eyelid) using a Desmarres eyelid retractor.

Chemical burns

Chemical burns occur as industrial and household accidents and also in criminal assault. They constitute a serious threat to vision and demand urgent attention.

Burns due to acid tend to cause limited damage because acids form insoluble protein complexes with conjunctival and corneal proteins, whereas alkali lyses cell membranes and forms soluble complexes which rapidly penetrate to the anterior chamber, and can affect the iris, ciliary body, lens and trabecular meshwork.

Burns tend to involve the lower part of the bulbar conjunctiva because the reflex closure of the lids, which follows the awareness of an approaching foreign substance, is preceded by an upturning of the eyeball (Bell's phenomenon). The immediate management is aimed at diluting and eliminating the chemical by rapid irrigation, ideally with a phosphate buffer, but often achieved most effectively by plunging the head into a basin of water and opening the eyes. Particulate matter such as lime must be sought and removed from the fornices and elsewhere under local anaesthetic.

To avoid bacterial infection a topical antibiotic is given, supplemented by a cycloplegic (atropine drops 1%) and a corticosteroid (prednisolone phosphate drops) if iritis is present. Damage to the bulbar and palpebral conjunctiva may lead to adhesions with obliteration of part of the conjunctival sac (*symblepharon*). Adhesions may be avoided by passing a lubricated glass rod across the fornices daily, or by inserting a scleral ring or moulded contact lens. The cornea is subject to extensive damage which may not be apparent in the early stages. The surest guide to the severity of the burn and the prognosis is the degree of limbal ischaemia at presentation. Vascularization, perforation, exposure and desiccation are the principle problems of severe burns. The risk of perforation is believed to be due to corneal collagen lysis by calcium– and zinc–dependent proteolytic enzymes which are formed by the damaged corneal epithelium and polymorphonuclear leucocytes. The chelating action of acetylcysteine, which directly affects the enzyme may be used to reduce this risk. Ethylenediaminetetraacetic acid (EDTA), and D-penicillamine also have been advocated, and topical and systemic ascorbic acid has been shown to be beneficial.

The late complications, however, pose difficult management problems including opaque vascularized cornea, deformed lid margins, limited ocular motility due to symblepharon, and dry eye from marked alteration of the tear film. Corneal grafting in this hostile environment is rarely successful, but attention to the lids and adequate tear supplements will enhance the effects of surgery.

If extensive symblepharon develops, the adhesions should be divided once the condition has become static (usually several months after the injury). An attempt is made to retain the conjunctival space by the immediate fitting of a contact lens or the sac is reformed by the use of a mucous membrane graft from the inner surface of the lower lip.

Conjunctivitis

Conjunctivitis, an inflammatory condition of the conjunctiva, is usually of an infective nature—bacterial or viral—and may be acute, subacute or chronic. Some cases, however, are of an allergic nature and others are related to certain skin disorders.

Infective conjunctivitis—acute or subacute conjunctivitis

This almost invariably affects both eyes simultaneously or within a short period of each other. It is the result of a variety of organisms (bacterial or viral) which are usually exogenous; it is therefore essentially a contagious disease fostered by crowded conditions and poor standards of cleanliness, although rarely the cause is endogenous.

It commences as a feeling of discomfort in the eyes. This often becomes intense, with a sensation of grittiness but without any deep-seated pain, except sometimes on exposure to bright light (*photophobia*). Characteristically there is a profuse discharge from the eyes, which may be watery, mucous, mucopurulent or purulent according to the severity of the condition and the nature of the organism. This discharge accounts for the stickiness of the eyelids, particularly after sleep, and for the excoriation of the lid margins in the later stages. Sometimes the discharge may cause rainbow effects as it passes across the cornea, but these, unlike the rainbows which occur in closed-angle glaucoma, disappear on blinking.

The degree of redness of the eyes also varies according to the severity and nature of the infection. It affects the bulbar and palpebral conjunctivae and is usually vivid. Its superficial situation in the bulbar conjunctiva may be demonstrated by movement of the reddened area on rubbing the margin of the lower lid against the bulbar conjunctiva (in contrast to the darker and deeper immovable type of redness which characterizes an episcleritis). The redness is less intense in the circumcorneal region (in contrast to the marked circumcorneal or ciliary injection which characterizes an iritis or closed-angle glaucoma). In severe cases the inflamed conjunctiva may be so congested that it becomes swollen (*chemosis*). Rarely the cornea becomes involved secondary to the conjunctivitis, although there are certain inflammatory conditions in which the conjunctiva and cornea are involved together (keratoconjunctivitis). *Conjunctival injection* is the term given to the redness which occurs in conjunctivitis and also in other inflammatory or non-inflammatory conditions, such as allergic disorders, or as a reaction to irritants such as foreign bodies, chemical agents, tobacco smoke and smog.

There are special features which characterize different forms of infective conjunctivitis according to the nature of the organism.

Bacterial infections

Moraxella lacunata. This diplobacillus causes a mild but fairly persistent catarrhal or occasionally mucopurulent conjunctivitis which is the result of the macerating effect of an enzyme secreted by the organism. The effect is usually limited to the regions of the lateral and medial canthi (hence the name *angular conjunctivitis*) because the action of the organism is inhibited to some extent by the lysozyme in the tears in the main part of the conjunctival sac. There is often a collection of froth-like secretion on the lid margins which produces a red and eczematous condition of the lids with a sensation of intense irritation and itchiness of the eyes.

Staphylococcus. S. aureus (coagulase positive) produces a conjunctivitis which is usually of the acute catarrhal type, but is occasionally of a chronic nature with a marginal keratitis in which small white infiltrates (*subepithelial keratitis*) occur at the limbus with a tendency to spread circumferentially; this keratitis may be a sensitivity reaction to the staphylococcus (or to some other antigen).

Recent work suggests that *S. epidermidis* (coagulase negative), with its several phage types, may be incriminated in a spectrum of acute and chronic disorders involving the cornea and conjunctiva, ranging from a mild follicular conjunctivitis to severe marginal corneal ulceration.

Haemophilus influenzae (Koch-Weeks bacillus). This organism is responsible for the large epidemics of mucopurulent conjunctivitis (pink eye) which are particularly common in closely confined communities.

Streptococcus pneumoniae (pneumococcus). Pneumococcal conjunctivitis commonly follows an infection of the tear sac (dacryocystitis) and tends to be associated with subconjunctival haemorrhage.

Neisseria gonorrhoeae (gonococcus). This organism is usually harboured by the abundant leucocytes within the secretion. The infection may occur in the newborn, causing a severe bilateral conjunctivitis (*ophthalmia neonatorum*) within a few days of birth, following a direct infection from the infected vaginal passage. Large amounts of purulent secretion accumulate under tension behind tightly closed swollen and red eyelids, necessitating great care during examination because of the tendency for pus to spurt into the examiner's eye when attempts are made to prise the lids open. In severe cases there is rapid involvement of the cornea with ulcer formation, which may lead to corneal perforation, loss of the anterior chamber and, frequently, damage to the anterior part of the lens (*anterior polar cataract*). Sometimes the perforation heals with restoration of the anterior chamber, although a fairly dense corneal scar persists. At other times the underlying iris becomes adherent to the cornea with the formation of a *leucoma adherens*. In severe cases the infection may spread rapidly to involve the whole eye (*endophthalmitis* or *panophthalmitis*) with a subsequent shrinkage of the eye (*phthisis bulbi*), which becomes blind. At one time it was customary to try and prevent ophthalmia neonatorum by the routine use of silver nitrate 1 or 2% drops (Credé 's method) or sulphacetamide 10% drops in the eyes of the newborn after the careful washing of the outer surfaces of the eyelids with a simple lotion. However, this prophylactic treatment has largely fallen into abeyance because it is not sufficient to prevent a severe infection such as gonococcal infection, and indeed it may mask the immediate effects of the infection so that its diagnosis (and therefore its treatment) are delayed. The only adequate prophylactic treatment for the child is to recognize and treat any infection in the mother during the pregnancy.

Ophthalmia neonatorum may also occur as a result of infection in the newborn infant by other organisms, such as *Haemophilus influenzae* (Koch-Weeks bacillus), *Streptococcus pneumoniae* (pneumococcus), *Staphylococcus, Escherichia coli,* or *Chlamydia* (TRIC agent). These cause a much less severe condition, often with only slight mucopurulent discharge from the eyes, except for the TRIC agent which may be as destructive as the gonococcus. There is sometimes an associated failure of canalization of the nasolacrimal duct (see p.212).

All cases of ophthalmia neonatorum—defined as 'a purulent discharge from the eyes of an infant commencing within 21 days from the date of its birth'—must be notified by the medical practitioner in attendance under the Public Health Regulations of 1926.

Gonococcal conjunctivitis may occur also in other age groups, particularly in the adult following the direct introduction of the infective agent into the eye from a source of infection, for example, gonococcal urethritis in the patient or some other individual. It usually remains confined to one eye provided the spread of infection is avoided. The conjunctivitis develops after an incubation period of two to five days and is very acute with abundant creamy purulent discharge, massive chemosis and swelling of the lids. In contrast to most other forms of conjunctivitis, the cornea is prone to develop ulceration of a severe type so that a perforation of the cornea and other complications (see Chapter 4) are likely.

Corynebacterium diphtheriae. This organism is liable to cause a severe conjunctivitis with the formation of a true membrane involving the mucosal and even the submucosal parts of the conjunctiva, with an occasional spread of the membrane onto the skin of the lid. Removal of the membrane is usually followed by haemorrhage. Later it may be replaced by scar tissue with obliteration of parts of the fornix (symblepharon) or with deformity of the eyelid, such as an entropion.

Diphtheroid bacilli (e.g. *Corynebacterium xerosis*) are not pathogenic in the conjunctiva. Other organisms, such as *Streptococcus haemolyticus, Streptococcus pneumoniae* (pneumococcus), *Neisseria meningitidis* (meningococcus) and *Haemophilus influenzae* (Koch-Weeks bacillus), are rarely associated with membrane formation as part of a severe conjunctivitis, and in these conditions the membrane is a false one because it is not incorporated in the underlying tissues.

Pseudomonas aeruginosa (Pseudomonas pyocyanea). This rarely causes a primary conjunctivitis, although conjunctivitis may occur following inflammatory changes of the cornea (see Chapter 4).

Micrococcus catarrhalis. This causes a mild form of conjunctivitis.

Treatment of bacterial conjunctivitis

Discomfort is relieved by the removal of crusts and excessive secretions by simple irrigation with bland saline or boracic lotion. Too frequent irrigations are undesirable because they dilute the lysozyme of the tears which is an effective antibacterial substance. The eyes should not be bandaged. Dark glasses may be necessary if there is photophobia.

Antibacterial treatment. There are many chemotherapeutic or antibiotic drugs which may be used locally in the eye in the form of drops during the day and in the form of ointment at night to prevent the adherence of the lids to one another. In gonococcal conjunctivitis in the neonate and in the adult, treatment must be both topical and systemic. Topically an intensive regimen is used: penicillin (6 mg/ml) every minute for thirty minutes, every five minutes for thirty minutes and then every thirty minutes until the condition is controlled. Intramuscular penicillin with oral probenecid comprises the systemic regimen. It is important to also treat the mother and the sexual partner(s) of the infected adult. Treatment of TRIC ophthalmia neonatorum is with topical tetracycline and systemic erythromycin.

There are a number of antibacterial drugs with a fairly wide range of activity available, such as chloramphenicol (0.5% drops or 1% ointment), bacitracin (1% drops or ointment), the aminoglycosides, particularly gentamicin, and neomycin. Polymyxin ointment (10 000 units/g) is effective against *Pseudomonas aeruginosa* and many other bacteria. Zinc sulphate drops (0.5 or 1%), often combined with adrenaline (1 in 1000) because of its vasoconstrictive effect, are specific against the effects of the enzyme of *Moraxella lacunata*. In general, the efficacy of topical medication and its penetration depend partly on the frequency of application, the degree of lipid solubility, the drug vehicle and the pH.

Note: There is a more recent tendency to omit the examination of the conjunctival secretion for the pathogenic organism as a routine procedure in cases of conjunctivitis because of the wide range of effectiveness of many of the modern drugs. However, a culture of the organism and its sensitivity to various drugs should be carried out whenever possible and certainly in all cases which fail to show a quick response to treatment.

Viral infections

Conjunctivitis caused by a virus is usually associated with the formation of follicles, hence the term *follicular conjunctivitis*. However, follicles occur in other conditions, for example allergic conditions, and they should not be considered as indicative only of a viral condition. The follicles represent proliferations of the normal lymphoid tissue which is present in the submucosal (adenoid) layer of the conjunctiva, and appear as pale, slightly raised patches of relatively small size arranged in regular rows within the palpebral and forniceal conjunctivae. More rarely a virus infection is associated with ulcerative or granulomatous changes.

Conjunctivitis may occur in virus conditions of the skin such as molluscum contagiosum or herpes zoster, in virus conditions of the cornea, such as epidemic keratoconjunctivitis, herpes simplex and herpes zoster (see Chapter 4), or in systemic virus conditions, such as measles and mumps; conjunctivitis in systemic conditions may be exogenous or endogenous.

Chlamydial infections

Paratrachoma (trachoma inclusion conjunctivitis—TRIC). This is produced by *Chlamydia,* an obligatory intracellular organism which has a reservoir in the genital tract and is, therefore, primarily a sexually transmitted disease. Neonatal ophthalmia is contracted during delivery and characteristically results in a mucopurulent papillary conjunctivitis. The adult variety tends to be a unilateral low-grade chronic conjunctivitis with a markedly follicular pattern, particularly in the fornices, associated with a fine punctate epithelial/subepithelial keratitis and limbal inflammation which may proceed to *pannus* (encroachment of vessels on to the cornea).

The organism may be isolated from the conjunctiva, cervix, urethra and rectum, and characteristic basophilic intracytoplasmic inclusions are found in conjunctival scrapings. Indirect immunofluorescent antibody techniques confirm the systemic nature of the infection, and allow accurate subtyping of *Chlamydia.*

Management involves topical and systemic treatment for three weeks with tetracycline or a sulphonamide drug; in infants, in whom oral tetracycline is contraindicated, erythromycin is used. It is important to also treat the sexual partner(s).

Trachoma. This term refers to the chronic scarring keratoconjunctivitis endemic in the Middle East, Asia and Africa that is a major cause of preventable blindness. The condition is caused by *Chlamydia* serotypes different to those causing paratrachoma and lymphogranuloma venereum (LGV) and has distinct epidemiological differences.

Whereas the paratrachoma serotypes have a genital reservoir, endemic trachoma has a purely ocular reservoir. Although direct eye to eye and fomite transmission occurs, the role of eye-seeking flies is paramount in the rapid, repetitive and indiscriminate spread of infection, which is facilitated by overcrowding and poor sanitation. Furthermore, the flies are vectors of bacterial and viral pathogens which compound the inflammatory response, contributing to blinding disease.

Clinically the condition presents, after an incubation period of about one week, as an acute bilateral conjunctivitis with intense discomfort, photophobia and redness of the eyes. There is an associated marked thickening of the palpebral conjunctiva resulting from papillary hypertrophy, with a gradual thickening and engorgement of the surface layers so that the conjunctiva assumes a rich velvety red appearance which obscures the underlying conjunctival vessels and tarsal glands. Follicular formations, which are localized accumulations of lymphocytes, plasma cells and epithelioid cells in the subconjunctival tissues, project through the surface of the conjunctiva to form round, translucent prominences suggestive of sago grains or frog spawn. These follicles occur to some extent over the whole conjunctiva, but are most obvious on the palpebral conjunctiva, particularly of the upper lid, and are responsible for the granular appearance which provides the name *trachoma* (from the Greek for *'roughness'*). The cornea is also involved, not simply because of the rubbing on the cornea of the granular undersurfaces of the upper lids, but also as the result of primary involvement which causes punctate epithelial erosions, punctate epithelial keratitis, and punctate subepithelial keratitis with the production of distinctive yellowish coloured subepithelial opacities. These changes occur particularly in the upper part of the cornea and are accompanied by superficial vascularization of the affected area with the formation of scarring (*superficial pannus*) which causes a disturbance of vision when it extends into the central parts of the cornea.

The infective state of trachoma tends to be self-limiting after a period of months or even years. Changes continue in the tissue of the lids because of the proliferation of scar tissue which occurs in the previously hypertrophied subepithelial tissues and within the tarsal plate, so that the palpebral conjunctiva, although becoming relatively white and smooth, develops radiating lines of scarring which are important diagnostic features of the disease. This scarring is liable also to lead to adhesions between the bulbar and palpebral conjunctivae, particularly of the upper lid, with partial obliteration of the fornices (*symblepharon*), and to entropion of the eyelids, particularly the upper one so that the eyelashes turn in and rub on the cornea. Trichiasis may also occur due to the development of aberrant lashes. Ptosis of the upper lid may follow an increase in the bulk of the lid or involvement of the levator muscle (or its associated smooth muscle). The corneal pannus may become less marked in time, but some permanent scarring is inevitable and the development of small irregular faceted scars, which are often difficult to detect, is liable to affect the vision markedly. The linings of the canaliculi may be involved, with the production of *epiphora*.

The diagnosis of trachoma is often easy because of the many distinctive clinical features, but it is confirmed in the laboratory by identification of the specific inclusion bodies within damaged epithelial cells in conjunctival scrapings, by the isolation of the organism, and by the presence of polymorphonuclear leucocytes and mononuclear cells (in the absence of eosinophils) in conjunctival scrapings, and by microimmunofluorescent antibody analysis of tears and serum.

Management of trachoma is on a community and individual basis. Clearly it is vital to break the cycle of transmission and this requires public health measures to improve sanitation and housing conditions, and mass campaigns of topical and systemic treatment with tetracycline or sulphonamide drugs to reduce the ocular reservoir of *Chlamydia*.

Individual management is aimed at eliminating *Chlamydia*, and treatment of sight-threatening attacks of bacterial infection; in the later stages surgical treatment may be required. It is often necessary to correct deformities of the lids such as entropion, trichiasis and lid shortening. If available, keratoplasty may be necessary for severe corneal scarring, although a contact lens may provide a useful level of vision without recourse to keratoplasty, the results of which may be prejudiced by the unhealthy state of the cornea, the lack of tears and the vascularization.

All these measures require a system to deliver primary eye care with regular surveillance and health education.

Other chlamydial infections. Conjunctivitis also occurs in *lymphogranuloma venereum (LGV)* and in *Reiter's disease,* in which a mild catarrhal conjunctivitis is associated with urethritis, polyarthritis and pyrexia.

Granulomatous conjunctivitis

This is characterized by the formation of granulomatous masses together with a generalized conjunctivitis of the affected eye, a regional adenitis, particularly of preauricular lymph nodes, and sometimes a pyrexia—a symptom complex known as *Parinaud's oculoglandular syndrome*. It may be exogenous or endogenous and occurs in association with certain diseases including (a) *syphilis*, in the form of a large painful ulcer (primary chancre) or of a localized inflammatory mass (gumma) of the underlying episcleral tissues or tarsal plate; (b) *tuberculosis*, in the form of a raised mass of the bulbar conjunctiva which may form indolent ulceration; (c) *viruses* such as lymphogranuloma venereum and infectious mononucleosis; (d) *leprosy*, in the form of nodules in the palpebral conjunctiva, particularly near the lid margins, or in the bulbar conjunctiva, usually near the limbus with subsequent involvement of the cornea (unlike other forms of granulomatous conjunctivitis this may be bilateral); (e) *tularaemia*; and (f) *fungus conditions* such as rhinosporidiosis. Treatment is aimed at the general disease, with local treatment to combat any secondary infection; sometimes it is necessary to excise the nodular lesions (which should, of course, be examined histologically).

Endogenous conjunctivitis

This occurs in certain systemic disorders, such as measles, influenza, glandular fever, leptospirosis and gonorrhoea (in its later stages), as a result of an endogenous infection. However, the exogenous type of conjunctivitis is more common than the endogenous type.

Chronic conjunctivitis

This is induced in various ways: (a) as the aftermath of a severe attack (or repeated attacks) of acute or subacute conjunctivitis, sometimes in association with excessive or prolonged use of topical drugs; (b) as the result of undue exposure of the bulbar conjunctiva in exophthalmos, proptosis, facial paralysis or ectropion; or (c) as the result of defective tear drainage through the lacrimal passages, which is usually associated with recurrent infection of the tear sac. The symptoms are similar to those of 'eyestrain'—tiredness and heaviness of the eyes, particularly after prolonged use, a sensation of grittiness, and a feeling of excessive heat in the eyes. The affected conjunctiva is hyperaemic and there is a persistent discharge. This discharge is sometimes of an infective nature but is usually merely an excess of the normal mucous secretions of the conjunctiva and often also of the sebaceous discharges from the tarsal (meibomian) glands of the eyelids; this accounts for the redness of the lid margins which is a common feature.

Treatment is aimed at removing the cause of the condition, the control of any infection, the discontinuance of harmful drugs, the relief of any nasolacrimal obstruction and the correction of any deformity of the eyelids.

Allergic or hypersensitivity keratoconjunctivitis

When normal body defences produce unwanted effects on host tissue, the term *allergy* or *hypersensitivity* is used. Such reactions may be divided into four types according to the pathological events which take place.

Type I or IgE mediated hypersensitivity

This occurs when tissue-based antibody is exposed to an allergen; mast cells (from the tissue) and basophils (from the blood) react by degranulating to release a number of vasoactive substances that mediate inflammation. Atopic patients, on exposure to pollens (as in hay fever) or other organic allergens, may develop an acute swelling of the conjunctiva, associated with rhinitis. These are IgE-mediated responses, as is the potentially more serious condition of *vernal keratoconjunctivitis*. This tends to affect young males with a history or family history of atopy, and occurs usually, but not invariably, during the spring and summer (the term *spring catarrh* is a misnomer). The predominant symptoms in the acute stages are discomfort, intense itching and stringy discharge. Conjunctivitis is a constant feature with the development of a slight milky translucence of the bulbar conjunctiva and the formation of giant, flat-topped papillae (cobblestones) in an inflamed, infiltrated palpebral conjunctiva, particularly of the upper lids on which there lies a stringy mucoid discharge. Marked follicular enlargement and congestion of the limbus may occur, especially in pigmented races.

Keratitis occurs in certain cases following an extension of the limbal and conjunctival lesions, with the formation of a vascularized pannus, which resembles the pannus of trachoma. Keratitis may also occur as a separate entity in the form of a punctate keratitis with minute dull grey spots, particularly in the upper part of the cornea, but not at the extreme periphery. Rarely, confluence of a punctate keratitis may produce a large area of epithelial loss. A transversely oval ulcer is formed onto which a fibrin type substance may be deposited which builds up in successive layers to form a hydrophobic plaque over which the epithelium cannot spread. These lesions may cross the visual axis, with the risk in the young (less than seven years) of amblyopia. The majority require surgical removal. Vernal keratitis is aggravated by the roughened undersurfaces of the upper lids and by deposits of any therapeutic agent which forms suspensions. Scrapings of the conjunctiva show an inflammatory exudate which contains lymphocytes, plasma cells, usually abundant eosinophils, and often damaged epithelial cells. The serum IgE level is elevated.

Treatment in the acute stage is aimed at reducing the intense inflammatory response by the administration of frequent (hourly) topical steroids, a cycloplegic, a mucolytic (acetylcysteine), and sodium cromoglycate drops, which prevent mast cell degranulation by stabilizing the cell membrane.

Very occasionally systemic steroids are required. Care should be exercised, however, in the long-term use of steroids because of the complications which may occur, particularly a form of glaucoma in the susceptible individual with topical steroids and cataract with systemic steroids.

In the long-term, it is important that sodium cromoglycate is instilled even if the child is free of symptoms. It should be noted that it is usually a self-limiting disease which seldom persists into adult life.

Type II or complement-dependent hypersensitivity

This occurs in the conjunctiva as part of a systemic process involving epithelial cells; for example, pemphigus and pemphigoid.

Pemphigus. In this condition there is widespread fragile blistering of the skin due to desmosomal disruption in the prickle cell layer as a result of deposition of an IgG antibody and complement. Papillary hypertrophy of the conjunctiva may occur but resolves without scarring.

Pemphigoid. By contrast, the immune reaction in pemphigoid occurs in a linear fashion on the basement membrane of the epithelial cells, producing a recurrent mucopurulent conjunctivitis with ulceration. There are secondary fibrovascular proliferative changes in the subconjunctival tissue resulting in early distortion of the canthi and later development of broad-based symblepharon with partial obliteration of the conjunctival sac. There are subsequent degenerative changes in the cornea because of exposure due to faulty closure of the eyelids and loss of the normal moisture of the eye. This latter follows destruction by fibrosis of the conjunctival mucous glands and obliteration of the lacrimal ducts which discharge the lacrimal fluid (tears) into the conjunctival sac from the main and accessory lacrimal glands. Suppuration of the degenerate cornea is a likely terminal event leading to an endophthalmitis and subsequent phthisis bulbi.

Treatment is aimed at maintaining a normal moist environment for the cornea. Periodic acute exacerbations are treated energetically with topical steroids. Surgical division of symblepharon and mucous membrane grafting tends to excite further inflammatory reaction and is very rarely successful.

Type III or immune-complex hypersensitivity

This is the result of an interaction between circulating antibody, circulating antigen and complement, and leads to an acute vasculitis. Bacteria (*Haemophilus influenzae*), viruses, atypical bacteria (mycoplasma) and drugs (sulphonamides and phenylbutazone) may induce this response, which is known as *erythema multiforme (Stevens–Johnson syndrome).* Even though evidence of skin involvement may be scarce, marked ocular involvement may be present, manifest as an occlusive vasculitis producing a conjunctival infarct that later scars. Long-term complications include mild symblepharon, aberrant lashes which abrade the cornea, metaplasia of the epithelium, and the development of the dry eye syndrome despite copious abnormal tears.

Management demands awareness of the condition during the acute stage when topical steroids can prevent most of the debilitating long-term sequelae. Mucous membrane grafts are more successful in this condition.

Type IV or cell-mediated hypersensitivity

This is produced by tissue-based, thymus-dependent (T) lymphocytes. There are numerous stimuli for this type of response, such as contact with topical drops, ointments or their preservatives and vehicles, or cosmetics, particularly those which are applied near the eye, such as mascara, or which are introduced into the eye by rubbing with the fingers, such as nail varnish. The condition is characterized by a profuse watery discharge with hyperaemia of the conjunctiva, follicle formation, and eczematous and swollen lids. Treatment requires identification of the allergic agent if possible. Topical medication should be avoided, although in some cases corticosteroid drops may be necessary; hydrocortisone will ameliorate the skin involvement.

Phlyctenular conjunctivitis is another disorder of cell-mediated immunity which is believed to be a response to mycobacterial, bacterial, fungal or chlamydial protein. It is characterized by discrete raised pink/creamy coloured micro-abscesses on the bulbar conjunctiva or cornea, especially near the limbus. These represent subepithelial aggregations of polymorphonuclear leucocytes with surrounding lymphocytes and plasma cells, and usually form ulcerated areas as a result of loss of the overlying epithelium. Pain, photophobia and mucopurulent discharge occur if the conjunctiva becomes secondarily infected. This condition readily responds to topical steroids.

Degenerations

Concretions

These occur in the crypts of the palpebral conjunctiva following a gradual accumulation of inflammatory or degenerative products. They usually remain as small white spots of little or no significance, but sometimes they become calcareous and project beyond the surface level and cause irritation. They may be removed readily by a sharp-pointed instrument such as a 21G needle using a surface anaesthetic (amethocaine 1% drops).

Pingueculae

These are yellow-coloured oval slightly raised masses which form on the bulbar conjunctiva on either or both sides of the cornea in the interpalpebral area; the slightly broader part of the lesion is directed towards the cornea. They occur almost universally, particularly after middle age, and represent hyaline degenerative changes. Treatment is by simple excision, although this is seldom indicated because the resultant scar tissue is likely to be as obvious as the pinguecula. Sometimes, however, a pinguecula extends to form a pterygium.

Pterygium

This degenerative condition of the conjunctiva is associated with similar changes in the cornea. It presents as a wing-shaped vascular thickening of the bulbar conjunctiva which begins on either or both sides of the cornea, more commonly on the nasal side. The part adjacent to the cornea (its head) encroaches onto the cornea and insinuates itself between the epithelium and Bowman's membrane. This encroachment occurs when there are superficial degenerative changes in the cornea of a primary nature, which are shown by the grey edge in the superficial corneal tissues distal to the spreading head of the pterygium. The main part (body) of the pterygium also extends in the opposite direction so that its terminal part (tail) reaches the region of the medial (or lateral) canthus. It occurs essentially following persistent exposure to wind and dust, so that it is common in parts of the world like the Middle East and Australia but may occur in any country.

Treatment. If a pterygium is threatening to involve the central part of the cornea or if it is cosmetically unsightly, it should be removed. It is usual to shave the head of the pterygium from the cornea (*superficial keratectomy*), and to remove the bulk of the pterygium by a subconjunctival approach; a fairly large portion of the conjunctiva near the limbus is also removed so that a bare area of sclera remains after the operation. This should prevent a further encroachment of the conjunctival tissues onto the affected part of the cornea before healing is complete. Postoperative beta-irradiation is useful in recurrent cases or sometimes following the first operation if the pterygium is fleshy and 'active' looking. The affected part of the cornea remains permanently scarred even after a successful operation, so it is essential to operate before the central part of the cornea is involved, although in advanced cases this complication may be overcome by combining the removal of the pterygium with a lamellar keratoplasty.

Pseudopterygium. When a fold of conjunctiva becomes adherent to a limbal corneal lesion like an ulcer, the appearance is similar to a true pterygium. However, it can be distinguished by passing a probe under it, demonstrating the bridge-like nature of the encroachment in a pseudopterygium.

Cysts

Lymphatic cysts

These appear as small worm-like dilatations of clear thin-walled vessels. They may be removed by simple excision (although care should be taken to localize them by a suture before opening the conjunctiva otherwise they may be obscured by haemorrhage). Simple incision is liable to be followed by recurrence.

Implantation cysts

These occur in the subconjunctival tissues following the implantation of a fragment of conjunctiva after injury or operation. If they become large, they are readily excised.

Tumours

Various tumours may arise in the conjunctiva, particularly at the limbus, but they are rare.

Papilloma

This is a benign epithelial tumour which appears as a small raised vascular mass with an irregular surface.

Epithelioma

This may occur spontaneously or in a previously inflamed or injured area. It forms a raised vascular mass which is often only locally invasive, but sometimes it may spread to the regional lymph nodes (preauricular and cervical) or it may even form distant metastases. The histological appearances are variable; it is usually a squamous cell carcinoma but may be a basal cell carcinoma or an intraepithelial epithelioma (Bowen's disease), in which the lesions appear as slightly elevated diffuse patches of highly vascular gelatinous tissue with a yellowish-grey colour, characteristically occurring in elderly men.

Reticuloendothelial tumours

Tumours such as the lymphomas and leukaemias may present as diffuse masses in the conjunctiva.

Tumours of vascular origin

Tumours of vascular origin, such as lymphangioma, angioma and endothelioma, are very rare.

Pigmentary disorders

These may be classified as benign or potentially malignant. Benign conditions include the pigmentary staining areas of conjunctiva which occur more commonly in dark-skinned races and are accentuated during hormonal variations (e.g. pregnancy, puberty or in Addison's disease), and the pigmented naevus (hamartoma) that completes its growth by adolescence (junctional naevus becoming subepithelial). Very rarely a naevus may become malignant.

Those disorders with malignant potential have been termed *precancerous melanosis*. They represent areas of pigmented tissue whose malignant progression (to malignant melanoma) is manifest by an increase in size and a change in pigmentation or vascularity. If these changes occur, the lesion merits excision biopsy. If it involves the lids, an exenteration (removal of the eye with its conjunctival covering, the lids and the contents of the orbit) may be necessary, but before carrying out such a drastic measure an attempt should be made to control the malignant process by irradiation or cryotherapy. Precancerous melanosis occurs particularly in middle age, more commonly in women, and may remain benign for an indefinite period, although it may show phases of progression and regression in different parts of the surface tissue because of its multicentric nature.

Granulomas

Formation of granulomas is liable to follow operative trauma if Tenon's capsule (the connective tissue enveloping the eyeball except for the area of cornea and limbus) is incorporated in the conjunctival wound or if there is a reaction to suture material (usually catgut, as used in a squint operation). They may also occur in the palpebral conjunctiva as extensions of meibomian cysts (*chalazions*).

Asymptomatic sarcoid granulomata may sometimes be found in the conjunctival fornices with the appearance of elongated follicles, and are readily accessible for diagnostic biopsy.

Dermoid and dermolipoma

These are benign growths which are congenitally determined.

Treatment

In general, benign tumours may be treated by simple excision, while malignant tumours require wide excision with postoperative irradiation.

Infestations

The adult worm of *Loa loa*, limited to certain regions of West Africa and transmitted by the biting fly, *Chrysops*, may be seen meandering in the subconjunctival tissues without inducing an inflammatory response. Topical anaesthesia immobilizes the worm for easy removal.

Deposition of certain fly eggs results in the development of the early larval stages within the conjunctiva (*ocular myiasis*) which generates a brisk inflammatory response.

4

The Cornea

Structure and function

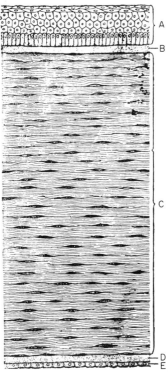

Fig. 18. The histological appearance of the cornea: A. epithelium; B. Bowman's membrane; C. stroma; D. Descemet's membrane; E. endothelium.

The structure of the cornea demonstrates a remarkable combination of rigidity for protection with transparency for the transmission and refraction of light. It forms the anterior one-sixth of the outer coat of the eyeball (the sclera forming the remaining five-sixths), and is composed of five layers as shown in Fig. 18.

Epithelium The delicate squamous surface epithelium is continuous with the conjunctival epithelium at the limbus. There is a transition of cell

43

type from the columnar cells adjacent to its basement membrane, through polyhedral cells, to attenuated, non-keratinizing, nucleated cells with few organelles at the surface. Basal epithelial cells show modifications of their boundaries known as *hemi-desmosomes*, which are attached to the underlying basement membrane and Bowman's membrane. Although similar firm attachments exist between other layers, it is only at the surface that there is a continuous lateral desmosomal attachment which prevents the ingress of tears. Furthermore, multiple foldings of the external cells (*microplicae, microvilli*) increase the surface area and are coated by the mucous layer of the precorneal tear film. The integrity of the epithelium is dependent on a free supply of oxygen, hence the oedematous changes which follow ill-fitting contact lenses. Defects of the epithelium heal readily by a rapid sliding process of the surrounding epithelial cells.

Bowman's membrane. This is a thin lamina of condensed stromal tissue which is fairly resistant to injury or disease, but once perforated it does not regenerate and is replaced by scar tissue.

Stroma. This represents 90% of the thickness of the cornea and is continuous with the sclera. It is composed of many lamellae which lie parallel to one another with little or no interlacing. Each lamella contains uniform collagen fibrils which extend across the cornea in parallel sheets. The stroma is avascular, but contains modified fibroblasts (*keratocytes*) which interdigitate between the lamellae and have extensive cytoplasmic processes. Individual collagen fibrils lie in a mucopolysaccharide ground substance and the regular interfibrillary distance is maintained by mutual repulsion of their ionic charge.

Metabolism is both aerobic (Embden-Meyerhof pathway) and anaerobic (hexose monophosphate shunt and tricarboxylic acid cycle), with the smaller molecular weight substances such as ions, sugar and oxygen being derived from the aqueous and the larger molecular weight aminoacids gaining access from the limbal circulation.

The rigid layering of the lamellae is of surgical importance because it facilitates the removal of a uniformly thick disc of corneal tissue (lamellar graft) along a precise plane of cleavage; it also permits a fairly marked swelling of the stromal tissues under certain pathological conditions. To a large extent the precise arrangement of the collagen fibrils in the stroma determines its transparency. If this is disturbed by mechanical stress following injury, by a sudden rise of pressure within the eye as in the acute phase of closed-angle glaucoma, or by oedema of the ground substance as in deep keratitis, there is a scattering of the light rays by interference, with a loss of transparency. The transparency of the stroma also depends on its avascularity, so that the entry of vessels into the stroma in certain disease conditions, often as a result of an increase in the spaces between the fibrils, leads to some loss of transparency.

Descemet's membrane. This is a thin lamina which separates the stroma from the underlying endothelium, by which it is secreted. It is fairly resistant to injury and disease.

Endothelium. This is a thin single layer of cells on the inner surface of the cornea which is continuous with the endothelial covering of the trabecular tissues in the filtration angle and with the surface endothelial layer of the iris. It has a protective function in controlling the access of the intraocular fluid (aqueous humour) into the stroma. It plays an active part in pumping fluid out of the cornea, so that a loss of the endothelium may result in a water-logging of the corneal stroma. In contrast to the epithelium, the endothelium does not exhibit replacement by mitosis, so that loss of cells, a normal event throughout life, is made up by enlargement and spread of the remaining cells. It follows that loss of endothelial cells as a result of injury, for example during an intraocular operation such as cataract extraction or as a result of degenerative changes, may indirectly result in oedematous changes in the epithelium and stroma (*bullous keratopathy*).

The recent development of the endothelial specular microscope allows a detailed in vivo examination of the morphology of the endothelium at a magnification of 120 times. In the contact specular microscope the objective cone applanates a thin hydrogel contact lens placed on the cornea. The area of each field examined is 1 mm^2. By modifying the incident light, the contour of the posterior endothelial surface may be seen in three dimensions—the relief mode. Examples of these are shown in Fig. 19.

The precorneal tear film

The precorneal tear film provides a smooth refractive surface on the front of the eye, and acts as a lubricant for the lids, as a vehicle for antibacterial and some nutritional components and as a means of flushing out surface debris. It can be divided into three layers. The most superficial contains the oily secretions of the meibomian glands which delay evaporation of the second or aqueous layer, which is contributed by the lacrimal and accessory lacrimal glands. The third layer covers the corneal epithelium and contains the macromolecule *mucin*, secreted by the goblet cells, which renders the otherwise hydrophobic surface hydrophilic. The inherently unstable tear film, is regenerated by blinking.

The corneal reflexes

Light from a window or electric light source is mirrored on the anterior surface of the cornea as a bright reflex—this is one of the *Purkinje–Sanson* images (the other images being formed by the posterior surface of the cornea and by the anterior and posterior surfaces of the lens)—

(a)

(b)

(c)

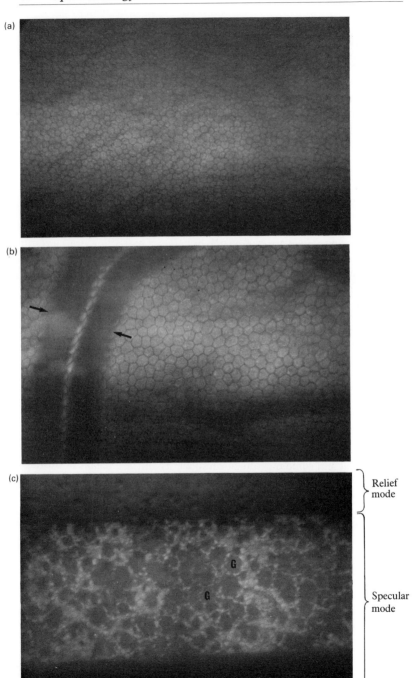

Relief mode

Specular mode

(d)

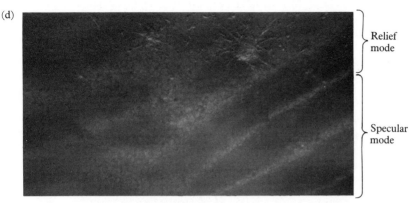

Relief mode

Specular mode

Fig. 19.   Endothelial specular microscopy (contact method). (a) Normal endothelial cells in area of 1 mm². (b) Corneal graft (p.62). Note (i) enlarged cells; and (ii) part of a posterior corneal ring (arrows), a reproducible wrinkling of the posterior corneal surface useful for relocation purposes. (c) Fuchs' endothelial dystrophy (p.67). Note multiple guttata (G), enlarged cells, and protrusion of guttata into the anterior chamber seen in the relief mode. (d) Heterochromic cyclitis (p.94). Note multiple keratic precipitates in specular mode with branching pattern of endothelial deposits in relief mode. All photographs are taken at the same magnification.

and the clarity and uniformity of these reflexes are dependent on the normal transparency and curvature of this corneal surface. These images are used in the determination of the anterior corneal radii (keratometry), a prerequisite for contact lens prescribing, and also used for corneal and anterior chamber depth measurements.

Corneal sensitivity

The normal corneal epithelium is very sensitive to touch. The sensation which is mediated is essentially one of pain, irrespective of the nature of the stimulus, and serves a protective function. Any prolonged infective condition of the epithelium impairs this sensation, thus rendering the cornea more liable to subsequent disease; this is noted particularly after recurrent bouts of herpes simplex and herpes zoster keratitis.

Diagnostic stains

Fluorescein 2% drops. This dye stains immature epithelial cells (exposed by the removal of the surface cells following injury or disease) a very bright shade of green, and areas of defective epithelium a less bright shade of green. Fluorescein also stains the precorneal tear film, especially the marginal strip adjacent to the lid margin. If excess dye is removed by irrigation with saline before examining the eye, fluorescein staining of the epithelium will not be confused with fluorescein in the precorneal fluid.

Rose Bengal 1% drops. This is a dye which stains fatty components of diseased epithelial cells, for example those damaged as a result of virus invasion or dessication.

Congenital anomalies

Microcornea

A small cornea occurs in a small eye (microphthalmos) which follows a developmental failure of the whole eye, but it may also occur in an otherwise normal eye. It produces a hypermetropic refractive error and its association with a narrow filtration angle may predispose to closed-angle glaucoma.

Megalocornea

A large cornea occurs in normal eyes of males only and may predispose to dislocation of the lens or to cataract formation. It causes myopia, but is distinguished from the enlarged cornea which occurs in high axial myopia by the absence of changes in the posterior segment of the eye (see p.12). It is distinguished from the enlarged cornea which occurs in buphthalmos by the absence of splits in Descemet's membrane.

Injuries

Abrasion

The cornea is highly susceptible to superficial injury because of the delicacy of its epithelium. It is usually the lower part of the cornea which is affected because the eye turns up during the instinctive closure of the eyelids as a protective response to an approaching object. An abrasion causes immediate and often severe pain, redness of the conjunctiva, particularly in the circumcorneal region, and intense lacrimation. The abrasion usually heals rapidly within 12 to 24 hours unless a secondary infection of the abraded area causes a corneal ulcer with all its subsequent complications.

Treatment. This consists of the prevention of secondary infection by antibiotic drops and of pupillary and ciliary spasm by cycloplegic drops (e.g. homatropine or cyclopentolate), and of the relief of pain by immobilizing the lids with a pad.

Recurrent erosion

Any form of corneal abrasion (classically the scratch from a baby's fingernail) may break down repeatedly, even months after an injury. It usually occurs on opening the eye in the early morning when an adhesion between the undersurface of the upper lid and the epithelial cells of the healed cornea area which formed during sleep is broken, stripping cells from that part of the cornea. It seems likely that some acquired defect renders these cells more 'tacky' than usual.

Treatment. Each recurrence is treated as an abrasion, and an attempt is made to avoid recurrences by the prolonged use of a lubricating agent (e.g. parolein drops) at night until the injured area is completely healed. Debridement of an area of unstable epithelium often allows more rapid healing, but it must be remembered that several months must elapse before any satisfactory re-adherence to the basement membrane occurs.

Very thin hydrogel contact lenses also facilitate epithelial healing by removing the traumatizing effect of blinking and producing rapid relief of pain.

Superficial foreign bodies

The cornea is a frequent target for foreign bodies which are swept by the wind into the eyes or directed into the eyes in occupations which use grinding machines. The foreign body usually lodges in the lower part of the cornea and causes immediate pain, redness, lacrimation and a gritty sensation on movement of the eyelids over the affected area. The foreign body is readily visible on focal illumination against the background of the iris, but sometimes it comes into view only on looking at the cornea in a particular direction or by the use of the slit-lamp microscope.

Treatment. It is sometimes possible for the patient to dislodge the foreign body by forcible and rapid movements of the lids over the corneal surface, a process aided by the intense lacrimation associated with the injury. However, this ability is short-lived because a rapid swelling of the corneal cells causes the foreign body to become firmly lodged, particularly when there is destruction of the epithelium. The foreign body is removed under a local anaesthetic (benoxinate 0.4% or amethocaine 1%). Except for very superficial foreign bodies, which can be wiped off the epithelium with a moist cotton wool bud, the safest and least traumatic method is to use a sterile needle (21G) under slit-lamp microscope control. After removal, treatment is as for a corneal abrasion (see above).

Deep foreign bodies

The cornea is fairly resistant to perforation because of the layering of its lamellae and because of the presence of Descemet's membrane, so that even a small sharp foreign body which enters the cornea at considerable speed may become lodged within the stroma without entering the eye. Sometimes a foreign body may be present in the stroma without causing any immediate discomfort because the surface wound is so small that it heals rapidly. Such a foreign body may be removed, but this demands the skill of an experienced surgeon, and in certain cases the surgeon may elect to avoid any interference because of the damage to the surrounding cornea that may follow.

Perforating wounds

This subject is covered in Chapter 17.

Ultraviolet light

Ultraviolet light may affect the eyes during its therapeutic or cosmetic administration, following a flash from a welder's arc, or following intense exposure to the glare of the sun (so-called *snowblindness*). There is a severe reaction in the conjunctiva and cornea, usually of both eyes; this occurs after an interval of a few hours since the reaction represents a photochemical response. There is marked hyperaemia of the conjunctiva, diffuse superficial oedema of the corneal epithelium (which stains vividly with fluorescein drops), intense photophobia, lacrimation, spasm of the eyelids (blepharospasm) and pain. The conditions responds to the immediate application of amethocaine 1% drops to relieve the pain, and adrenaline drops 0.01% to relieve the congestion. The condition should be prevented by wearing protective tinted goggles during any likely exposure to ultraviolet light, but the associated reduction in clarity sometimes engenders a casual attitude to their use in certain industrial procedures.

Keratitis

Keratitis is the name applied to inflammatory conditions of the cornea, whether exogenous (bacterial, viral, mycotic or drug-induced) or endogenous (syphilis, onchocerciasis, leishmaniasis or leprosy). Because of its avascularity, there is a limited pattern of visible response. The majority, however, produce spots on the cornea (*punctate keratitis*), and it is only by careful examination of associated features in the tarsal and bulbar conjunctiva, lids and glands that one can distinguish cases of a viral nature, those with a bacterial component (e.g. the keratitis that may be associated with staphylococcal blepharoconjunctivitis), those of a non-infective nature (e.g. *keratitis sicca* occurring in excessive dryness of the eye, *rosacea keratitis* associated with acne rosacea, or *neurotropic keratitis* which follows lesions of the ophthalmic division of the trigeminal nerve) or those of a traumatic nature (e.g. the neuroparalytic keratitis—*exposure keratitis*—which follows paralysis of the facial nerve, the keratitis which follows exposure to ultraviolet light, and the keratitis which follows persistent trichiasis).

Small superficial spots only visible with staining are called *punctate epithelial erosions,* deeper epithelial lesions are called *punctate epithelial keratitis* and stromal spots are called *subepithelial keratitis.*

Bacterial keratitis

A bacterial infection of the normal cornea occurs only rarely. A compromised cornea, whether from previous corneal disease (e.g. trachoma or herpes simplex), impaired sensation (e.g. herpes zoster or leprosy), impaired lid function leading to exposure (e.g. in seventh nerve palsy) or poor or deficient tears (e.g. in keratoconjunctivitis sicca or pemphigoid) allows easier access for micro-organisms.

Keratitis can be caused by many bacterial organisms which have been discussed in Chapter 3, such as *Staphylococcus, Streptococcus, Neisseria gonorrhoeae* (gonococcus), *Pseudomonas aeruginosa, Proteus* and *Escherichia coli,* and it is usually associated with some degree of conjunctivitis.

The characteristic lesion of a superficial bacterial keratitis is a corneal ulcer which may be single or multiple; because of its infective nature it is sometimes termed a *catarrhal ulcer.* This appears as a grey circular area on the surface of the cornea, often initially without any loss of corneal substance, but invariably with oedema of the surrounding corneal epithelium which dulls the normal brightness of the cornea within and around the affected area and distorts the normal corneal reflex. The affected area may be determined by using fluorescein drops. The eye becomes red in the circumcorneal region (*circumcorneal injection*) and the deep vessels here may also be involved (*ciliary injection*); a generalized redness occurs when there is an associated conjunctivitis. The ulcer causes severe pain, lacrimation, photophobia, blepharospasm, and sometimes spasm of the pupil (miosis) as a result of stimulation of the abundant sensory nerve endings within the corneal epithelium. Most catarrhal corneal ulcers have a marginal distribution, but infection with *Streptococcus pneumoniae,* or more rarely with *Pseudomonas aeruginosa,* tends to cause the formation of a more centrally placed ulcer which often shows irregularly spreading edges (hence the term *acute serpiginous ulcer*). Rarely the ulcer is confined to the epithelium so that it heals without leaving any significant scar, but usually there is involvement of the corneal stroma which leads subsequently to fibrosis and permanent scarring. The scar may be small (a *nebula*) or large (a *leucoma*), and sometimes it may be marked only by a slight depression (a *facet*). In the later stages, particularly when the ulcer is near the limbus, vessels from the conjunctival circulation pass over the limbus to the affected area (*superficial vascularization*) and these tend to persist for a prolonged time. Sometimes the ulcer fails to heal, particularly when it is in the central part of the cornea. It then extends through the stroma to the level of Descemet's membrane, which may protrude through the ulcerated area as a thin vesicle (*descemetocele*) because of the pressure of the intraocular fluid, even when this pressure is normal. Later this vesicle may rupture (*corneal perforation*), although as a rule Descemet's membrane is remarkably resistant to perforation. This type of severe deep ulcer usually occurs when there is considerable sepsis, and an associated collection of purulent inflammatory cells in the anterior chamber may form a mass in the lower part of the anterior chamber (*hypopyon keratitis*).

In a corneal perforation, aqueous humour is expressed from the anterior chamber through the corneal opening at the moment of perforation and the patient is often aware of warm fluid running down the cheek. It is rare for corneal perforation to heal with normal restoration of the anterior chamber; it is often followed by serious complications. Part of the iris may be expressed through the perforation (*iris prolapse*) leading eventually to an extensively thickened and scarred cornea containing iris tissue (*corneal staphyloma*). Parts of the iris may remain in contact with the inner aspect of the perforation without actually prolapsing (*anterior synechiae*), and in such cases there is often an extensively scarred area of cornea (*leucoma adherens*). A corneal perforation is also liable to result in the lens coming into contact with the cornea so that an *anterior subcapsular cataract* occurs. Occasionally in elderly people there may be an extensive choroidal haemorrhage following the sudden lowering of the intraocular pressure (*expulsive choroidal haemorrhage*) and this is fostered by an abnormality of the choroidal vessels or of the elastic lamina of Bruch's membrane. It is also possible for adhesions to form between the peripheral part of the iris and the filtration angle (*peripheral anterior synechiae*) so that secondary glaucoma may develop. Sometimes a corneal ulcer may lead to an anterior uveitis and even to inflammation of the whole eye (*panophthalmitis*) with subsequent shrinkage of the eye which then becomes blind and degenerate (*phthisis bulbi*).

Treatment

Various antibiotic preparations have reduced the incidence of bacterial keratitis because of their widespread use in the treatment of superficial injuries and infections of the eyes in factory first-aid departments, hospital casualty departments and in general practice. In established cases, the immediate priority is to identify the organism using Gram's stain in tissue removed from the margins of the ulcer. At the same time a variety of culture media (aerobic, anaerobic, enriched and fungal) are innoculated for confirmation of the infecting organism (or primary identification if no organism is seen using Gram's stain) and to determine antibiotic sensitivities.

Because of the devastating effect bacterial keratitis may have on vision, a broad-spectrum antibiotic regimen is given immediately on an intensive basis until the sensitivities are known, when the treatment may be altered accordingly. An example of such a regimen is gentamicin and methicillin as a subconjunctival injection and as hourly drops.

The use of atropine drops reduces pain by eliminating the spasm of the sphincter muscle of the iris and of the ciliary muscle of the ciliary body, and prevents the formation of posterior synechiae.

If topical steroids are used to aid resolution of the inflammatory process and to reduce the degree of eventual scarring, this should be with great caution for fear of encouraging fungal or viral replication, or even perforation if the ulcer is deep.

Delayed healing, despite correct therapy, should raise the possibility of a fungal infection.

A bandage contact lens may be useful in incipient perforation or descemetocele; occasionally a corneal graft in the acute stage is necessary as a protective measure but with little prospect of the graft remaining clear.

When the vision is affected by severe scarring, a corneal graft operation may be performed when the condition is no longer active; sometimes a contact lens may be of value in improving the vision, particularly when the residual scar causes corneal distortion.

Viral keratitis

The commoner forms of viral keratitis are due to adenovirus, herpes simplex virus, herpes zoster virus and molluscum contagiosum virus.

Adenovirus

This virus produces a keratoconjunctivitis. Although it does occur sporadically, it may occur in epidemics where direct transmission by medical personnel is often involved. The sporadic type typically produces a pharyngitis with fever and a follicular conjunctivitis with only mild keratitis (*pharyngoconjunctival fever*), while epidemic keratoconjunctivitis, usually caused by adenovirus type 8 or 19, presents with an intense follicular conjunctivitis, proceeding to a fine epithelial keratitis, and leading to relatively circumscribed areas of infiltrate of the superficial stroma (*subepithelial punctate keratitis*). Vision may be seriously affected and infiltrates can take up to two years to clear. In the early stages there is tender preauricular lymphadenopathy, and scrapings of the conjunctiva show an abundance of mononuclear cells, few eosinophils, few polymorphonuclear leucocytes and an absence of inclusion bodies. No specific treatment is available, but topical antibiotics prevent secondary bacterial infection and topical steroids may be used in severe keratitis or pseudomembrane formation.

Herpes simplex

Herpes simplex demonstrates a range of ocular morbidity that can be roughly divided into three types: (a) the primary infection, characterized by an ulcerative blepharitis, follicular conjunctivitis, a vesicular rash and in 50% some degree of corneal involvement; (b) recurrent epithelial keratitis; and (c) stromal disease or keratouveitis and its complications.

Primary epithelial disease is associated with multiple small vesicular formations (*fine punctate keratitis*) which stain vividly with Rose Bengal; they also stain with fluorescein although only after they rupture to form minute superficial areas of ulceration. More rarely the punctate areas may be coarse, stellate, areolar or even filamentary in nature. These early punctate epithelial lesions become associated with subepithelial lesions of a greyish-white colour which tend to be permanent. Sometimes there are associated herpetic vesicles of the skin of the face, particularly on the eyelids or the side of the nose. These lesions are prone to recur, especially during some other infection, for example of a respiratory nature, presumably due to a lowering of the natural immunity to the virus.

A distinctive form of recurrent herpes keratitis is the *dendritic ulcer* in which vesicles coalesce to form an irregular line of superficial ulceration with many small extensions from the main stem, each of which ends in a 'bud-like' formation. There is a tendency for this to lead to a deep stromal type of keratitis (*disciform keratitis*), which begins as oedema of the stroma, particularly centrally, with keratic precipitates producing haziness and impaired vision; these features may be permanent, although they usually become less marked after a prolonged time. The oedematous process favours the entry of deep vessels from the episcleral plexus into the cornea, thus leading to further scarring. Their deep nature is indicated by their disappearance beyond the limbus in contrast to more superficial vessels which may spread to the cornea from the conjunctival vessels (Fig. 20). Deep vessels usually persist indefinitely within the cornea, although after many months or even years circulating blood may be absent; these 'ghost vessels' appear as thin white lines which are distinguished from prominent corneal nerves by their sites of entry at the limbus and by their fairly regular course within a particular layer of the stroma. There may be an accompanying iritis, often with elevation of the intraocular pressure. These changes in the stroma may represent an immunological response due to the virus meeting an antibody which enters the cornea from the limbal circulation. The more superficial epithelial changes may persist during the active period of the deep ketatitis, and it is likely

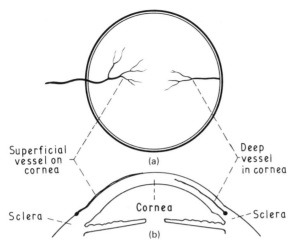

Fig. 20. Corneal vascularization—superficial vessels from the conjunctival circulation and deep vessels from the ciliary plexus as shown on (a) surface view and (b) vertical section of the cornea.

that the abnormal condition of the stroma prevents the overlying epithelium from healing (*metaherpetic ulcer*) so that it remains defective despite an absence of any active disease within its cells.

Treatment. Primary ocular herpes simplex is treated with topical antiviral agents to the eye and skin lesions, and with a cycloplegic if there is secondary ciliary spasm. In recurrent epithelial disease, especially dendritic ulcers, physical removal of the viral load by gentle wipe debridement with a cottonwool bud followed by ten days of topical antiviral drug administration allows resolution, usually without scarring.

In recent years a number of antiviral agents have become available whose activity is based on their ability to interrupt the synthesis of viral DNA. However, in so doing they may interfere with host epithelial DNA and this accounts for the high incidence of epithelial toxicity.

Because of poor stromal penetration, idoxuridine (IDU) and adenine arabinoside (Ara-A) are used more for epithelial disease, while trifluorothymidine and particularly acycloguanosine (acyclovir), which have good penetration, are used in stromal disease and keratouveitis. None of these agents has preventive properties, which at present are only shown by interferon, but this is not yet widely available.

Topical steroids, with frequent supervision, are used in the immunological condition of disciform keratitis but because they enhance viral replication, an antiviral agent must be given concomitantly. When topical steroids are used, it is essential to continue their use for many weeks or even months with a gradual reduction in amount, otherwise a recrudescence is likely; the possibility of steroid-induced glaucoma must also be borne in mind.

Indolent ulceration may benefit from a bandage hydrogel contact lens or temporary tarsorrhaphy (closure of the lids by uniting the lid margins with sutures), while in the later stages permanent scarring may necessitate a keratoplasty to restore the vision of the eye, sometimes preceded or followed by beta-irradiation or laser photocoagulation to diminish the vascularization.

Atopic patients are especially liable to bilateral and severe herpes simplex keratitis and its complications.

Herpes zoster

Herpes zoster is the result of reactivation of the chickenpox virus (varicella) that has remained latent in the posterior root ganglia since the primary infection. Though it may occur at any age, the majority of cases occur in elderly patients and there is an association with impaired immunity and diseases of the reticuloendothelial system. Ophthalmic herpes zoster represents reactivation of virus in the trigeminal ganglion.

The rapid development of severe neuralgic pain over part or the whole of the area of distribution of the ophthalmic division of the trigeminal nerve (the scalp, the forehead, the upper lid and the side and tip of the nose) is usually the first manifestation. It persists for several hours or even days, before redness and swelling of the affected area with the formation of characteristic vesicles develop. There is marked variation in the area and severity of skin involvement, and although vesicular involvement of the lid margins and tip of the nose usually indicates ocular involvement (because the nerve supply of the tip of the nose—the external nasal nerve—is the terminal branch of the sensory nerve of the eyeball–the nasociliary branch of the ophthalmic division of the trigeminal nerve), the severity of the rash bears no relationship to the severity of the ocular involvement. The acute manifestations are a mucopurulent conjunctivitis, an episcleritis and quickly fading superficial keratitis or deeper nummular keratitis that may persist indefinitely with consequent disturbance of vision. Scleritis and optic neuritis are rare features, while transient ophthalmoplegias may occur. Prolonged iritis results in iris atrophy and an insidious secondary glaucoma may follow.

Impaired corneal sensation often leads to indolent ulceration (*neurotrophic keratitis*), which is best managed by a liberal central tarsorrhaphy.

Immediate management often requires admission to hospital because the patients exhibit marked malaise in addition to pain. Screening for immunodeficiency and reticuloendothelial disease is done at this stage.

Antiviral agents such as idoxuridine 4% or acycloguanosine are useful early in the evolution of the skin vesicles, but have no place in the ocular regimen. The mainstay of treatment is topical steroids—cream for the skin and drops and ointment for the eye. Prophylactic antibiotics may be given as well as cycloplegics, and careful attention must be directed to the difficult problem of the alleviation of pain. Long-term follow-up is desirable to pre-empt the complications of insidious disease.

Molluscum contagiosum

The DNA virus responsible for molluscum contagiosum produces pale, umbilicated lesions, which, if on the lids or lid margin, may produce a low-grade chronic follicular conjunctivitis and superficial keratitis. Resolution follows their incision and curettage, the contents showing characteristic intracytoplasmic eosinophilic inclusions.

Measles

While a mucopurulent conjunctivitis with occasional keratitis and iritis characterizes measles in the well-nourished, the prolonged anaemia in the undernourished and immune-deficient leads to marked keratitis and corneal necrosis, an ideal environment for bacterial superinfection. Thinning, scarring and even perforation contribute to this major cause of blindness in developing countries.

Mycotic keratitis

Fungal infection of the cornea may affect eyes already compromised by bacterial or viral infection, particularly if topical steroids have been part of the treatment regimen, in which case *Candida albicans* is most often implicated. Direct innoculation of the cornea by vegetable matter is the usual history in cases due to the filamentous fungi such as *Aspergillus* and *Fusarium*.

These ulcers run an indolent relapsing course and present as slightly elevated grey/white lesions with subepithelial extensions giving them a crenated edge, satellite lesions and recurrent hypopyon, despite treatment. Diagnosis rests upon corneal scrapes deep into affected tissues, cultures from which allow species identification and sensitivity, permitting rational specific chemotherapy.

The imidazole group of drugs—clotrimazole, miconazole, econazole and ketoconazole—are useful against the filamentous organisms, while the addition of 5-fluorocytosine makes effective treatment for *Candida*. For *Actinomyces*, penicillin remains effective.

Penetrating keratoplasty in unresponsive cases removes the fungal load and pre-empts spontaneous perforation and the risk of endophthalmitis.

Other forms of keratitis

Interstitial keratitis

This deep keratitis presents as a white cloudiness of the stroma following an oedematous process, often localized initially but becoming more generalized. Severe loss of vision may be the only symptom for several days or even weeks, although usually there is also severe pain, photophobia and blepharospasm because of an intense iritis. Oedema of the stroma favours the ingrowth of vessels into the cornea from the deep episcleral plexus of vessels at the limbus (these vessels cannot be traced beyond the level of the limbus because of their deep origin), which causes a patchy pink appearance (*'salmon patches'*). The iritis is often associated with the production of keratic precipitates (KP) and often also of posterior synechiae, although these may be masked by the gross disturbance of corneal transparency. The oedematous and vascularized state of the corneal stroma causes the formation of dense scar tissue; this is permanent to some extent, although it gradually becomes less diffuse so that small 'windows' of partial clearing may permit a reasonable return of vision, particularly for close reading—a factor of great importance from an educative point of view when the condition occurs in a child. The corneal vessels also become less obvious in time and eventually are free of circulating blood (*'ghost vessels'*). Sometimes, however, the condition may recur, or in later life degenerative changes may occur in the cornea. In this way the vision in interstitial keratitis may show three phases: (a) extremely poor in the early and acute stage; (b) considerable improvement some years later; and (c) a gradual deterioration in advancing yers.

In the more localized forms of interstitial keratitis, the disease occurs characteristically near the limbus, although it may spread later to the more central parts of the cornea when it tends to be more persistent. Sometimes the changes are limited to several large punctate foci in the posterior third of the corneal stroma.

Some cases of interstitial keratitis are associated with congenital syphilis with or without the other stigmata of the disease (e.g. Hutchinson's teeth and saddle-shaped depression of the nose); the keratitis usually occurs between the ages of 5 and 18 years. Only one eye is involved initially but the other is almost inevitably attacked some weeks or months later. It may also occur in acquired syphilis, tuberculosis, leprosy, leishmaniasis, trypanosomiasis, onchocerciasis, lupus erythematosus, mumps and infectious mononucleosis, when it is commonly confined to one eye. It is essentially an endogenous condition.

Other forms of interstitial keratitis include *disciform keratitis*, which follows herpes of the cornea (see above), and *keratitis profunda*, which is associated with an anterior uveitis (see Chapter 6).

Treatment. Topical steroids reduce the ravages of the disease, particularly when they are applied early. The pupil is dilated with atropine to prevent the formation of posterior synechiae. Treatment is also directed to the cause of the condition—for example, systemic pencillin is given in massive doses in syphilis. When the degree of permanent scarring is sufficient to cause marked impairment of vision, a keratoplasty may restore useful vision, despite the presence of vessels within the diseased cornea, provided perfect apposition is achieved between the donor and host cornea with a precise method of suturing.

Mooren's ulcer

This is a chronic, indolent, but often painful type of ulceration which occurs without any obvious infective element in an elderly person. It is usually unilateral initially, but there is a tendency for the other eye to be involved later. The lesion begins as a concentric depression of a wide area of the cornea at the limbus. There is a characteristic undermining of the edge of the depression away from the limbus, so that there is an overhanging thickened portion of cornea which spreads gradually (hence the term *chronic serpiginous ulcer*) across the whole cornea, leaving behind a somewhat attenuated but densely scarred and vascularized cornea.

Treatment. This is often fairly hopeless; keratoplasty is of limited value because the donor cornea is liable to become scarred and vascularized by spread of the disease from the affected host cornea, and such an operation is often not feasible in an elderly and debilitated patient. The main aim is to limit the spread of the disease early—before the central cornea is affected—by using systemic steroids and immunosuppressive agents. The protection of the cornea by a conjunctival flap over the affected area may be of value, and sometimes beta-irradiation is an effective procedure.

Neuroparalytic keratitis

This is a degenerative condition which follows exposure of the eyeball in conditions such as facial paralysis due to, for example, Bell's palsy and leprosy. The lower part of the cornea is more commonly affected because the upper part is protected by the fact that the eye turns up when an attempt is made to close the partially paralysed lids (Bell's phenomenon).

Treatment. The main aim is to protect the eye by an adequate tarsorrhaphy. A lateral tarsorrhaphy is effective in limiting the exposure of the cornea and has the merit of not interfering with the vision, but a central tarsorrhaphy is necessary in severe cases.

Mustard gas keratitis

Mild exposure to mustard gas causes an immediate and intense conjunctival irritation which usually subsides within a few days or weeks; in more severe exposures there is associated corneal involvement with the development of superficial ulcerated areas which become scarred and vascularized and may even lead to perforation. Other characteristic changes in the cornea become evident later (sometimes as long as 30 years later) with the formation of multiple ulcers in association with areas of stromal collapse, and with the entry of vessels into the superficial parts of the cornea which have varicosities with a tendency to cause haemorrhages. This is essentially a degenerative condition as a result of the changes which occur in the cornea following contamination with this radiomimetic substance. The vision is affected by the scarring and by the corneal irregularities and distortions, which tend to cause repeated alterations in the refractive error.

Treatment. The keratoconjunctivitis is treated along the usual lines (pp.31 and 52), but a more specific form of treatment is the use of a flush-fitting contact lens; this lessens the discomfort of the eye, protects it from repeated attacks and improves the visual acuity by eliminating the effect of the continually changing corneal irregularities.

Acne rosacea keratitis

This disorder of facial skin with ocular accompaniments tends to occur in young and middle-aged adults, particularly in females; it is less common in childhood and old age. Characteristic dilatation of the vessels of the forehead, cheeks, and nose in a 'butterfly-wing' distribution is the earliest feature, followed by the formation of papules and pustules; hyperplasia of the sebaceous epithelium may result in rhinophyma.

There is usually a chronic blepharoconjunctivitis and recurrent meibomian cysts, but the principal lesion occurs on the cornea as a marginal keratitis, particularly of the lower (and more exposed) region, with the formation of fairly large, tongue-shaped, greyish-white, superficial infiltrations spreading from the limbus towards the more central part of the cornea with leashes of superficial vessels from the limbal circulation. Sometimes fine or coarse forms of epithelial keratitis also occur, with the later occurrence of subepithelial opacities of a slightly yellow colour. The condition generally pursues a relatively mild but chronic course with periods of recession and recrudescence, but sometimes it is severe with widespread involvement of the cornea and consequent disturbance of the vision and even an associated deep keratitis. A generalized feeling of discomfort of the eye and eyelids is associated with photophobia when there are active corneal lesions.

The pathogenesis of the condition is not clear, though it is suggested that there is a local sensitivity to circulating androgens. In addition, there is chronic colonization of the sebaceous glands with *Corynebacterium acnes* or other micro-organisms, which induce a chronic inflammatory response. This releases bacterial lipases which increase the local concentration of free fatty acid, which is toxic to epithelial surfaces.

Treatment. Treatment is directed at the systemic disorder with long-term tetracycline, initially 1 g/day reducing to 250 mg once or twice daily for at least six months. For children, erythromycin is used. Except in cases of severe keratitis, where topical steroids are very effective, topical treatment is of little benefit.

Keratoconjunctivitis sicca

This term refers to the effects of a reduction in the aqueous component of the precorneal tear film, and although it may occur as a congenital anomaly (Riley-Day syndrome—a disorder of the autonomic nervous system), the majority of cases are associated with a systemic disorder with an autoimmune basis, such as rheumatoid arthritis, systemic lupus erythematosus, thyroiditis, and primary biliary cirrhosis. The triad of dry eye, dry mouth, and arthritis (usually rheumatoid) is known as *Sjögren's syndrome.* An elevation of IgG and IgM antibodies to salivary duct epithelium is usual, while lymphocytic infiltration of lacrimal and salivary glands is uniformly present, suggesting a destructive autoimmune process of the glandular tissues which leads ultimately to atrophy.

Intractable burning and foreign body sensation dominate the symptoms. Examination shows a poor marginal tear strip, debris in the precorneal tear film, and scattered foci of desiccation (*dry-spot formation*) on the corneal and conjunctival epithelium. These are well demonstrated by a vital dye such as Rose Bengal. Excess mucus may attach to areas of abnormal epithelium (cornea only) to produce filaments (*filamentary keratitis*).

Treatment. The dryness is relieved by artificial tears (e.g. methylcellulose 1% drops, which have the advantage of a more persistent action than a lotion such as saline because of their slightly oily nature). A mucolytic (e.g. acetylcysteine 10% drops) is useful in filamentary keratitis. Sometimes sealing of the lacrimal puncta by cauterization may help to conserve any available moisture of the eye, but this is reserved for those without any hope of spontaneous recovery, otherwise there might be subsequently a troublesome epiphora.

Ophthalmia nodosa

This is essentially a foreign-body reaction to the presence of fine hairs which may be animal (e.g. from a caterpillar) or vegetable (e.g. from a cactus) in origin. These hairs tend to migrate in the tissues so that they produce flat-topped yellow nodules in different ocular tissues—the conjunctiva, the cornea and the iris—with accompanying inflammatory changes. The lungs may be affected similarly.

Certain other forms of keratitis—the keratitis that may accompany phlyctenular keratitis and vernal keratoconjunctivitis—are discussed on pp. 36 and 38 and sclerosing keratitis is discussed on p.71.

Keratoplasty (corneal grafting)

This operation consists of the replacement of a diseased area of cornea (the host cornea) by part of the cornea from another human eye (the donor cornea) which is usually obtained from a cadaver (a *homograft*). The Human Tissue Act of 1953 allows an individual to bequeath his or her eyes for such a purpose. It is essential for the eyes to be enucleated within a few hours of death, otherwise the cornea is unsuitable for transference when use is made of natural tissue. However, fresh cornea may be preserved in specific nutritive media either at 4°C for four days or at 36°C for one month. It is essential for the donor cornea to be transparent and to be free from disease. Sometimes the donor cornea is obtained from an eye removed because of a disorder not involving the integrity of the cornea and not liable to be transmitted to the host eye (e.g. malignant disease confined to the posterior segment of the eye); this precludes the use of an eye with a retinoblastoma. The cornea, unlike other parts of the body, accepts this transference of tissue because the absence of vascularization reduces the occurrence of the immunological reactions which are responsible for the rejection of other transplanted tissues; this unique property of the cornea is lost to some extent when the host cornea is vascularized as a result of disease. The donor cornea may be provided by the patient himself (an autograft) in the rare event of a person having one potentially sighted eye with a diseased cornea and another irrevocably blind eye with an intact cornea.

There are two main forms of keratoplasty: *lamellar keratoplasty* which involves the transplantation of the anterior half or two-thirds of the cornea (usually about 0.4mm) so that the anterior chamber remains intact during the operation, thus preserving host endothelium, or *penetrating keratoplasty* which involves the transplantation of the whole thickness of the cornea. A keratoplasty is usually performed to restore vision when the cornea is scarred, but sometimes it is also performed for therapeutic reasons; for example, to prevent the spread of a Mooren's ulcer, to restore the integrity of the anterior chamber after the rupture of a descemetocele, to accelerate the healing of the cornea after severe chemical burns, or to remove a diseased portion of cornea which has suffered repeated attacks of disciform ulceration. A lamellar keratoplasty is only valid as an optical procedure when the diseased condition of the cornea is confined to the anterior part, but it is of particular value as an emergency procedure to maintain the integrity of a diseased cornea; in such a case a penetrating keratoplasty may be performed subsequently for optical purposes.

Keratoprostheses

In an extensively diseased cornea when a keratoplasty is unsuccessful, an attempt may be made to substitute the central part of the scarred and vascularized cornea with various forms of acrylic keratoprostheses. An ingenious example is the osteoodontoprosthesis, which represents a narrow disc prepared from one of the canine teeth of the patient together with bone from the socket of the tooth; the outer ring of bone becomes adherent to the edge of the diseased cornea and the acrylic lens is placed within an inner ring of dentine. The use of dentine is based on the unique properties of a tooth which shows a ready acceptance of foreign material (dental fillings).

Keratomalacia

Keratomalacia results from a lack of vitamin A and occurs in infants and preschool children suffering from severe protein-energy malnutrition, amongst whom it is a major cause of blindness and subsequent sociodisability; it is an extremely rare condition in Western countries. The surface epithelium of the cornea becomes dry and insensitive so that it loses its normal lustre, and this is followed by a rapid opacification of the whole cornea, which may slough and perforate without any obvious inflammatory changes (*colliquative necrosis*). Other changes in the eye are dryness of the conjunctiva (*xerophthalmia*) with the formation of small, triangular, foam-like white areas near the limbus (*Bitôt's spots*) and night blindness (p.22).

Treatment. Massive doses of vitamin A are effective and must be provided with great urgency as a water-miscible intramuscular preparation of 100 000 International Units and as an oral oily preparation.

Of course, prevention of the condition is vital, and this demands an energetic search amongst communities with poor nutrition to establish prevalences, and health care facilities to provide nutritional supplements and continuing surveillance.

Note: It has been suggested that vitamin B deficiency (ariboflavinosis) causes a superficial vascularization of the cornea near the limbus, but this occurs only when there is an associated element of trauma.

Pigmentary disturbances

Blood-staining. This occurs after leakage of blood in a keratitis which is associated with intracorneal vascularization. It also occurs when haemorrhage in the anterior chamber (*hyphaema*) develops in association with a secondary glaucoma (p.313).

Copper. The Kayser–Fleischer ring is a green-brown ring due to copper deposition which occurs in the region of Descemet's membrane in the peripheral part of the cornea near the limbus. It develops at an early stage of Wilson's disease (hepatolenticular degeneration), an inborn error of metabolism of recessive inheritance in which there is abnormal copper metabolism with low serum copper and caeruloplasmin levels.

Melanin. A thin brown horizontal line—the so-called Stähli-Hudson line—may develop in the lower central part of the cornea after middle age, particularly in an area of scarring; this is usually an infiltration of melanin but sometimes it may be derived from blood (haemosiderin). Melanin pigment on the posterior surface of the cornea, sometimes in the form of a Krukenberg's spindle, is described on p.83.

Silver pigment. Small black particles are deposited in the region of Descemet's membrane in silver poisoning (argyrosis).

Iron pigment. Small brown particles are deposited in the corneal stroma when an iron foreign body is retained within the eye (siderosis, see pp. 177 and 349).

Copper pigment. Small brown particles are deposited in the corneal stroma, particularly in the peripheral parts and on the endothelium, when a copper foreign body is retained within the eye (see p.349).

Toxic and metabolic disturbances

Lignac-Fanconi syndrome

This is an inherited defect of amino acid metabolism; it is characterized by dwarfism and renal rickets. Deposits in the cornea, possibly cystine in nature, cause photophobia, and are apparent on slit-lamp microscopy as shiny rod- or needle-shaped crystals in the superficial stroma. Deposits may also occur in other ocular tissues: the conjunctiva, sclera, uvea and rarely the retina may be affected. Cystine storage disease (cystinosis) is a related disorder.

Synthetic antimalarial drugs

Drugs such as mepacrine and chloroquine are liable to cause the deposition of whitish-grey particles in the corneal epithelium and the most superficial layers of the stroma; these may cause a subjective awareness of coloured haloes (a symptom which is generally indicative of closed-angle galucoma). Chloroquine, which is used in the treatment of certain skin disorders such as lupus erythematosus and also in malaria, is liable to cause a pigmentary disturbance in the retina (see p.136). It is rare for these effects to occur when the drug is used in small doses (e.g. as a prophylactic measure) except in unduly susceptible individuals. The corneal changes are reversible when the drug is discontinued, but the retinal changes are irreversible.

Tumours

Tumours of the cornea represent local extensions of conjunctival tumours, which are described on pp. 40 and 41. Those of particular note are the limbal dermoid, Bowen's disease and melanomas.

Degenerations

Fatty degeneration

This occurs most commonly in the ageing eye. Circumscribed circular deposits of lipid material develop in the peripheral part of the corneal stroma, the so-called *arcus senilis (gerontoxon)* which is separated from the limbus by a narrow zone of unaffected cornea; in contrast to the similar but rare condition which occurs in infants, *arcus juvenalis (embryotoxon)*, when the deposits extend to the limbus. An arcus senilis develops gradually during adult life, usually starting in the lower part of the cornea and then the upper part before extending round the sides to form a complete ring; it never affects the transparency of the central cornea. It is almost invariably present in the elderly, but its presence before the age of 40 years may indicate a hyperlipidaemia with sometimes a predisposition to coronary heart disease; between the ages of 40 and 60 years it may be an indication of significantly raised serum cholesterol and phospholipid values.

Fatty degeneration may develop in an old corneal scar (following previous infection or injury) especially in the presence of corneal vascularization, or it may occur in a more generalized form in an extensively diseased eye. Sometimes active ulceration may develop in a fatty area, the so-called *atheromatous ulcer*, and a marked secondary infection may lead to a severe hypopyon keratitis, which is often a terminal event because of the poor response of such a diseased eye to treatment.

Extensive infiltration of the cornea by mucopolysaccharides and perhaps also by lipids is a feature of *gargoylism (Hurler's disease; dysostosis multiplex)*; this condition occurs in early infancy and produces characteristic general changes in the skull (widely spaced orbits and frontal bossing), in the abdomen (swelling due to involvement of the liver and spleen) and in the skeleton (dwarfism). The corneal changes may be very extensive and lead to gross loss of vision.

Sometimes small aggregations of lipid material containing calcium form fine white rings in the anterior part of the corneal stroma (*Coats' white rings*) usually at the site of a previous minor injury.

Calcareous degeneration

This occurs in eyes which are seriously damaged by long-standing disease such as keratitis, iridocyclitis and glaucoma; it is a characteristic feature of uveitis which occurs in early childhood, particularly in the presence of a rheumatic diathesis as in Still's disease. Deposition of calcium occurs between the epithelium and Bowman's membrane and later destroys this membrane with subsequent involvement of the anterior corneal lamellae. The calcareous changes occur particularly across the lower part of the cornea which is exposed when the lids are open, hence the term *band-shaped degeneration* but it is more usually termed *band keratopathy*. It may occur also in association with hyperparathyroidism, excessive vitamin D intake, and rarely as an isolated event (idiopathic type) in the elderly.

Treatment. The calcareous area in the central part of the cornea may be scraped away with a sharp knife and the operated area heals with or without the use of a lamellar corneal graft; obviously, however, such an operation is of no value when the rest of the eye is grossly diseased. The calcareous area may also be removed by a chelating agent such as disodium edetate.

Salzmann's dystrophy

This is a degeneration, rather than a dystrophy, which occurs as a result of chronic corneal inflammation in, for example, trachoma, rosacea keratitis and exposure. It results in grey nodular elevations on the surface of the cornea, often in a circinate pattern that may obscure vision.

Dellen

These represent shallow saucer-like excavations (dimples, facets) of the surface layers of the cornea (the epithelium and to some extent Bowman's membrane) near the limbus, each with a well-defined edge and with faint opacification of the floor. They are sometimes of a transient nature, persisting for only a few days or changing in extent within a few days. They occur simply as the result of the dehydration of the peripheral cornea which follows an elevated limbal lesion that interferes with adequate tear application. Treatment is directed to the limbal lesion.

Dystrophies

Hereditary dystrophies

These usually become evident in the early years of life, before or at puberty, and occur particularly in males, There are different forms: the *granular* or *nodular form* (the so-called *Groenouw's dystrophy*), the *lattice form*, and the *macular form*. The granular and lattice forms are inherited as dominant and the macular form as recessive conditions.

The opacified areas gradually extend from the central to the peripheral parts of both corneas, with a gradual impairment in the vision; the granular form usually shows the slowest progress, and reasonable vision may be retained until middle age. Histochemical examination has identified a proteinaceous deposit in the granular form, an amyloid deposit in the lattice form, and a localized corneal mucopolysaccharidosis in the macular form.

Treatment. A corneal graft is the only effective form of treatment, but it should be delayed until the vision is severely affected because, although the absence of vascularity favours a corneal transplant, there is a tendency for dystrophic changes to develop later in the donor cornea, particularly in the macular form.

Fuchs' dystrophy

This was originally described as an epithelial dystrophy, but the earliest changes occur in the endothelium which develops a bronzed appearance interspersed with black vacuoles representing localized thickenings of Descemet's membrane (*guttata*); the later epithelial changes are accompanied by opacities in the stroma which follow an oedema caused

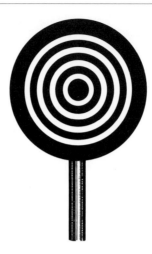

Fig. 21. Placido's disc.

by impairment of the endothelial barrier and pump mechanism. This condition, which seldom occurs before late middle age, is bilateral and progresses slowly, but ultimately the vision is impaired considerably; unfortunately it progresses more rapidly after any form of intraocular operation, particularly a cataract extraction, even when any corneal endothelial damage is minimal (see Chapter 9). Hypertonic solutions such as 5% sodium chloride drops may temporarily deturgesce the cornea, but ultimately a full thickness corneal graft is required.

Keratoconus (conical cornea)

This is a form of corneal dystrophy affecting mainly the central part of the cornea, which gradually becomes attenuated, bowed forwards and scarred. It is believed to be the result of an abnormal corneal stromal ground substance. There is a strong association with atopy and 60% of patients are born to mothers over 30 years old. It is a bilateral condition, often asymmetric in its expression, that usually starts around puberty. Progress is unpredictable; the vision becomes impaired by the development of a form of myopic astigmatism which is not susceptible, except in the early stages, to correction by ordinary spectacle lenses because of its irregular nature. The condition is detected to some extent by retinoscopy because of the distortion of the normal reflex from the fundus, but it is confirmed by demonstrating corneal thinning, and later conical ectasia, stromal scars and a fine brown line (Fleischer ring) in the epithelium delineating the base of the cone. In established cases the corneal curvature irregularity can be demonstrated by the distortion of the corneal reflection by means of Placido's disc (Fig. 21). The vision deteriorates markedly when ruptures develop in Descemet's membrane in the affected area so that the aqueous passes freely into the corneal stroma with consequent permanent scarring (*acute hydrops cornea*).

Treatment. Provided opacification has not occurred, many cases respond well to the use of contact lenses which restore the vision to a normal level by eliminating the effect of the abnormal curvature of the anterior corneal surface.

A perforating keratoplasty is also an effective method of treatment because of the avascularity of the diseased cornea, but this should be attempted only after contact lenses have been tried. The nature of the corneal changes necessitates a fairly large graft of 7 mm, or even more, in diameter. Sometimes a permanent mydriasis follows such an operation and this may be an indication that the changes which occur in keratoconus are not confined to the cornea.

5

The Sclera

Structure and function

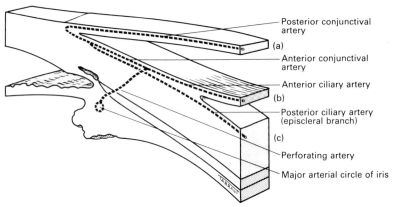

Fig. 22. Section through the episcleral and scleral tissues. (a) Conjunctiva. (b) Muscle and Tenon's capsule. (c) Sclera.

The sclera forms five-sixths of the protective outer coat of the eye and its dense fibrous tissue is continuous anteriorly with the stromal part of the cornea (which forms the remaining one-sixth). Its outer surface is covered by loose vascular tissue (the *episcleral tissue*) containing the deep episcleral vascular plexus; this is separated from the overlying conjunctiva by a thin layer of more dense fibrous tissue (*Tenon's capsule*) which contains the superficial episcleral vascular plexus (Fig. 22). Being virtually avascular, but freely permeable, the sclera derives its nutrition from both the superficial (episcleral) and deep (choroidal) vascular systems. Multiple interlamellar adhesions, the random arrangement of its fibres and its fully hydrated nature make the sclera opaque.

Injuries

The sclera is fairly resistant to injury but perforation may occur directly, for example by metallic fragments which strike at high speed or by injury with a sharp instrument, or indirectly as a rupture of the sclera following a severe concussion of the globe.

70

Episcleritis and scleritis

Since it is mesodermal in origin, the sclera is often involved in connective tissue disorders, most of whose manifestations are immunologically based, whether as a tissue-specific reaction or as a site of immune complex induced vasculitis.

It is important to distinguish *episcleritis*—inflammation of the superficial episcleral vascular plexus—and *scleritis*—involvement of the deep episcleral plexus—because the former is a benign, self-limiting condition, while the latter frequently has an ocular and general morbidity. Examination in daylight gives an excellent indication of the degree of scleral involvement, while slit-lamp examination (especially with red-free light), shows the extent of the involvement.

Episcleritis

This may be a diffuse or nodular area of localized redness with mild ocular discomfort that resolves without treatment in a few weeks. The nodular variety tends to be more protracted and may require systemic treatment with non-steroidal anti-inflammatory drugs (indomethacin, ibuprofen).

While the majority of cases remain unexplained, recurrent episcleritis commonly occurs as a sequel to ophthalmic herpes zoster and has been associated with gout.

Scleritis

Though the majority of cases of scleritis have no known aetiological basis, one-third have rheumatoid arthritis, and polyarteritis nodosa and Wegener's granulomatosis account for a further 10%. Herpes zoster may be complicated by recurrent scleritis.

Anterior scleritis presents as a diffuse or nodular scleral swelling with overlying episcleritis. It is typically associated with deep pain which radiates to the forehead and sinuses, and the eye is tender to palpation through the lid. The congestion is of a deeper hue than in episcleritis; the presence of patches of white tissue indicates non-perfusion and is termed *necrotizing scleritis*, which carries a worse prognosis for the eye.

A form of necrotizing scleritis not associated with surrounding inflammation, and seen as areas of scleral translucence, occurs almost exclusively in seropositive rheumatoid arthritis of long-standing. It is known as *scleromalacia perforans* because it may be followed by areas of scleral perforation.

Anterior scleritis may be complicated by uveitis, glaucoma and keratitis. The latter is often a *sclerosing keratitis* adjacent to the active scleral disease or causing peripheral corneal thinning. Keratitis occurs especially in Wegener's granulomatosis, a condition of necrotizing angiitis involving the lungs, sinuses and kidneys, though a purely ocular form may occur.

Posterior scleritis, by contrast, usually presents with little pain, but with impaired vision due to an exudative retinal detachment, limitation of ocular movements and proptosis. Rarely it may present as closed-angle glaucoma, as a result of shallowness of the anterior chamber due to an annular choroidal detachment. A-scan ultrasonography showing retrobulbar oedema and B scans showing scleral thickening are of great value in diagnosis.

Treatment. Scleritis requires systemic medication in the form of non-steroidal anti-inflammatory agents (indomethacin, ibuprofen) in high doses, since the drug has to penetrate relatively avascular tissue. Occasionally, high doses of systemic steroids are required, especially in necrotizing disease (though not in scleromalacia perforans). Immunosuppresive agents, such as cyclophosphamide, may have to be used.

Surgery is rarely required as perforation is uncommon, but non-epithelialized scleral defects and marked corneal thinning benefit from scleral/corneal grafts.

Blue sclera

A blue discoloration of the sclera may occur as a pathological entity in osteogenesis imperfecta (fragilitas ossium), an hereditary condition associated sometimes with deafness and a marked tendency, particularly in childhood, to develop fractures after relatively trivial injury. It should be noted, however, that under normal conditions the sclera may appear to have a slight bluish tint. This is caused by the choroidal pigment shining through an unduly transparent sclera, a phenomenon often seen during operation when the sclera becomes translucent following dehydration.

Staphyloma of the sclera

This is an area of thinned sclera which bulges outwards with the underlying uveal tissue. Different parts of the sclera may be involved: an *intercalary staphyloma* occurs immediately in front of the ciliary body and is lined by the root of the iris, a *ciliary staphyloma* is lined by the ciliary body, and an *equatorial staphyloma* is lined by the equatorial part of the choroid. The equatorial region of the sclera is weak because it marks the exit from the choroid of the four large vortex veins. These staphylomas usually follow prolonged periods of glaucoma and characteristically occur in blind eyes.

Posterior staphyloma is a feature of high axial myopia and is associated with extensive choroidoretinal changes around the optic disc and in the macular area (see p.13).

6

The Uveal Tract

Structure and function

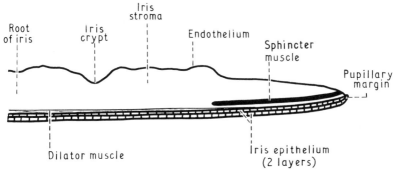

Fig. 23. The structure of the iris.

The uvea forms the middle coat of the eyeball. It has three different parts—the iris, the ciliary body and the choroid—in anatomical continuity.

The iris

This forms a forwards projection from the ciliary body in front of the lens; it is more or less circular and a central opening forms the pupil. The *anterior chamber* lies between its outer surface and the inner surface of the cornea, and the shallow *posterior chamber* between its inner surface and the outer surface of the lens.

The pupils average about 4 mm in diameter but, because of the balancing influences of the opposing parasympathetic and sympathetic impulses, they vary considerably in size under normal conditions, quite apart from the variations which occur during changes of illumination. In the infant they are relatively small, they increase in size during childhood and adolescence, and in later life again tend to become small. In hypermetropia they are usually smaller than in myopia. In emotional states they tend to become large due to increased sympathetic tone. In sleep they are small. In heavily pigmented (brown) eyes they are smaller than in lightly pigmented (blue) eyes. Normally the pupils of the two

73

eyes are more or less equal in size and an obvious difference in size (*anisocoria*) is usually of pathological significance.

The iris is composed of an outer endothelial layer, a stromal layer, and two inner layers of pigment epithelium (Fig. 23).

The thin endothelial layer on its outer surface is continuous with the corneal endothelium and with the endothelial lining of the trabecular spaces in the filtration angle of the anterior chamber. It is absent over the *iris crypts* which are irregular areas in which the superficial part of the stromal layer is defective.

The thick stromal layer is continuous with the stroma of the choroid and contains blood vessels running radially, except at the *collarette*— the junction between its thicker portion (the ciliary part) and its thinner portion (the pupillary part)—where they run circumferentially (the minor arterial circle of the iris). It contains two muscles in its deeper part: the *sphincter muscle* which runs circumferentially in the pupillary part and causes a constriction of the pupil, and the *dilator muscle* which runs radially in its ciliary, and to some extent pupillary, parts and dilates the pupil.

In infancy there is no pigment within the stroma so that the iris appears blue; this may persist indefinitely, but usually after a few years pigment is deposited so that it assumes varied patterns of colour— green, yellow and brown—which may be uniform or mottled. *Heterochromia iridis* is an iris which has one sector different in colour from the rest. *Heterochromia iridum* is a difference in colour between the two irides, for example one blue and the other brown. It may occur normally or pathologically (heterochromic cyclitis, p. 94).

Of the two layers of pigment epithelium, the outer one is continuous with the outer pigment epithelial layer of the ciliary body and is concerned with the formation of the sphincter and dilator muscles, and the inner one is continous with the inner non-pigmented epithelial layer of the ciliary body.

The pupillary reflexes (Fig. 24)

The sphincter muscle is innervated by the parasympathetic fibres of the oculomotor nerve (third cranial nerve) which arise in the parasympathetic parts of the oculomotor nucleus (nuclei of Edinger-Westphal and Perlia) in the midbrain. These fibres relay in the ciliary ganglion and subserve the constriction of the pupil to light and to a near stimulus. The parasympathetic parts of both oculomotor nuclei are stimulated by light stimuli from each retina because the afferent pupillary (visual) fibres from each eye pass to both sides of the midbrain; therefore a light stimulus to one eye produces a constriction of the pupil of the stimulated eye (*direct reaction to light*) and of the pupil of the other eye (*consensual reaction to light*). The parasympathetic parts of the nucleus are also concerned with the constriction of the pupil during accommodation (the *accommodation*

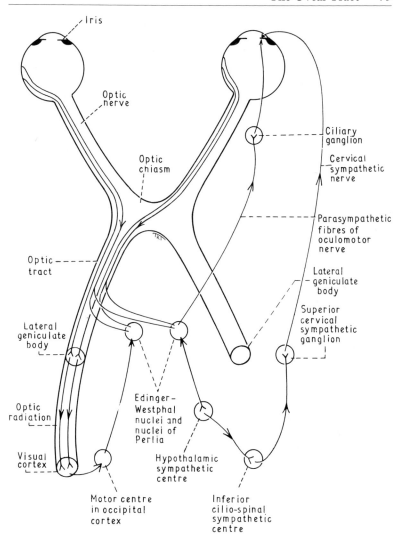

Fig. 24. The nerve pathways of the pupillary light and accommodation reflexes.

pupil reflex) and during convergence (the *convergence pupil reflex*); these are initiated by a centre in the occipital cortex which is controlled by the visual cortex (part of the psycho-optical reflex, see pp. 222 and 225). The dilator muscle is innervated by sympathetic fibres; these travel in the cervical sympathetic nerve from the ciliospinal centre (in the upper part of the spinal cord), are relayed in the superior cervical ganglion and pass to the eye via the sympathetic plexus around the internal carotid artery and the nasociliary branch of the ophthalmic division of the

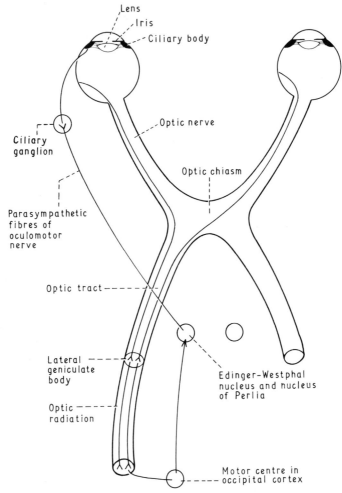

Fig. 25.   The nerve pathways of the accommodation reflex.

trigeminal nerve. The ciliospinal centre is controlled by a sympathetic centre in the hypothalamus; this can also produce a dilatation of the pupil by sending inhibitory impulses directly to the parasympathetic nuclei so that dilatation of the pupil follows relaxation of the sphincter; this is the type of dilatation which follows psychical stimuli.

The ciliary body

The stroma contains the ciliary muscle (longitudinal, oblique and iridic fibres) which on contraction causes a forward movement and thickening of the ciliary body, thus producing an accommodative change in the lens by a relaxation of the suspensory ligament (see pp. 9 and 10).

The accommodation reflex (Fig. 25)

The ciliary muscle is innervated by the parasympathetic fibres of the oculomotor nerve (third cranial nerve) which arise in the parasympathetic parts of the oculomotor nucleus and are relayed to the eye in the ciliary ganglion. The accommodation reflex is initiated from a centre in the occipital cortex which is controlled by the visual cortex (part of the psycho-optical reflex, see pp. 222 and 225) and produces a contraction of the ciliary muscle. The relaxation of the muscle may be the result simply of an inhibition of the parasympathetic system, but it is likely that the sympathetic nerves, which pass to the ciliary muscle by a route similar to those which supply the dilator muscle of the pupil (Fig. 24), are responsible for this.

The anterior part of the stroma contains the major arterial circle of the iris. The inner surface, which shows many ciliary processes containing highly vascularized tissue, is lined by two layers of epithelium: an outer layer of pigmented epithelium which is continuous with the pigment layer of the retina, and an inner layer of ciliary epithelium which is continuous with the terminal part of the rest of the retina at its margins (the *ora serrata*). The ciliary epithelium is concerned with the formation of aqueous humour by processes of dialysis and secretion.

The choroid

This is a vascular coat composed of arteries and veins with a layer of capillaries (the *choriocapillaris*) on its inner surface, which is separated from the underlying retina by Bruch's membrane; these capillaries nourish the outer half of the retina. The outer surface of the choroid is separated from the overlying sclera by a potential space (the *suprachoroidal space*).

Congenital anomalies

Persistent pupillary membrane

Late in fetal life the pupil is formed by the complete disappearance of a central circular area of the vascularized mesodermal tissue which covers the anterior surface of the lens. There is also a partial disappearance of this tissue over the pupillary part of the iris as far as the collarette (see p. 74), but sometimes small strands remain (*persistent pupillary*

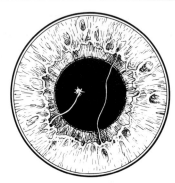

Fig. 26. Strands of persistent pupillary membrane and an epicapsular star on the anterior lens capsule.

membrane) which pass across the pupil. Sometimes one end of the strand lies free in the anterior chamber or is attached to the anterior lens capsule with the formation of small golden pigment deposits (the so-called *epicapsular stars*) (Fig. 26). None of these changes interferes significantly with vision.

Iridocorneal dysgenesis

The iris may be involved as part of the developmental disorder of mesenchyme known as the *anterior chamber cleavage syndrome*, where iris atrophy or adhesions to the cornea are associated with posterior corneal and anterior lens opacities (p.302).

Aniridia

In this familial condition, the iris fails to develop except for small rudimentary stumps in the region of the filtration angle. It is usually bilateral but seldom occurs to the same degree in both eyes. There is marked photophobia because of the unrestricted entry of light, and usually a mainly pendular type of nystagmus (see p.266); there is also a likelihood of glaucoma in early adult life (or even in childhood) because of angle closure by iris root remnants. Abnormal foveal development and a progressive vascularization and opacification of the peripheral cornea may occur. Dominantly inherited cases have strong penetrance, and there is an association between sporadic cases and Wilm's tumour. The photophobia is relieved by dark glasses or goggles; sometimes a specially shielded contact lens may be of value. The treatment of the glaucoma is discussed in Chapter 15.

Coloboma of the uvea

In this familial condition, a failure of closure of the fetal cleft causes a *coloboma* (an apparent absence or defect of ocular tissue) in the lower part of the eye. This may involve the iris, ciliary body and choroid, either together or alone. The extent of choroidal coloboma is variable; it may affect the peripheral part only or a whole sector so that it approaches the lower border of the optic disc. The affected area appears white because of the exposed sclera. The retina is also involved, except for a few retinal vessels which pass across the coloboma. Sometimes there is also a coloboma of the optic disc. The condition is usually bilateral, although each eye may be involved in different ways and to different extents.

Choroideraemia

This is a rare condition with sex-linked inheritance in which there is a progressive atrophy of the choroid and of the retinal pigment epithelium. This starts in the periphery and spreads to the whole fundus (except the macula) by middle age, so that the fundus appears white, although the overlying retinal vessels persist and the macula and optic disc are normal in colour. There is a progressive loss of peripheral vision with a marked night blindness, but there may be retention of central vision. The established disease is confined to males, but affected females may show modified 'pepper-and-salt' degenerative changes in the periphery of the fundus. Rarely an apparent choroideraemia results from a confluence of areas of gyrate atrophy (see p.96).

Albinism

Oculocutaneous albinism. Different inheritance patterns dictate the form of albinism as it affects the eye. Oculocutaneous albinism has a Mendelian-type recessive inheritance, and is subdivided into tyrosinase positive and tyrosinase negative depending on the ability of a hair bulb to elaborate melanin in the presence of tyrosine. Tyrosinase-negative patients show a permanent deficiency of pigment throughout the body (white hair, white eyelashes, pink skin, etc.). The eye appears pink because of the absence of pigment in the uveal tract and in the retina, which also causes a scattering of light so that there is photophobia and almost invariably a pendular nystagmus. The fundus appears unduly pale with a prominence of the retinal and choroidal vessels against the white background of the sclera. The eyes invariably become myopic. There is often a macular dysgenesis so that visual acuity is usually severely affected. Tyrosinase-positive oculocutaneous albinism, by contrast, has some potential for melanin formation, with the formation of freckles or tanning, while the irides may become hazel coloured, though translucent. The ocular features are similar to tyrosinase-negative patients, but the visual acuity is less impaired. A squint, more often divergent, is a common feature; in some cases the development of a squint is inevitable because of the absence of fusion. This is the result of a more or less complete decussation of the optic nerve fibres from the two eyes in the optic chiasma – the normal hemi-decussation is essential for a fusion of the two retinal images in the visual cortex.

Ocular albinism. This is an X-linked form of albinism with clinical features confined to the eyes. It may be overlooked because of the absence of the general features of albinism and also because some pallor of the fundus is a normal finding in childhood. The ocular changes are similar to those of tyrosinase-positive oculocutaneous albinism. The female carrier, however, with normal visual acuity, has peripheral retinal changes showing a mixture of normal and depigmented retinal pigment epithelium. The photophobia may be relieved by dark glasses or goggles. A flush-fitting shielded contact lens, which prevents light from entering the eye except by a small central aperture, is also of value. It is possible that the fitting of such lenses shortly after birth before the development of nystagmus may prevent its occurrence, although the photophobia and nystagmus do not prohibit a reasonable level of corrected vision, particularly for close reading, so that a normal education is possible.

Injuries

Iris

Hyphaema

Haemorrhage into the anterior chamber from the iris may follow blunt or perforating injury (see Chapter 17). The haemorrhage is often completely absorbed within a few days but, since a small traumatic hyphaema may be followed some hours, or even days, later by further haemorrhages, such cases should be admitted for observation. A secondary glaucoma, which may lead to a blood-stained cornea that takes many weeks to clear, may occur if clotted blood fills the anterior chamber and occludes the pupil (*pupil block glaucoma*), or if degenerating red blood cells (erythroclasts) clog the filtration angle. If necessary the hyphaema should be evacuated through a small paracentesis opening near the limbus in the lower outer quadrant of the eye; this may be reopened on subsequent days by depressing the outer lip of the incision to release further haemorrhage.

If the haemorrhage is clotted, a wide corneoscleral incision is made for careful irrigation and evacuation. Fibrinolytic agents have no proven value.

Spontaneous hyphaema may occur from a juvenile xanthogranuloma of the iris, severe uveitis, and intraocular neoplasms.

Traumatic mydriasis

A paralysis of the sphincter may follow blunt trauma so that the pupil becomes dilated and shows no response to light or near stimuli. There is usually a gradual recovery within a few weeks or months, but this is often only partial; involvement may sometimes be sectorial.

Iridodialysis

This represents a tear in the iris, usually at its junction with the ciliary body. It is seldom advisable to attempt to repair this defect because of its proximity to the filtration angle.

Iridoschisis

In this condition there is a generalized disruption of the iris stroma so that free ends of strands of iris tissue pass into the anterior chamber. It follows forcible entry of aqueous into the iris as the result of blunt trauma of the eye. A similar condition occurs in elderly people and is simply the result of degenerative changes in the absence of trauma (see p.96).

Ciliary body

The ciliary body is seldom affected by injury except a perforating one (see Chapter 17), but sometimes severe contusion of the globe causes a temporary reduction in the intraocular pressure (hypotonia) following a diminished production of aqueous from the ciliary body.

Choroid

Severe blunt trauma may cause a rupture of the choroid. In the early stages this is usually masked by choroidal haemorrhage, which appears dark red in colour because it lies deep to the retina, although some haemorrhage may also pass into the retina. Later it appears as a narrow crescentic white area, which often runs concentrically with the optic disc, due to exposure of the underlying sclera; any retinal vessel passing over it appears normal. A disciform neovascular membrane may develop from the margin of a choroidal rupture.

Uveitis

An inflammation of the whole uveal tract is termed *panuveitis* *(endophthalmitis)*. When it is confined mainly to the anterior segment it is termed *anterior uveitis* or *iridocyclitis* (sometimes separated into *iritis*—an inflammation of the iris, and *cyclitis*—an inflammation of the ciliary body); in the posterior segment it is termed *posterior uveitis* or *choroiditis*. Uveitis is usually a primary disorder, but it may follow some other infection (e.g. interstitial keratitis, p.58; scleritis, p.71). The majority of cases of uveitis have an immunological basis. The term covers a number of pathological entities related to the individual tissues of the area—in other words, uveitis may be a neuritis, a myositis or a vasculitis.

Anterior uveitis (iritis, cyclitis or iridocyclitis)

This condition usually starts fairly acutely with severe pain (often likened to the pain of toothache), intense photophobia, and a mild to severe degree of blurred vision. The condition is frequently confined to one eye. There are many clinical features:

Redness. There is some general *conjunctival injection* as in conjunctivitis, but there is also intense redness in the circumcorneal region with involvement of the deep episcleral vessels (*ciliary injection*); similar redness also occurs in closed-angle glaucoma (see p. 310).

Lacrimation. This is usually profuse, particularly on exposure to light, but, unlike in conjunctivitis, it is not mucopurulent.

Tenderness. The eyeball is very sensitive on palpation.

Exudation. Exudate containing protein and inflammatory cells enters the anterior chamber so that the aqueous becomes visible (*aqueous flare and cells*) instead of being optically 'empty' as in the normal eye. Cells may also be visible in the *retrolental space*, which lies between the posterior surface of the lens and the anterior face of the vitreous. The exudation in the anterior chamber causes *keratic precipitates* (KP) to form on the posterior surface of the cornea. The cells in the anterior chamber circulate because of movement of the aqueous upwards over the surface of the iris and downwards behind the inner suface of the cornea; this movement is induced by thermal currents (Fig. 27) caused by the temperature of the anterior chamber being higher than the air outside the eye. Therefore the KP usually assume an axial distribution in the lower part of the cornea (Fig. 28). The KP are often variable in size and colour. The large non-pigmented KP ('mutton-fat' KP) are characteristic of the granulomatous forms of uveitis found in tuberculosis or sarcoid. Sometimes, however, they may be small with a widespread distribution over the cornea, even in its upper part (Fig.

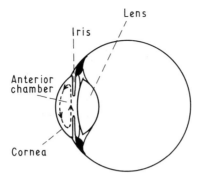

Fig. 27. The convection currents of the aqueous humour in the anterior chamber.

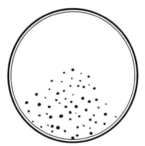

Fig. 28. An axial distribution of keratic precipitates (KP).

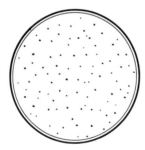

Fig. 29. A widespread distribution of keratic precipitates (KP).

29), as in heterochromic cyclitis (p.94) or in the Posner–Schlossman syndrome (p.94). KP tend to become pigmented after some time so that pigmented KP are usually indicative of long-standing disease, although in a few cases they may be pigmented from the outset. Old KP tend to become crenated; they persist long after the active stage of inflammation.

Note: Fine particles of iris pigment may be deposited on the posterior surface of the cornea in any form of iris atrophy (e.g. in old age, pigmentary glaucoma or after prolonged glaucoma), even in the absence of uveitis; they sometimes have a spindle-shaped vertical distribution (*Krukenberg's spindle*).

The exudation also produces other effects. It may form a purulent deposit in the lower part of the anterior chamber (*hypopyon*), and in severe cases there may also be some haemorrhage (*hyphaema*). It readily causes adhesions between the posterior surface of the iris and the anterior surface of the lens (*posterior synechiae*), particularly when the pupil is allowed to remain constricted. When the whole pupillary area is involved there is a *seclusion* of the pupil (360° attachment of the pupil margin to the anterior lens capsule). This is liable to be followed by a bulging forwards of the main part of the iris (*iris bombé*) because the aqueous cannot pass into the anterior chamber from the posterior chamber, which leads to secondary glaucoma. Adhesions may develp between the anterior surface of the iris and the posterior surface of the corneoscleral junction in the filtration angle (*peripheral anterior synechiae*); this leads to secondary glaucoma when a sufficiently large area of the filtration angle is occluded by the synechiae. The exudate may become organized on the anterior surface of the lens in the pupillary area (*occlusion* of the pupil), a condition which may also lead to secondary glaucoma. Organized exudate may form from the ciliary body into the anterior part of the vitreous (*cyclitic membrane*), which may be associated subsequently with a retinal detachment.

The intraocular pressure. The intraocular pressure of the eye is seldom affected in the early stages of uveitis, although sometimes the pressure may be slightly lower than normal. In the later stages, particularly after repeated attacks, secondary glaucoma may ensue in various ways as discussed above.

Nodule formation. The formation of nodules is characteristic of the granulomatous forms of the disease (see below).

Cataract. Prolonged uveitis predisposes to cataract.

Atrophic changes. It is not uncommon for an eye to recover more or less completely from an attack of iridocyclitis, particularly after the use of modern therapeutic methods. However, repeated severe attacks ultimately lead to atrophic changes of the iris with a decrease in pigmentation and sometimes with more generalized atrophic changes (*atrophia bulbi*), scarring and vascularization of the subepithelial parts of the cornea (*band keratopathy*), chronic inflammatory changes in the uveal tract leading ultimately to calcareous and even osseous changes, cataract and shrinkage of the globe. Shrinkage may also follow a severe septic inflammation of the whole eye (*panophthalmitis*); this is termed *phthisis bulbi*.

Posterior uveitis (choroiditis)

This seldom produces symptoms other than blurring of vision; this may vary from a very slight lack of definition to a well-marked diffuse haze. In the active stage there is an outpouring of inflammatory cells (exudation) into the vitreous, which causes blurring of vision; these cells may be visible also in the retrolental space, but they are seldom present to any significant extent in the anterior chamber. The vitreous exudate is liable to form persistent opacities. In the acute stage the affected area of the choroid is swollen and fluffy white due to intense inflammatory changes, although this may be difficult to observe if the vitreous haze is intense or if the area lies in the periphery. Using fluorescein angiography (p.109), there is initial masking of choroidal fluorescence followed by diffuse leakage of the dye, so that there is a pronounced fuzziness around the edges of the lesion when the focus of choroiditis is active. There is also some leakage of dye into the underlying oedematous retina, which is particularly evident when there is an involvement of the macular area. The underlying retina is involved and produces a scotoma in the visual field due to a destruction of the deeply placed visual receptor cells (rods and cones). Later the scotoma is associated with a sector-shaped field defect which extends from the region of the scotoma to the periphery of the field. This is due to destruction of the superficially placed retinal nerve fibres which pass through the affected area from the sector of the retina peripheral to the lesion. The surrounding retina is oedematous to varying degrees. After several weeks the acute stage subsides and one or more atrophic areas of the choroid and retina develop, so that the sclera is visible as a white, often fairly circular focus, surrounded usually by varying amounts of pigmentary aggregation.

The area of involvement may be localized (*focal choroiditis*), widespread (*diffuse choroiditis*), or multiple (*disseminated choroiditis*); it may occur in the macular region (*central choroiditis*), adjacent to the optic disc (*juxtapapillary choroiditis*), or in the peripheral region (*anterior choroiditis*).

The final visual result depends on the area of the retina involved; direct implication of the macular area usually destroys the central vision, but even indirect implication by oedema, as in a juxtapapillary choroiditis, tends to be followed by fine pigmentary disturbances at the macula which affect the central vision to some extent. Involvement of a peripheral retinal area may leave little or no subjective awareness of the defect.

Pars planitis (chronic posterior cyclitis)

In the form of uveitis which involves the peripheral part of the uvea (the *pars plana* of the ciliary body), there are certain distinctive features: (a) a tendency to affect young people; (b) often bilateral, scanty inflammatory changes in the anterior chamber; (c) exudative inflammatory changes of the pars plana associated with a peripheral retinal perivasculitis; (d) marked inflammatory disturbance of the anterior part of the vitreous with dust-like opacities which may eventually form confluent exudates (*'snowball' opacities*) on the surface of the peripheral retina related to a detached posterior vitreous; and (e) oedema of the macular region which may cause cystoid degenerative change (see p.145).

Panuveitis (endophthalmitis)

A generalized uveitis occurs classically in sympathetic ophthalmitis (p.94), syphilis, occasionally in Still's disease (p.93), and in other non-specific forms. It presents with blurring of vision. Sometimes in the early stages, the apparently mild state of the anterior uveitis (fine KP, slight flare and relatively few cells in the aqueous humour) is in contrast to the marked oedema of the retina, particularly surrounding the optic disc, due to widespread posterior uveitis; this is revealed in the later stages by the development of scattered areas of choroidoretinal atrophy. The papilloedema may be followed by secondary optic atrophy, presumably as a result of damage to the capillary circulation of the disc during the active stage; the ultimate visual prognosis is poor. Sometimes, particularly in infants, the retina becomes detached as a result of proliferation of the inflammatory products in the underlying choroid; this disorganized mass of retinal and uveal tissue may be termed a *pseudoglioma* and must be distinguished from a retinoblastoma (see p.146).

Treatment In addition to topical treatment for uveitis, systemic steroids, adrenocorticotrophic hormone (ACTH) or cytotoxic or immunosuppressive agents may be necessary for the satisfactory control of the inflammatory process.

Aetiology of uveitis

In only a minority of cases can the aetiology of uveitis be readily identified, such as the acute inflammatory response to trauma and direct infection. However, evidence is accumulating to suggest that a variety of immune phenomena, such as immune complex deposition in the highly vascular uveal tissue, autoimmunity as a result of the ocular tissues becoming antigenic following infection or trauma, or an abnormal immune response, may be the stimulus to inflammation.

Although the biological mediators of inflammation, such as histamine, prostaglandins, immunoglobulin, complement degradation products and leucocytes, result in the features described above, there are certain clinical patterns which allow identification of the original aetiology; these are outlined below.

Bacterial infection

Tuberculosis

Tuberculous uveitis may occur directly (primary) or indirectly (secondary).

Primary infection. Direct ocular involvement by *Mycobacterium tuberculosis* produces an extensive lesion in the anterior uvea, particularly in the region of the root of the iris with involvement of the ciliary body, or in the posterior uvea. This is serious because the inflammatory and caseous changes may cause perforation of the globe before the onset of the usual reparative processes of fibrosis.

Secondary infection. Indirect ocular involvement by tuberculosis from some remote source is more common. The uveitis may be anterior (with the formation of characteristically large 'mutton fat' KP) or posterior. Its intensity is variable because it depends on the tissue immunity, which is lowered in states of malnutrition or in the presence of active disease.

Diagnosis. The Mantoux skin test measures the sensitivity to intracutaneous injections of dilute tuberculin, but this test is becoming of less value because of the widespread use of BCG vaccination. A positive reaction indicates a tuberculous focus, but this is only significant in the child because a positive reaction is common in the adult due to an old and quite inactive lesion. It should be noted also that it is a measure of skin and not necessarily uveal sensivitity. A radiographic examination may show an active or inactive focus of the disease in the chest.

Treatment. Multiple drug regimens for the treatment of the systemic disease are combined with topical anti-inflammatory agents as described below.

Syphilis

Congenital syphilis An anterior uveitis occurs with an interstitial keratitis (p.58), but also as a separate entity, particularly in the very young. More rarely a posterior uveitis, affecting the peripheral parts of the choroid, occurs with or without an anterior uveitis. Both eyes are usually involved. The infection is apparent in the first year of life as a diffuse pigmentary change in both fundi, the so-called 'pepper and salt' appearance. The management of congenital syphilis is discussed on p.59.

Acquired syphilis. An anterior uveitis may occur in the secondary or tertiary stages of syphilis and, without effective systemic treatment, is prone to recurrence; occasionally the affected iris shows patches of dilated capillary blood vessels, the so-called *roseolae*. Posterior uveitis may also occur in the secondary or tertiary stages as a retinal perivasculitis. In the serological diagnosis of syphilitic conditions of the eye, it is evident that reliance can no longer by placed solely on the Wassermann reaction (WR) or the Kahn Test. There are two main aims in such serological tests: first, the detection of antibodies against *Treponema pallidum* using living or dead suspensions—these include the Treponemal Immobilization (TPI), the Reiter protein complement fixation test (RPCFT), the fluorescent treponemal antibody test (FTA-200), and the fluorescent treponemal antibody test (FTA-ABS); and second, the detection of antibody-like substances ('reagins')—these include the complement fixation tests such as the Wassermann reaction (WR) and the cardiolipin WR, flocculation tests such as the Kahn test and Price's protein reaction (PPR), and the Venereal Diseases Reference Laboratory (VDRL) slide test. It is recommended that the cardiolipin WR, the VDRL slide test and the RPCFT should be used as routine tests, with the inclusion of other tests such as the TPI and FTA-ABS only when these three tests prove to be inconclusive. Treatment with penicillin is now less likely to succeed because of increasing antibiotic resistance; management must therefore be dictated by a specialist in this field.

Leprosy

Uveal involvement in leprosy is a major cause of blindness in individuals who are already beset with sensory and skeletal disabilities. Iritis may also be a feature of corneal ulceration secondary to lagophthalmos (facial nerve palsy) and impaired corneal sensation (trigeminal nerve involvement). The iritis of leprosy has two forms: acute and chronic.

Acute form. This is a manifestation of a type III immune complex hypersensitivity, and occurs in lepromatous leprosy as part of a lepra reaction; release of large quantities of antigen by treatment may also result in widespread deposition of immune complexes.

Chronic form. This form is limited to multibacillary or lepromatous leprosy. The organism has a preference for small non-myelinated nerves and a cool environment. Thus the uvea, especially if there is impaired lid closure because of lagophthalmos, is an ideal site for replication. Neuritis of the iris results in an insidious inflammation manifest as small lepromas on the iris nerves (*pearls*), a faint flare and a few cells in the anterior chamber. The dilator pupillae fibres are preferentially affected, which results in their atrophy and dysfunction, leading to a very constricted pupil; this, combined with axial corneal or lens opacities, results in a marked impairment of vision.

It takes years for the evolution of the iritis and management is therefore directed at early recognition and early treatment of the systemic disease.

Brucellosis (*Malta fever or undulant fever*)

Granulomatous anterior uveitis, sometimes recurrent, or posterior uveitis with disseminated nodular foci of exudative choroiditis, may be features of brucellosis.

Viral infection

Viruses responsible for the exanthemata may produce mild iritis, while herpes simplex and herpes zoster both produce iritis usually in assocation with keratitis. Cytomegalovirus may cause disseminated choroiditis and occurs in immunocompromised individuals.

Fungal infection

Patients with immune deficiency are more susceptible to fungal dissemination in which uveitis may be a feature; it also occurs in drug addicts using intravenous drugs.

Histoplasmosis

This is a fungal condition which occurs particularly in parts of the United States. It causes small disseminated peripheral foci of choroiditis, a juxtapapillary choroiditis, and sometimes isolated spherical yellow-white nodules in the choroid, usually without any obvious pigmentary disturbance. The vitreous remains clear and anterior uveitis is rare. There is often also a disciform type of choroidal haemorrhage in the submacular or peripapillary area. Foci of disease may occur in the lungs. A skin test using fresh antigen provides a positive result in the majority of cases.

Infestations

Toxoplasmosis

This follows an infestation by *Toxoplasma gondii*. This has been long recognized in animals, particularly rodents and birds, and it has been recently discovered that the sexual phase of the life cycle occurs in cats.

Thirty per cent of the population in the UK have serological evidence of past subclinical infection. The majority of cases are transmitted by the oral route, either by ingestion of oocysts derived from cats or by eating uncooked meat containing pseudocysts which contain the parasites. Infection may be acquired congenitally by transmission from the mother (who may never show any signs of the disease) to the fetus, and the earlier in pregnancy that the infection occurs, the greater the consequences for the fetus. It is believed that all cases of ocular toxoplasmosis are the result of congenital infection.

Central nervous system. In the early stages of pregnancy a meningoencephalitis of varying intensity occurs, leading in some cases to convulsions and even death. Later there may be hydrocephalus, epilepsy, spasticity, comatous attacks or mental retardation. Foci from previous cerebral involvement are often visible on radiographic examination of the skull because they become calcified.

Digestive system. Involvement of the liver may be associated with jaundice.

Lymphatic system. Involvement of the spleen may cause splenomegaly.

Eye. Isolated patches of acute choroidoretinitis are prone to occur with a predilection for the central part of the fundus, so that the macula may be implicated directly or indirectly by a spread of oedema from an adjacent focus. Later the focus appears as a white atrophic area with usually dense, surrounding pigmentation. There is a tendency to recurrence after a prolonged interval, and a frank choroidoretinitis in the older child or adult may be the result of a previously undetected congenital lesion. It follows that aetiologically there are two types of lesion: one which is the direct result of the organism in the absence of any immunity, and the other which is a hypersensitivity reaction to protozoal antigen released from pseudocysts within the retina in the presence of immunity. Although the effects of the posterior uveitis are marked, the predilection of the organism for nervous tissues makes it likely that it is primarily an infection of the retina with secondary involvement of the underlying choroid.

Other ocular defects such as cataract, nystagmus, microphthalmos and ophthalmoplegia are more rare.

Serological diagnosis. The antibody titre in the blood may be determined by a methylene blue test: the dye stains *Toxoplasma* deeply when it is incubated with normal serum, but less deeply when there are antibodies in the serum. A high titre (e.g. 1 in 64000 or 1 in 32000) may persist for several years after an infection. A low titre (e.g. 1 in 32) is not diagnostic unless repeated tests show a rising titre with an active choroiditis.

Complement fixation and immunofluorescent tests are also useful; these tests confirm exposure to toxoplasmosis at some time, but have no value during ocular disease exacerbations unless the test is negative, indicating no exposure to the organism.

Treatment. Treatment to reduce the consequences of the acute inflammatory reaction is only given for lesions that threaten the macula, or are adjacent to the optic disc or to arteries. Anterior uveitis is treated topically but chorioretinitis requires a combination of a systemic steroid and an antiprotozoal drug such as clindamycin, tetracycline or pyrimethamine; the latter causes marrow depression, so weekly blood counts are necessary and folinic acid must be given concurrently.

Onchocerciasis

Onchocerca volvulus, the cause of 'river blindness' in Africa and South America, is a roundworm transmitted in larval form (microfilariae) by the blackfly *Simulium damnosum*. Mature worms live in the subepidermis and may be detected clinically as nodules. The microfilarial progeny invade the eye to produce keratitis, anterior and posterior uveitis and optic neuritis. Live microfilariae do not excite a destructive immunological reaction, but dead ones do, so that great caution must be used during treatment lest the ensuing hypersensitivity creates a destructive endophthalmitis. Chronic infiltration results in secondary glaucoma, cataract and optic atrophy.

Sarcoidosis

This multisystem disease is characterized by the formation of non-caseating granulomas in the lymph nodes as non-tender lymphadenopathy, in the lung as bilateral hilar lymphadenopathy (BHL)—often in association with erythema nodosum of the skin—or as a diffuse lung infiltration that may lead to fibrosis, in the salivary glands (Heerfordt's disease or uveoparotid fever when the uveitis is associated with fever, splenomegaly, polyneuritis and involvement of the parotid gland, when there may also be a facial paralysis; or Mikulicz's syndrome when the uveitis is associated with involvement of the lacrimal gland in addition to the salivary glands), and less commonly in the bones, usually with overlying skin lesions and hypersensitivity to vitamin D.

Acute anterior uveitis, frequently with BHL and erythema nodosum, is the commonest ocular finding. Chronic iritis with band keratopathy also occurs, while posterior uveitis, manifest as a focal vasculitis or chorioretinitis, is not uncommon. Optic nerve papillitis or infiltration simulating papilloedema may also be present.

Although the aetiology remains unknown, there is evidence of a partial defect of the cell-mediated or T-lymphocyte immune system. This anergy is confirmed by a negative response to Mantoux testing. Chest X-ray is positive in 80% of cases. The Kveim test—the formation of a granuloma at the site of an intradermal injection of a suspension of sarcoid granuloma—is helpful. However, it carries the risk of serum hepatitis, and is invalidated by the concurrent use of systemic steroids, the drug of choice in systemic and ocular sarcoidosis except for an isolated anterior uveitis when topical agents should suffice.

Keratoconjunctivitis sicca and conjunctival forniceal granulomata (which may be biopsied) are other presentations of ocular sarcoid.

Arthropathies

The seronegative arthropathies—Still's, Crohn's, Reiter's and Behçet's disease, ankylosing spondylitis, ulcerative colitis and psoriasis—are associated with uveitis.

Some of these disorders are associated with genetically determined antigens that are present on most nucleated cells but are most readily identified on leucocytes; these are known as the *histocompatibility antigens* and form the human leucocyte antigen system of classification (HLA).

There is a strong association between acute anterior uveitis and the possession of HLA-B27, between Behçet's disease and HLA-B5, between histoplasmosis and HLA-B7, and between Vogt–Koyanagi–Harada's disease and HLA-BW225.

A major association exists between HLA-B27 and ankylosing spondylitis. Furthermore, most patients with Crohn's disease, ulcerative colitis, psoriasis and Reiter's disease who have features of ankylosing spondylitis—most commonly a sacroiliitis—possess HLA-B27.

All patients with this antigen do not develop acute anterior uveitis, but it appears that its possession confers a hereditary susceptibility, possibly to an infective agent, by modulating the immune response.

Apart from Behçet's disease, the seronegative arthropathies with uveitis predominantly affect the anterior segment. Specific features of these conditions are considered below.

Still's disease

In this condition of childhood a seronegative form of rheumatoid arthritis is associated with a persistent bilateral uveitis of insidious onset, initially non-granulomatous but later developing granulomatous features. It particularly affects children with pauciarticular disease (less than four joints affected) who have positive serum antinuclear factor. Most of the inflammatory changes take place in the anterior segment, but occasionally there may be posterior involvement with macular oedema. Sometimes an identical form of uveitis develops in the absence of any arthritic changes, although these may develop later. Cataract is prone to develop even relatively early in the disease, but is readily amenable to lensectomy. Optic atrophy may follow secondary glaucoma, while band-shaped keratopathy is a characteristic feature.

Management requires regular surveillance of children with arthritis to detect the clinical features of a symptomless iritis; when present, topical steroids, mydriatics and occasionally pulsed systemic steroids are required. The risk of suppression of the pituitary–adrenal axis must be considered.

Reiter's disease

In Reiter's disease—a postinfective (after a genitourinary infection or dysentery) arthropathy—a scleritis may develop in addition to anterior uveitis. There is a close association with HLA-B27.

Behçet's disease

This disease occurs particularly in Japan and the Mediterranean areas, and affects the 20 to 40 age group; it has a distinct HLA association. It presents as a severe relapsing uveitis, with episodes of recurrent oral and genital ulceration, and more rarely thrombophlebitis, polyarthritis, carditis and central nervous system disease. The uveitis appears as an iritis, but the severity of this often masks more widespread inflammatory changes within the eye as a result of an obliterative arteritis, which is manifest as choroiditis, retinal vasculitis or optic neuritis. Systemic steroids and chlorambucil are presently the only suitable agents for treatment of this condition.

Vogt–Koyanagi–Harada's syndrome

This is a self-limiting condition with a spectrum of signs, the most constant being a granulomatous panuveitis and optic neuritis associated with serous retinal detachment; other features include alopecia, vitiligo, poliosis (whitening of the hair and eyelashes), vertigo, dysacousis and meningism. Current evidence suggests that it is an autoimmune disorder directed at pigmented tissue, with histological appearances akin to sympathetic uveitis.

Other forms of uveitis

Some forms of uveitis are not associated with any systemic disorder.

Heterochromic cyclitis

Heterochromic cyclitis is a distinctive uveitis which occurs most commonly in young adults, usually in one eye only, with a mild but persistent course. There is a gradual depigmentation and atrophy of the iris stroma so that alteration in the colour of the iris of the affected eye is a characteristic feature of the condition. It is interesting that there is a complete absence of any posterior synechiae, despite the persistent nature of the uveitis. The KP are small, white and somewhat crenated, with a widespread distribution over the entire posterior corneal surface (as in the Posner–Schlossman syndrome—see below). A few cells occur sporadically in the anterior chamber and in the retrolental space, with the formation sometimes of fine opacities in the anterior part of the vitreous. The vision is relatively unaffected until, after an interval of several years, a posterior cortical cataract ensues with eventually widespread cataractous changes; the removal of the cataractous lens is usually a satisfactory procedure. Sometimes glaucoma occurs in the affected eye with pathological cupping of the optic disc and consequent visual field loss, probably because of deposits of inflammatory material in the filtration angle. A peripheral choroidoretinitis may also occur.

Posner–Schlossman syndrome (glaucomatocyclitic crisis)

The Posner-Schlossman syndrome is a distinctive form of anterior uveitis in which an apparently mild form of iritis— characterized by small, white, somewhat crenated KP which are widespread over the entire posterior corneal surface (as in heterochromic cyclitis)—is associated with a high intraocular pressure, although, unlike congestive glaucoma, mistiness of vision and the appearance of haloes are seldom marked and the condition remains confined almost invariably to one eye.

Sympathetic ophthalmitis

Sympathetic ophthalmitis occurs only after a perforating injury, including surgery, of the eye, particularly involving the ciliary body. Its nature is unknown; it may be viral in origin (there is certainly no consistent evidence of any bacterial agent) with an associated cell-mediated immune response to a soluble retinal antigen in the injured eye—the *exciting eye*—and in the uninjured eye—the *sympathizing eye*. The uveitis of the sympathizing eye, which becomes intense after a mild start, occurs some weeks, months, or even years after the injury and is associated with an intense uveitis of the exciting eye. Thus an injured eye which remains inflamed some weeks after a perforating injury is potentially dangerous unless it is removed before the onset of inflammation in the uninjured eye. Its removal after this is of no value in arresting the uveitis of the sympathizing eye; indeed its removal then is most unwise because it may finally retain more vision than the sympathizing eye, although the vision of both eyes is likely to be poor unless there is a rapid and sustained response to intensive treatment with steroids. It follows that it is most unwise to retain a severely injured eye which shows persistent inflammatory changes some weeks after the injury despite intense anti-inflammatory treatment when the long-term visual prognosis is poor.

Phacoanaphylactic uveitis (lens-induced uveitis)

Phacoanaphylactic uveitis occurs as an allergic response to lens material liberated during an extracapsular cataract extraction, following a rupture of the lens capsule, or following seepage through the abnormally permeable lens capsule in a hypermature cataract; the allergic response is usually induced by previous exposure to lens material, for example, after an extracapsular extraction in the other eye. The uveitis is intense, and, when lens material is present, it is usually necessary to remove it.

Treatment of uveitis

1. Maintenance of full pupillary dilatation during the active stage. This prevents the formation of posterior synechiae which lead to complications (see Chapter 15). This may be achieved by mydriatics—atropine 1% drops or ointment, hyoscine 0.25% or 0.5% drops, cyclopentolate 1% drops, or phenylephrine 10% drops—but sometimes it is necessary to inject Mydricaine (a solution of atropine, procaine and adrenaline), which has a most powerful mydriatic effect, into the subconjunctival tissues after adequate surface anaesthesia with amethocaine 1% drops because it causes fairly severe discomfort.
2. Restriction of the inflammatory response. This is achieved using topical steroids (e.g. prednisolone drops hourly or two-hourly) in anterior uveitis, and systemic steroids (e.g. prednisolone 40 mg daily) in posterior uveitis. During prolonged systemic steroid therapy, care should be taken to recognize any marked increase in fluid retention, any significant rise in the blood pressure, or any glycosuria, and therapy should be preceded by chest X-ray.
3. Relief of pain and photophobia. This is achieved by the application of heat, the prevention of pupillary movement by maintaining full mydriasis, the use of dark glasses (or even an eye pad), and various analgesics.
4. Control of any septic element. Chemotherapeutic agents or antibiotics are used topically, subconjunctivally or systemically in hypopyon iritis.

5. Eradication of any known cause of the uveitis. For example, any systemic condition, such as syphilis or gonorrhoea, should be treated.

The treatment of complications are discussed elsewhere; for example, for secondary glaucoma, see Chapter 15 and for cataract, see Chapter 9.

Rubeosis iridis

In rubeosis iridis, networks of new vessel formations develop on the anterior surface of the iris, particularly in certain retinal diseases such as diabetic retinopathy, thrombosis of the central retinal vein, retrolental fibroplasia and long-standing retinal detachment (all discussed in Chapter 8). It is possible that the new vessels are a response to a 'vasoformative factor' from the diseased peripheral retina, and this 'stimulus' may be diminished by destroying the retina beyond the equator using photocoagulation or cryotherapy. Rubeosis iridis is liable to cause obliteration of the filtration angle by the formation of peripheral anterior synechiae, and intractable secondary glaucoma may result.

Degenerations

Iris

Iris atrophy is usually secondary to prolonged anterior uveitis or glaucoma, or may follow herpes zoster ophthalmicus or trauma. Rarely it occurs as part of a unilateral condition, known as the iridocorneal-endothelial syndrome, where iris atrophy, sometimes with full-thickness hole formation, is associated with pupil distortion, marked corneal endothelial abnormalities and peripheral anterior synechiae that lead to a secondary glaucoma. Another form of iris atrophy—iridoschisis—is usually traumatic in origin (see p.81).

Choroid

Gyrate atrophy. In this familial condition due to an inborn error of ornithine metabolism, circular or irregular areas of choroidal atrophy occur in the peripheral parts of both fundi, with atrophic changes in the overlying retina; the affected areas appear white because of the exposed underlying sclera. Later these areas become confluent and it is suggested that ultimately choroideraemia may develop (complete absence of the choroid), but it is more likely that this occurs only as a congenital anomaly (see p.79). The condition is associated with myopia, cataract and vitreous changes.

Central areolar choroidal dystrophy. In this familial condition irregular areas of choroidal atrophy occur in the central parts of both fundi but, unlike gyrate atrophy, the degenerative changes are confined to the choriocapillaris, the overlying retinal pigment epithelium and the photoreceptors; the exposed choroidal vessels appear ophthalmoscopically to be sclerosed, hence this condition is also known as *central areolar choroidal sclerosis*, but there are seldom sclerotic changes histologically.

Disciform degeneration. This follows the formation of a fibrovascular membrane under the retina, usually in the submacular area, which may bleed into the subretinal space. It has been suggested that the neovascular membrane follows degeneration of the choroidal vessels, particularly the capillary layer (the *choriocapillaris*). However, it is more likely that the primary lesion is a disruption of the elastic lamina of Bruch's membrane as a result of the ageing process, so that the

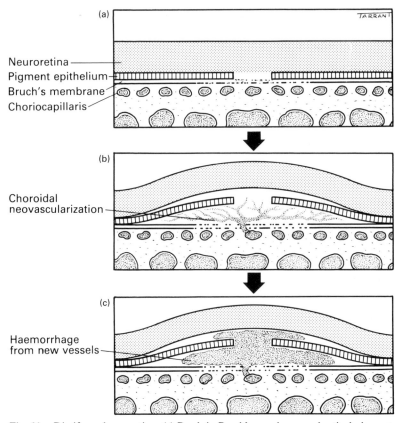

Fig. 30. Disciform degeneration. (a) Break in Bruch's membrane and retinal pigment epithelium. (b) Choroidal new vessels penetrating Bruch's membrane to produce pigment epithelial and neuroretinal elevations. (c) Haemorrhage from choroidal neovascular membrane organizes into a disciform scar.

(a)

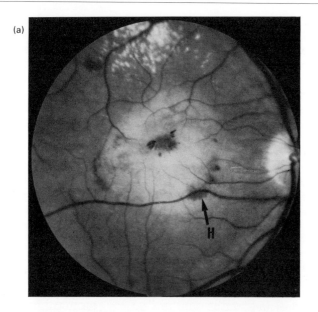

(b)

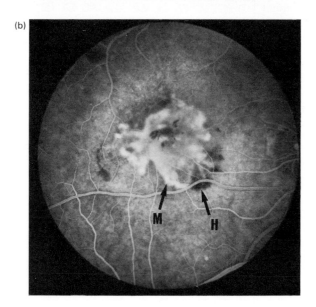

Fig. 31. Disciform macular degeneration. (a) Red-free photograph. (b) Fluorescein angiogram. Note the neovascular membrane (M) at the macula, and the deep retinal haemorrhage (H) and pigment epithelial detachment obscuring the underlying fluorescence.

haemorrhage follows a failure of the elastic lamina to support the choroidal capillaries (Fig. 30). Sometimes the subretinal extravasation is more exudative than haemorrhagic and produces detachment of the pigment epithelium. Fluorescein angiography demonstrates a rapid filling of the neovascular membrane, with subsequent leakage of the dye from the choroidal vessels into the area of detached pigment epithelium, with a surrounding dark non-fluorescent area which represents the haemorrhage (Fig. 31). Inevitably there is a disruption of the function of the overlying retina. Ophthalmoscopically the lesion appears as a dark swelling without any obvious haemorrhage, unless this tracks into the overlying retina. Eventually the deep haemorrhage usually absorbs with atrophic changes in the retina and choroid, but it may become organized, with the formation of a raised, often pigmented, mass of tissue (*Fuchs' black spot*).

Anterior segment necrosis (ischaemic ocular inflammation)

A peculiar form of anterior uveitis may result from a disturbance of the blood supply to the anterior segment of the eye (*ischaemic ocular inflammation*), particularly when there is undue interference with the recti muscles which contain the anterior ciliary arteries. This may occur in extensive retinal detachment surgery, in certain muscle transplant procedures (as a general rule it is unwise to detach or involve more than two rectus muscles, even in childhood), or in ipsilateral carotid/ophthalmic artery disease. It may also occur simply as the result of long-standing ocular disease. Other features include diffuse episcleral redness, corneal oedema with a wrinkling of Descemet's membrane, neovascularization of the iris, atrophy of the iris with an irregular semidilatation of the pupil which responds poorly to light and drugs, cataract, and a greyness of the peripheral part of the retina with haemorrhages. The response to anti-inflammatory measures is poor. Blindness may ensue when the condition is a true 'necrosis', but ischaemia is usually compatible with retention of some form of vision.

Tumours

Melanoma

This tumour probably has a neuroectodermal origin in the uveal tract. It may be simple (*benign melanoma, pigmented mole, naevus*), often present in early life, or malignant (*malignant melanoma*).

Iris

A simple melanoma presents as a localized pigmented mass on the surface of the iris or within the stroma, and it is composed largely of spindle cells; it is different from an iris freckle which is simply a proliferation of normal stromal melanocytes. A change to malignancy is indicated by an increase in its size so that it may project into the anterior chamber, sometimes with an area of corneal contact, or into the posterior chamber where it lies against the lens. It may also extend to the tissues of the filtration angle and the anterior part of the ciliary body.

Treatment. When malignancy is suspected, the tumour should be excised completely, together with a strip of normal iris (*iridectomy*) and also with a portion of the ciliary body (*iridocyclectomy*) when necessary. Early and adequate local excision carries a good prognosis and avoids the removal of the eye.

Choroid

A simple choroidal naevus appears as a bluish-grey mass under the retina. Its benign nature is shown by certain features: (a) no obvious increase in size over a prolonged period; (b) no marked elevation of the retina over the affected area; (c) a retention of visual function in this area of retina (because the benign tumour does not involve the choriocapillaris which supplies the outer part of the retina); and (d) the absence of any surrounding serous retinal detachment. In fluorescein angiography there is an area of non-fluorescence corresponding to the area of the tumour because this screens the background fluorescence of the choroid. In a change to malignancy, which seldom occurs before middle age, these features are lost; of particular importance is the development of an area of retinal detachment, apart from the detached retina overlying the tumour, because of fluid in the subretinal space. The formation of this fluid confirms the active nature of the choroidal lesion, and the free nature of the subretinal space determines the fact that, although the serous detachment is usually adjacent to the tumour, it may be remote from it because the fluid from the tumour gravitates to the lower part of the subretinal space. There is a disturbance of retinal function over the tumour and in the area of serous detachment, but sometimes this is not noticed by the patient until the central vision becomes affected. A few haemorrhages may occur in the retina in the area of the tumour.

A ^{32}P test may be of value in certain cases; the radioactive phosphorus is taken by mouth and its concentration over the surface of the affected and unaffected eyes is determined with a Geiger counter 24 hours later. An excessively high uptake over the affected area is of diagnostic importance, but the results are sometimes inconclusive, particularly as they depend largely on a comparison of values between corresponding parts of the affected and unaffected eye. It follows that the result of any one test should not unduly sway clinical judgement. Transillumination of the globe by shining a bright light into the eye through the sclera may reveal a shadow over the affected area, but this test is not always reliable. In fluorescein angiography there is a filling of the vessels of the tumour with the dye and throughout the substance of the tumour there is an abnormal pooling of fluorescein, with a finely flecked fluorescence at the border of the tumour as the result of leakage of the dye. Recently the non-invasive technique of ultrasound has been developed, which can reliably identify a solid mass and also determine if there has been penetration through the sclera (see Fig. 69c, p.276). The main lesions which may be confused with a malignant melanoma are subretinal haemorrhage (p.97), simple retinal detachment (p.137), and metastatic carcinoma (see below).

A malignant melanoma usually remains confined to the eye for a considerable period before involving the extraocular tissues by direct spread through the sclera or before forming more distant metastases (classically in the liver, but sometimes in the skin or in other regions) as a result of blood spread. Indeed the tumour in the eye may become so large that it causes a secondary glaucoma (caused sometimes by obliteration of the filtration angle by the formation of new vessels on the surface of the iris) so that the eye becomes blind and painful; it follows that sometimes an 'unknown' blind eye should be removed if it is not possible to examine the fundus ophthalmoscopically in case it harbours a malignant melanoma.

Treatment. Enucleation of the eye is the treatment of choice, and, provided there is no evidence of extraocular extension at operation or on histological examination of the eye and there are no metastases within a few years, there is a good prognosis. However, there is evidence that the pressure on the globe which is inevitable in its removal may cause a dissemination of malignant cells, and in recent years a more conservative approach is being adopted, particularly in the elderly person. Sometimes if the other eye has poor vision (or has been lost by injury or disease) it may be justified to try to control the tumour by irradiation (e.g. the application of a cobalt disc) or by photocoagulation of the affected area.

Haemangioma (angioma)

A haemangioma may occur in any part of the uveal tract—very rarely in the iris and ciliary body but less rarely in the choroid. A haemangioma of the iris, because of its vascular nature, causes periodic bleeding (*hyphaema*). A haemangioma of the choroid may not become evident until adult life despite its congenital nature. It is usually situated near the optic disc. It grows slowly with the formation of a raised mass and eventually with the development of a remote serous retinal detachment in the lower part of the eye. In fluorescein angiography the tumour shows a brilliant early fluorescence because of its vascular nature, with a coarsely flecked fluorescence at the border of the tumour because of leakage of the dye; both these features are usually more prominent than in a malignant melanoma of the choroid.

Quite frequently a haemangioma of the uveal tract is associated with a *naevus flammeus (port-wine stain)* affecting the skin of the face in the distribution of the ipsilateral trigeminal nerve (fifth cranial nerve). Similar abnormal vessels occur in the episcleral region near the limbus so that glaucoma may ensue following obliteration of the filtration angle. Similar lesions in the ipsilateral cerebral cortex may cause hemiplegia, epilepsy and mental deficiency (the *Sturge–Weber syndrome*, one of the phakomatoses, p.149).

Neurofibroma

This tumour occurs rarely in the choroid, usually as a manifestation of von Recklinghausen's disease, one of the phakomatoses, but small iris fibromas are a more common feature. A diffuse or plexiform neurofibroma involving the anterior chamber angle can result in buphthalmos.

Metastatic carcinoma

The choroid is a common site for carcinomatous metastatic deposits from a primary focus in the lungs or breast, and it is usually an indication of widespread dissemination. The lesion responds readily to irradiation and, unless the patient is moribund, this should be carried out because it permits the retention of useful vision and prevents the complications which may follow a later total retinal detachment, such as a secondary glaucoma. Removal of the eye is seldom justified unless it becomes blind and painful.

Cysts

A spontaneous cyst of the iris as a result of a separation of the two pigmented layers following an accumulation of fluid, sometimes of an inflammatory nature, is extremely rare. An implantation cyst on the surface of the iris is slightly more common and may follow a proliferation of epithelial tissue which is introduced into the eye from a corneal wound at the time of a perforating injury or operation; sometimes this cyst becomes sufficiently large to necessitate its removal, otherwise glaucoma may ensue. A congenital iris cyst is a rare event.

Anomalies of the pupillary reflexes

These follow lesions of the afferent or efferent parts of their nervous pathways.

Lesion of the afferent pupillary (visual) pathway in the retina or optic nerve.

This causes a defect in the pupillary constriction in response to light of both the affected eye (direct light reflex) and the unaffected eye (consensual light reflex) because the afferent pupillary fibres from each eye are transmitted to the parasympathetic parts of the oculomotor nuclei on both sides of the brainstem. The defects are complete if the lesions are complete and partial if the lesions are partial. In contrast, the consensual light response of the affected eye and the direct light response of the unaffected eye are normal. Constriction of the pupil of the affected eye which occurs as a consensual response is followed by dilatation of the pupil when the light stimulus to the unaffected eye is discontinued and the dilatation continues even when the affected eye is stimulated by light (*Marcus Gunn pupillary phenomenon* or *relative afferent pupillary defect*).

Lesion of the afferent pupillary (visual) pathway in the optic chiasm or optic tract

This causes defects similar to those described above, but only when the retinal area that corresponds to the affected part of the pathway is stimulated because of the partial decussation of the afferent pupillary (and visual) fibres in the optic chiasm (see Chapter 16); this 'hemianopic' pupil response is difficult to determine clinically because of the scattering of light on illuminating any part of the retina.

A lesion of the afferent visual pathway caudal to the exit of the afferent pupillary fibres from the optic tract does not interfere with the pupillary light reflexes; it follows that total blindness caused by lesions of both cortical visual areas is compatible with unimpaired pupillary light reflexes.

Lesion of the efferent parasympathetic pupillary pathway

This causes a defect in the pupillary constriction of the eye on the side of the lesion to a light stimulus of the ipsilateral eye (direct light reflex) and to a light stimulus of the contralateral eye (consensual light reflex), but there is no defect in the light responses of the other eye. There is also a defect in the pupillary constriction of the eye on the side of the lesion to a near stimulus (accommodation and convergence pupillary reflexes). This represents an *internal ophthalmoplegia*.

Lesion of the efferent peripheral sympathetic pupillary pathway

This causes little interference in the pupillary reaction to light because the main effect of the hypothalmic sympathetic centre is an indirect one on the parasympathetic nucleus, so that pupillary dilatation follows an inhibition of the nucleus rather than peripheral sympathetic stimulation. However, it causes other characteristic features (*Horner's syndrome*): a somewhat constricted pupil (*miosis*) resulting from the unopposed action of the sphincter muscle of the pupil, a narrowing of the palpebral fissure (*ptosis*) from a failure of the superior (and inferior) palpebral smooth muscles, decreased sweating of the ipsilateral forehead (*anhidrosis*) and (occasionally) decreased pigmentation of the affected iris. The *enophthalmos* which is sometimes described is more apparent (following the narrowing of the palpebral fissure) than real, because there is no effective smooth muscle in the orbit which alters significantly the position of the eye. Conversely, an irritative lesion of the sympathetic pathway (e.g. the early stages of a neoplasm in the upper part of the chest involving the cervical sympathetic chain) produces the opposite effects: a somewhat dilated pupil (*mydriasis*), a widening of the palpebral fissure, and an increased sweating of the ipsilateral forehead.

Myotonic pupil (Adie's pupil)

This is more common in females and usually occurs in early adult life. It is almost invariably confined to one eye initially, but eventually becomes bilateral in some cases. The pupil is somewhat dilated with an apparent absence of any response to light, directly or consensually, except for slight worm-like heavings of the pupil margin. The pupil constricts to a near stimulus, but this is slow, becoming effective only after a considerable time. There is also a slowness of the pupil to revert to its usual size after removing the near stimulus; this retention of some form of near response distinguishes the myotonic pupil from the dilated pupil which follows the administration of a mydriatic such as atropine. In addition, the myotonic pupil, unlike the atropinized pupil, constricts after the instillation of methacholine 2.5% drops or pilocarpine 0.1%, thus demonstrating denervation hypersensitivity. Sometimes the tendon reflexes (particularly the knee and ankle jerks) are defective, but there are no other neurologic complications and, although the site of the lesion is unknown, the most likely area is the ciliary ganglion. Because of myotonic involvement of the ciliary muscle, the majority of patients have demonstrable accommodation abnormalities.

Argyll Robertson pupil

This is characterized by a persistent but somewhat irregular miosis with an absence of (or, in the early stages, with an impaired) response to light, directly and consensually, and with a brisk response to a near stimulus. It is almost invariably bilateral, although the degree of miosis may be unequal. It occurs in lesions affecting the pretectal region of the midbrain (hence its bilateral nature) in a wide variety of cerebral disorders (encephalitis, vascular abnormalities, traumatic lesions) but characteristically it occurs in neurosyphilis (tabes dorsalis and general paralysis of the insane); in the juvenile form of neurosyphilis the pupils may be involved in a similar way except for an absence of miosis.

Hippus

This term applies to a state of pupillary unrest with constant slight fluctuations without any change in illumination. It has been described in some cases of disseminated sclerosis and chorea.

Anomalies of accommodation

Paralysis

This occurs in lesions of the part of the oculomotor nucleus or nerve subserving the intrinsic ocular muscles of the ciliary body, but it is rare.

Insufficiency

This occurs commonly at any age and is usually precipitated by some emotional factor, such as overwork or worry, or by some debilitating disease which causes a functional (not an organic) disorder. Blurred reading vision is associated with symptoms of eyestrain, such as aching and redness of the eyes and headaches, and there may also be weakness of convergence. These may be relieved partly by the correction of any refractive error, but it is essential to treat the underlying cause. It also occurs naturally with age, but this is of an entirely different nature (*presbyopia*, p.17).

Spasm

This may also occur at any age because of emotional factors. The persistent excess of accommodation causes a blurring of vision in the distance because of an induced myopia, an inability to read small print unless held close to the eyes, and the symptoms of eyestrain. There may be an associated spasm of convergence which results in a latent or even manifest convergent squint, and an associated spasm of the sphincter of the pupils with miosis. The treatment is directed to the underlying cause.

Influence of drugs on the pupils and the ciliary body

The mydriatic and cycloplegic effects of drugs such as atropine and hyoscine, and the miotic and cyclospastic effects of drugs such as eserine and pilocarpine, are discussed elsewhere (see pp.16, 308 and 309).

7

The Retina

Structure and function

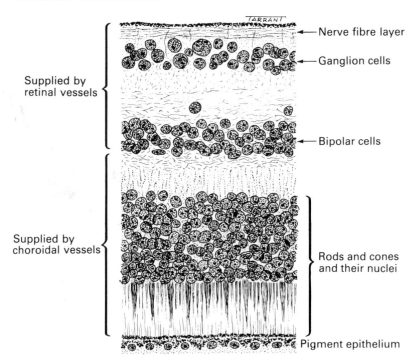

Fig. 32. The minute structure of the retina (after Duke-Elder).

The retina forms the inner coat of the eye and is concerned with the reception of the images of the fixation object (central vision) and of the other objects in the visual panorama (peripheral vision). It has two main parts (Fig. 32)—the pigment epithelium (the outer layer) and the neural part (the inner layers)—a distinction of importance because the two parts lie in apposition without any form of union, except around the optic disc and in the extreme periphery at the *ora serrata*, so that there is a potential space between them (this is the site of the subretinal fluid in a retinal detachment). The peculiarity of 'apposition without adherence' is the result of the development of the retina in the embryo by an invagination of the primary optic vesicle to form the secondary

107

optic vesicle; the invaginated portion forms the neural part of the retina and the uninvaginated portion forms the pigment epithelium. An abnormal closure of the cleft of the secondary optic vesicle results in the formation of a uveal coloboma (see p.78).

The neural part is complex, but functions as three main layers:

1. *An outer layer of rods and cones* which lies immediately beneath the pigment epithelium; their nuclei form the outer nuclear layer.

Under conditions of bright illumination the *rods* are concerned with an appreciation of light and movement, but under conditions of dim illumination their function is enhanced. The rods contain visual purple (*rhodopsin*) which is bleached on exposure to light and becomes reformed as a photochemical response which is dependent on an adequate supply of vitamin A and on adequate contact between the rods and normally functioning pigment epithelium. The rods are responsible for *scotopic vision.* They are present throughout the retina, particularly in the more peripheral parts, but are absent from the fovea.

The *cones* are concerned with an appreciation of form and colour under conditions of bright illumination (*photopic vision*). They are present throughout the retina but particularly in the fovea, where there are no rods, and in the parafovea, where there are few rods. (The fovea and parafovea combine to form the *macula.*)

2. *A middle layer of bipolar cells* which provide the connecting link between the rods and cones and the ganglion cells. It forms the inner nuclear layer.

3. *An inner layer of ganglion cells* which give rise to the nerve fibres which pass along the innermost part of the retina (*nerve fibre layer*) to the optic nerve head, optic nerve, optic chiasm and optic tract to reach the lateral geniculate body. This layer is absent directly over the fovea which is, therefore, less thick than the rest of the retina.

Blood supply

The *central retinal artery*, which is a branch of the *ophthalmic artery* (a branch of the internal carotid artery), enters the eye through the optic nerve head within the optic cup and divides into four main branches, which supply each retinal quadrant—the *superior temporal, inferior temporal, superior nasal* and *inferior nasal arteries.* Each of these arteries (or their branches) acts as an end artery so that its occlusion causes a loss of function in a retinal sector. They supply only the inner half of the retina (as far as the bipolar cells); the outer half, containing the rods and cones, is supplied indirectly by the capillaries of the choroid (the choriocapillaris) (Fig. 32). The fovea is devoid of retinal vessels and is nourished exclusively by the choriocapillaris. Sometimes a small artery passes to the retina, usually its macular part, from the circle of Zinn within the sclera, which is derived from the ciliary circulation. This is termed a *cilioretinal artery* and ophthalmoscopically it appears as a small artery which emerges from the border of the optic disc (in contrast to the main retinal arteries which emerge from the optic cup). An identical appearance occurs when a small retinal artery leaves the main retinal artery in the optic nerve behind the lamina cribrosa, and is therefore not visible ophthalmoscopically, to pass independently to the retina. It is not possible, therefore, to determine purely ophthalmoscopically the true incidence of a cilioretinal artery.

The *central retinal vein* leaves the eye in company with the central retinal artery and has similar branches in each retinal quadrant.

Electrodiagnostic methods of assessing retinal function

The electroretinogram (ERG). This records the sum of the action potentials generated by the retinal receptors and bipolar cells in response to a flash of light.

The electro-oculogram (EOG). This records the changes of ocular potential caused by metabolic activity, mainly in the retinal pigment epithelium.

These electrodiagnostic methods provide evidence of abnormal responses in lesions involving the circulation of the choroid or involving the pigment epithelium, receptor cells or bipolar cells of the retina. They are of particular value when it is not possible to view the fundus because of a dense opacity of the media such as a cataract, or in certain abiotrophic, degenerative or vascular lesions of the retina at a stage when there are no obvious ophthalmoscopic changes. However, the electroretinogram (ERG) provides a mass response so that half the retina must be involved before the result is abnormal. The electro-oculogram (EOG) may also be used in assessing the movements of the eye because any movement causes a shift in the ocular potential.

Fluorescein angiography

In recent years the method of fluorescein angiography has assumed an important role in the assessment of certain retinal and choroidal disorders. Fluorescein (5 ml of 10% solution) is injected intravenously (into the antecubital vein of the arm), and the appearance of the dye in the fundus by way of the central retinal and posterior ciliary arteries, and its final disappearance are recorded by a camera containing high-speed monochrome film which photographs the fundus at regular intervals (about once every second). The technique allows detailed examination of the retinal vasculature; normal retinal vessels have tight endothelial junctions that prevent leakage of the loosely protein-bound dye, whilst the choroidal system and new vessels do not have this property and therefore leak. Haemorrhage and pigment mask underlying fluorescence, while defects in the pigment epithelium allow choroidal fluorescence to be seen.

To fluoresce, the dye has to be stimulated by light of wavelength 475 nm by interpolating an appropriate filter into the illumination system. In order to view and record this fluorescence, a barrier filter to all but the fluorescent light, wavelength 520 nm, is placed in front of the film.

In the normal eye the following sequence of events is recorded: (a) a *choroidal flush* which lasts for less than a second; (b) an *early retinal arteriolar phase* which spreads outwards from the optic disc; (c) a *late retinal arteriolar phase* in which the whole arteriolar tree is brightly fluorescent; (d) a *retinal capillary phase* which appears first as a reticular pattern in the late retinal arteriolar phase and persists beyond that phase; (e) an *early retinal venous phase* which appears in the late retinal arteriolar phase as a layering or streaming along the venous walls; (f) a *late retinal venous phase* at a stage when the retinal arterioles lose their fluorescence; and (g) finally a fading of the brightness of the venous fluorescence but with a persistence of some fluorescence because of a recirculation of the dye, particularly within the optic disc. In addition, the outline of the choroidal vessels is visible against the background of scleral fluorescence.

Congenital anomalies

Opaque nerve fibres

The optic nerve fibres in the retina are normally non-myelinated so that they are not visible ophthalmoscopically; the myelinating process which spreads along the optic nerve from the central nervous system in the fetus, and even for a short time after birth, terminates at the lamina cribrosa in the deeper part of the optic nerve head. Rarely the myelination extends into part of the retina so that the nerve fibres in the affected area become visible as an opaque white, slightly striated patch with 'feathery' edges which characteristically tends to obscure partially the retinal vessels in the affected region because of the superficial position of the optic nerve fibres; this is in direct contrast to other white patches such as exudates, colloid material or choroidal atrophy which lie deep to the retinal vessels. Opaque nerve fibres are usually contiguous with the optic disc, but rarely an isolated patch may occur in another part of the retina. There is some depression of visual function in the affected area; rarely when the opaque nerve fibres are extensively present in the central part of the fundus there is a marked and permanent loss of vision.

Abnormal pigmentation

The uniform 'redness' of the normal fundus on ophthalmoscopic examination is caused by the blood within the underlying choroidal circulation. The pattern of the choroidal vessels is obscured by the dense pigmentation of the retinal pigment epithelium, but if this pigmentation is less dense than usual these vessels become visible to some extent so that the fundus has a tigroid appearance (the so-called *'tigroid' fundus*). A marked deficiency or even a complete absence of pigmentation, as in albinism, gives the fundus a pale pink appearance due to the exposure of the underlying choroid and sclera. Sometimes in the normal fundus, pigment accumulates in discrete patches in the deeper parts of the retina—the so-called *'cats paw' pigmentation* ('bear's paw' pigmentation in the United States).

It should be noted that a slight darkening of the parafoveal and paramacular areas as compared with the rest of the retina is normal, with the fovea standing out as a glistening white spot, but this darkening is of uniform nature; this is in contrast to the irregular pigmentation which occurs in, for example, macular dystrophy.

Abnormal vascularization

Normally the extensive network of hyaloid vessels which fills the vitreous in the fetus disappears shortly before birth, but occasionally parts of these vessels persist as congenital remnants. A hyaloid artery covered by glial tissue may project from the optic disc into the vitreous (*Bergmeister's papilla*).

Embryopathic pigmentary retinopathy

A congenital anomaly of the pigment epithelium may follow certain maternal infections (e.g. syphilis, rubella and influenza) in the first three months of pregnancy. Involvement of the pigment epithelium in both eyes may result from interference with its normal development rather than destruction of established pigment epithelium, as occurs in inflammatory conditions. There is irregular pigmentation of the fundus; in some areas the pigment cells are more or less devoid of pigment and in other areas they contain an excess of unusually large pigment granules. This anomaly also accounts for the appearance in the fundus of small bluish pigmented spots—the so-called *pepper-and-salt* changes. It is doubtful if the condition leads to any serious visual disturbance unless the macular area is implicated significantly, but rarely involvement of the macular area may lead in later childhood to the development of a disciform type of macular degeneration with a marked loss of central vision.

Coloboma of the retina

Coloboma of the retina occurs in association with coloboma of the choroid (p.78); sometimes branches from the retinal vessels in other parts of the retina pass over the coloboma.

Retinal dysplasia

This is a developmental disorder, sometimes of a familial nature, which is present at birth even in full-term infants. A greyish-white tissue in the vitreous represents the elevated malformed retina which may become adherent to the posterior surface of the lens. The condition is usually bilateral and the eye may be slightly microphthalmic with a shallow anterior chamber. It is frequently associated with other malformations such as cardiovascular defects, cleft palate, hare lip, hydrocephalus, mental retardation, polydactylism and intestinal malrotations. This condition is different from retinal aplasia (p.143).

Injuries

Commotio retinae (Berlin's oedema)

Blunt trauma of the eye (e.g. a hit from a fist or stone) may cause oedema of the retina underlying the area of the injury or of the retina opposite to this area as a result of a contrecoup effect. The affected area appears cloudy and swollen with fine radiating lines of 'tension' on its surface. This appearance is striking when it affects the macular area (the usual site of involvement of the contrecoup effect following an injury to the front of the eye) because the foveal region, which does not share in the oedematous process owing to the absence of a nerve fibre layer, stands out as a red circular area against the white background of the surrounding swollen retina. Pigmentary changes usually occur in the retina after the subsidence of the oedema and some permanent disturbance of the vision follows macular involvement.

Solar retinopathy

An oedematous condition of the macula may follow exposure to infrared light from the sun. This is induced very rarely by normal exposure, but it occurs more commonly on observing the eclipse of the sun (eclipse blindness); a pigmentary stippling of the macula remains on resolution of the inflammatory process.

Non-accidental injury syndrome (battered-baby syndrome)

Retinal haemorrhages, particularly in the form of an extensive preretinal haemorrhage involving the central fundus, are a feature of this distressing condition in which child abuse also leads to fractures of the long bones and subdural haematomas, sometimes of a repeated nature. The retinal changes may be so severe as to cause a retinal detachment with haemorrhage in the subretinal space, so that it resembles Coats' disease histologically, and there may be subsequent optic atrophy. The retinal changes are prone to occur when the baby is spun around at high speed (the so-called *aeroplane spin*). Other ocular abnormalities may occur; injuries to the eyelids, posterior subcapsular cataract, peripheral choroidoretinal atrophy, vitreous haemorrhage, and cortical blindness as the result of diffuse cerebral damage. The establishment of the cause of these lesions is often difficult because the history is almost invariably misleading, but the sociological importance of the recognition of the nature of the syndrome is obvious.

Retrolental fibroplasia (retinopathy of prematurity)

Retrolental fibroplasia in the premature baby almost invariably affects both eyes within a few weeks of birth, particularly when the birth weight is less than 1.35 kg and when there has been exposure to excessive concentrations of oxygen; it is suggested that a concentration of less than 30% in the atmosphere is safe, but the main determining factor is the concentration of oxygen in the arterial blood. The oxygen causes a sequence of events in the immature retinal vessels: vasoconstriction which leads to vaso-obliteration occurs during the exposure to oxygen and vasoproliferation occurs after removal from the oxygen.

The earliest ophthalmoscopic changes occur in the periphery of the retina which appears grey with a disappearance of the fine retinal vessels in that area, although these must be interpreted with care because some degree of greyness is normal in the very young, and the retinal vessels do not extend to the most peripheral part of the retina in the premature child. The proliferation of vasoformative tissue usually progresses to the formation of vascularized fibrous strands from the retina into the anterior part of the vitreous, which lead to areas of retinal detachment. Eventually the retina becomes totally detached and disorganized with the formation of a retrolental membrane which obscures any view of the fundus, usually with total blindness. Subsequently new vessels may develop on the surface of the iris. The shallowness of the anterior chamber, a characteristic feature of this condition, favours development of secondary glaucoma as the result of obliteration of the filtration angle by peripheral anterior synechiae. Sometimes, however, the early changes in the retinal periphery subside without any invasion of the vitreous so that some visual function is retained, although the eye often becomes myopic. A retinal fold may pass from the optic disc to the periphery of the fundus with a disruption of central vision when it passes temporally through the macular area; this retinal fold is more likely to pass temporally than nasally because in the premature child the lack of vascularization of the peripheral retina is more marked in the temporal region.

The sequence of events and the characteristic clinical features seldom cause any difficulty in diagnosis, but conditions which show similar features are persistent hyperplastic vitreous (p.186) and persistent vascular sheath of the lens (p.167), retinoblastoma (p.146), endoph-thalmitis (pseudoglioma) (p.86) and Coats' disease (see below); recently a dominantly inherited condition, *exudative hyalo-retinopathy,* with appearances very similar to retrolental fibroplasia, has been described, which may be complicated by vitreous haemorrhage.

There is no effective treatment, but fortunately it may be prevented by exercising great care that premature babies are not exposed to excessive concentrations of oxygen. This is a difficult policy to enforce in the presence of acute respiratory distress syndrome of the newborn, and the avoidance of an undue concentration of oxygen within the oxygen tent (e.g. not more than 30%) is not wholly reliable because the only valid criterion is the repeated estimation of the oxygen level in the arterial blood, which involves a highly specialized technique in the neonatal period.

Massive retinal fibrosis

This occurs in early childhood and is a protrusion from the retina of a greyish-white fibrous mass; it is the result of organization of a massive deep retinal haemorrhage occurring at birth because of some predisposing factor such as prolonged labour, premature delivery, precipitate birth or asphyxia. It does not lead to a true retinal detachment because a proliferation of the retinal pigment epithelium into the mass unites the affected area with the underlying choroid, but a gradual contraction of the lesion progressively involves the surrounding retina. It is an uncommon condition considering the relative frequency of retinal haemorrhage, even after a normal delivery (perhaps in the region of 10%). There may be associated intracranial haemorrhages; death may ensue if these are severe, and surviving infants frequently show some permanent malformation of the central nervous system such as cerebral spastic paralysis or mental retardation.

Metastatic retinitis

A metastatic infective embolus may occur in the retina in any septicaemic disease of childhood. It causes a localized inflammatory reaction which may remain undetected because it is often symptomless (except for loss of vision, which is not appreciated by a child), but subsequent organization of the affected tissue leads to retinal detachment with the appearance of a white mass behind the pupil. There is usually an associated cloudiness of the vitreous so that the retinal lesion appears as an indistinct white haze. The immunosuppressed individual or the drug-addict who takes drugs intravenously may develop a septic retinitis, often due to fungal infection.

Coats' disease

Coats' disease is a rare condition which comprises various clinical entities in which a localized retinal detachment, usually in the central part of the fundus, follows an exudative or haemorrhagic extravasation in the outer retinal layers and in the subretinal space. Sometimes it occurs in telangiectasis (*retinal telangiectasis of Reese*) or aneurysm formations (*multiple miliary retinal aneurysms of Leber*) of the retinal vessels. It occurs particularly in male children between the ages of 5 and 15 years, but also sometimes in the female and in the young adult. It is usually unilateral. The extravasation becomes organized and cholesterol crystals accumulate within the mass; these are regarded usually as a secondary change, but recently it has been suggested that they are the result of an abnormal effect of the lipoproteins in the blood plasma and that they may have some primary influence. The vision is seriously affected when the macula is involved. Rarely a secondary uveitis or glaucoma develops in advanced cases. The conditions which sometimes show similar features are retinoblastoma (p.146), pseudoglioma due to an endophthalmitis (p.86), angiomatosis retinae (p.148) and infestation of the retina by *Toxocara canis* (p.141).

There is no effective treatment for the established condition, but photocoagulation or cryotherapy of the abnormal retinal vessels may limit the extent of the retinal involvement.

Retinal vasculitis

Retinal vasculitis is essentially an inflammation of the retinal veins (*periphlebitis* or *phlebitis*), but the occasional involvement also of the arteries (*periarteritis* or *arteritis*) dictates the use of the term *vasculitis*. Recent evidence suggests the condition is an immunological disorder either an immune complex vasculitis or autoimmunity to retinal antigens that may be isolated to the eye, or part of a systemic immunological disease such as sarcoidosis, Behçet's disease, Wegener's granulomatosis, lupus erythematosus and occasionally multiple sclerosis.

It is characteristically a condition of young adults, and affects males more than females. The brunt of the disease occurs in the periphery of the retina, with irregular dilatation of the retinal veins, the formation of widespread haemorrhages within the retina and near its surface (preretinal haemorrhage), zones of sheathing along the affected veins, and inflammatory cells in the vitreous. The condition is usually self-limiting after months or even years, but it is only in mild cases that the visual prognosis is reasonably good because of the relative sparing of the central retina; peripheral retinal haemorrhages are liable to extend into the vitreous with subsequent organization and new vessel formation from the retina (*retinitis proliferans*) which may lead to localized or even extensive areas of retinal detachment. The condition is frequently bilateral, but the two eyes may be affected unequally.

More rarely the disease affects the retinal veins within the optic nerve head, with a massive dilatation of the retinal veins along their whole length from the optic disc to the periphery, and marked oedema of the retina surrounding the optic disc and also sometimes of the macular area. There are comparatively few retinal haemorrhages, so that vitreous haemorrhage and subsequent retinitis proliferans are unlikely to occur unless there is an associated peripheral form of the disease. Fluorescein angiography has shown that there are two main stages of vascular decompensation. First, venous decompensation occurs—the leakage of the dilated retinal veins is shown by perivenous fluorescence—but the capillaries which are also dilated are not permeable and there are no microaneurysms. These changes occur when there is only a moderate retinopathy with haemorrhages and cottonwool spots and absence of marked retinal oedema so that the central vision remains good. Second, capillary decompensation occurs, with an extensive leakage of fluorescein. These changes occur when there is marked retinopathy with obvious retinal oedema and significant impairment of vision, particularly when there is *cystic maculopathy*. Eventually an increase in retinal tissue pressure may cause some areas of capillary closure with the development of ischaemic changes, resulting in the formation of new vessels. This condition, which is usually confined to one eye, gradually subsides over a period of months but with a persistence of some degree of retinal vein dilatation, some postoedematous blurring of the optic disc, and a variable disturbance of the macular area.

The central form of retinal vasculitis may mimic a central retinal vein thrombosis (p.127), but in this latter condition the dilatation of the retinal veins and oedema around the optic disc are associated with widespread retinal haemorrhages and there is often evidence of hypertensive or arteriosclerotic changes in the retinal vessels of the unaffected eye. The two conditions appear, therefore, to be different, but it is suggested that central retinal vasculitis represents a form of central retinal vien thrombosis occurring in the presence of an otherwise normal vascular system, so that there is a potential for the development of collateral channels; this is confirmed by the later development in some cases of central retinal vasculitis of a typical central vein thrombosis with its unfortunate sequelae. There are other conditions which show similar features but should not cause confusion: plerocephalic oedema (p.156) is bilateral (as a general rule) and the dilatation of the retinal veins is confined to an area around the optic disc; papillitis (p.153) is characterized by a marked loss of vision in the acute stage; and fulminating hypertensive retinopathy (p.119) is bilateral and shows other obvious features of widespread arterial and venous disease.

Treatment must be directed at the primary condition; bearing in mind the evidence for an immunological disorder, steroids, immunosuppresive and cytotoxic agents form the systemic treatment. Photocoagulation or cryotherapy may be used to treat areas of ischaemic retina in order to reduce the stimulus for new vessel formation.

Central serous choroidopathy (central serous retinopathy)

In central serous choroidopathy there is an elevation of the neuroretina (serous detachment in the macular area). It occurs usually in the young adult and may affect both eyes. It causes a general depression of the clarity of the central vision, particularly for colours, with distortion and micropsia, with the elevation of the retina inducing a *pseudohypermetropia*, but it seldom impairs the level of the visual acuity to a marked extent. The condition clears spontaneously in a few weeks, sometimes completely, but often with some distortion of vision caused by a fine pigmentary disturbance of the macula which follows the oedema; any recurrence causes a further visual deficit.

This condition is dealt with here because until recently it has been regarded as a central serous retinopathy, but it is now believed to be due to a focal choroidopathy of unknown cause resulting in a defect of the overlying Bruch's membrane and pigment epithelium, through which choroidal fluid is permitted to enter the subretinal space and produce a local detachment of the neuroretina, giving a characteristic fluorescein angiographic appearance. Occasionally, an indolent serous detachment is associated with a congenital pit or excavation of the optic disc.

Treatment. The majority of cases settle spontaneously, but if the condition persists for more than a few months, the site of leakage can be photocoagulated with the laser after its determination by fluorescein angiography.

Blood dyscrasias

Changes are liable to occur in the retina in various disorders of the haemopoietic system.

Anaemia

In severe anaemia the fundus appears relatively pale. Small scattered superficial haemorrhages tend to occur in the retina, often in association with a low-grade retinal oedema which increases the pallor of the fundus.

Leukaemia

In leukaemia the retinal veins are usually markedly dilated, but they appear less red than normal and the associated retinal haemorrhages often have a pale centre due to local infiltration with leukaemic cells. The retina usually shows a moderate degree of retinal oedema, particularly near the optic disc.

Polycythaemia

In polycythaemia the retinal veins are uniformly dilated and appear dark in colour. There are usually associated haemorrhages in the retina and in the advanced stages of the condition the retina becomes oedematous.

Macroglobulinaemia

Macroglobulin within the blood causes an increased blood viscosity with a consequent sludging of the circulation. A well-marked engorgement of the retinal veins is generally associated with optic disc swelling and retinal haemorrhages, and sometimes the central retinal vein becomes occluded. Pathologically the most striking feature is the development of capillary microaneurysms in the peripheral retina, which may be a response to anoxia.

Vascular retinopathy

Most of the changes in the retinal arteries and veins in disorders of the cardiovascular system follow an underlying hypertension, but atheroma and involutionary sclerosis may occur in the absence of hypertension.

Atheroma

Atheroma may develop in an artery as a patchy subendothelial fatty degenerative lesion, with or without an associated hypertension, particularly in the middle-aged or elderly. Its development may be a response to a diminished blood volume in an artery which is unable to compensate for this because of an associated fibrosis. The patch of atheroma tends to lead to a partial or even total occlusion of the artery as a result of thrombus formation of the atheromatous area. Ophthalmoscopically the affected artery appears as an opaque white mass obscuring part of the blood column.

Involutionary sclerosis

Involutionary sclerosis is simply an ageing process in the arteries, not necessarily associated with hypertension; it almost invariably presents after the sixth decade of life, although sometimes occurs at an earlier age. It affects particularly the larger vessels, but sometimes also the smaller branches. Fibrosis of the larger vessels is followed by a rise in the systolic level of the blood pressure, provided the heart is sufficiently sound to maintain the peripheral circulation, but without any rise in the diastolic pressure because of the absence of any increase in the peripheral resistance (in fact this is reduced because of the relative rigidity of the larger arteries).

Ophthalmoscopically the retinal arteries appear relatively straight and diffusely narrow with acute-angled branchings and a diminution in the intensity of the colour of the blood column, but without any obvious loss of transparency of the vessel walls; this is in contrast to the normal fundus in which the retinal arteries are wide and sinuous with prominent blood columns and wide-angled branchings. Similar changes in the arteries supplying the optic disc account for the very slight pallor which may occur in an elderly person in the absence of any other disease.

Hypertensive retinopathy

Hypertension is usually the result of an increased resistance of the peripheral circulation following generalized and widespread *arteriolar hypertonus*—a sustained physiological contraction of the affected vessels (in contrast to a spasm which is a sudden and violent type of contraction of limited duration). It is associated with a rise in the systolic and diastolic levels of the blood pressure, although the increase in the diastolic level tends to be less marked if there is a rigidity of the larger arteries as a result of fibrosis, or if there is a reduction in the area of the peripheral circulation which is capable of exerting hypertonus (also a result of fibrosis); therefore to some extent a pre-existing sclerosis may diminish the changes which occur in the vessels in hypertension.

It follows that the changes which occur in the arteries vary considerably in different groups of hypertensives and these are reflected in the appearances of the fundi.

Hypertension in the absence of a pre-existing sclerosis

This usually occurs in the younger age group. The different stages in its development are:

Diffuse hypertonus. In the early stages the marked hypertonus of the peripheral arteries in conjunction with a resilience of the larger arteries causes a marked increase in the systolic and diastolic levels of the blood pressure. Ophthalmoscopically the normal, fairly wide, sinuous and well-coloured retinal arteries become uniformly narrow, straight and relatively pale. There may be some congestion of the retinal veins immediately distal to the point of an arteriovenous crossing, but there is no concealment of the underlying vein...

Hypertrophy and hyperplasia. In the late stages reactive changes of hypertrophy and hyperplasia occur in the arterial walls; at first they are irregularly placed but later they become more widespread. Ophthalmoscopically the retinal arteries remain narrow and straight but the blood column becomes more pale and shows a slightly irregular outline. There is also concealment of the underlying retinal veins at the arteriovenous crossings (nipping).

Fibrosis (arteriosclerosis). This is the inevitable outcome of a persistent hypertension. The abnormal changes of hypertrophy and hyperplasia within the walls of the arteries are affected by a reactive sclerosis, although this fibrosis is seldom evident in the most peripheral retinal branches. Sometimes these changes may be followed by an occlusion of the central retinal artery or one of its branches (see p.122). Ophthalmoscopically the affected parts of the retinal arteries become irregularly dilated, curvilinear and red with increased surface reflexes, often termed *copper wiring*; eventually these changes may become widespread. The most peripheral parts of the retinal arteries usually remain narrow, straight and pale.

Fulmination. This usually occurs very rapidly in severe cases of fulminating or malignant hypertension, when the peripheral arteries are affected by a marked hypertonus in association with some focal necrosis. Ophthalmoscopically the retinal arteries have a fairly normal calibre near the optic disc, but the blood column is irregularly reduced in size and markedly pale. There are parallel zones of concealment where the arteries cross retinal veins, and later the arteries show marked tortuosity suggesting an elongation of their length. The more peripheral vessels remain straight and narrow. The retinal veins are usually congested with the development of areas of white sheathing within their walls.

There are other changes which may be present in the retina in hypertension:

Haemorrhages. Small haemorrhages of capillary origin occur in the superficial or deep parts of the retina in the more advanced hypertensive cases, and sometimes they lie in radiating lines in the macular area. Occasionally a large haemorrhage occurs at the site of a necrotic arteriole which shows a thrombotic column (straight and deep red in colour) in its proximal part, although this is usually separated from the parent stem by a white thread (*silver wiring*) which persists indefinitely even after disappearance of the thrombotic column; the distal part of the arteriole is not visible because it is devoid of blood.

Small round hard-edged white exudates. These occur in the deeper part of the retina, particularly around the optic disc and in the central fundus. They probably represent haemorrhages which have been altered by phagocytosis.

Soft white (cottonwool) exudates. These occur in the superficial parts of the retina in relation to the thrombosed arterioles (pale infarcts) following focal retinal ischaemia; they represent areas of axoplasmic hold-up.

Oedema. This occurs in the retina around the optic disc as a swelling, and often spreads to other parts of the retina. It is particularly noticeable in the macular area (*'macular fan'*).

Hypertension in the presence of pre-existing sclerosis

This usually occurs in the older age group. The changes in the arteries are irregular: the parts unaffected by fibrosis show hypertonus and the parts affected show dilatation, and the later development of hypertrophy and hyperplasia is less extensive because it does not occur in the parts affected by the fibrosis. Ophthalmoscopically the arterioles show irregular changes: the parts unaffected by fibrosis become hypertonic so that the blood column is narrow and less red in colour, and the parts affected by fibrosis become passively dilated so that the blood column is wider and more intense in hue and, because of the elongation of the affected vessel walls, there are areas of localized tortuosity. Eventually the whole arteriole system becomes diffusely wide, red and tortuous by a confluence of the fibrotic areas. Concealment of the retinal veins at the arteriovenous crossings is not a prominent feature, but the veins immediately distal to the crossings may be dilated, slightly dark and tortuous—features indicative of venous congestion. In the later stages any or all of the changes which have been described in fulminating hypertension may occur, but usually only after a fairly prolonged interval; the occurrence of arteriosclerosis provides some defence against necrotizing changes in the arterioles—the so-called *defence by sclerosis*.

Treatment

The treatment of hypertension involves many different considerations, such as the state of cardiac function, the presence of any pulmonary oedema and the possibility of renal disease. Various antihypertensive drugs which decrease the sympathetic effect on the blood vessels may be used; some act on the ganglia (ganglionic blockers) and others on the fibres (adrenergic blockers) or the central nervous system. It is important, particularly in the under 50s, to look for renal disease (glomerulonephritis, renal artery stenosis) and for phaeochromocytoma. An especially severe retinopathy occurs during toxaemia of pregnancy (p. 132).

Obstruction of the central retinal artery

A cessation of the circulation in the central retinal artery affects the vision in a variety of ways. The vision may be lost suddenly, completely and permanently (*amaurosis*) without any previous visual disturbance, or this may be preceded by transient episodes of blurred vision or even of total loss of vision, particularly when it results from carotid artery insufficiency (see below). Sometimes, however, a small area of central vision is maintained: (a) in the presence of a cilioretinal artery which is independent of the central retinal artery; (b) when a branch of the central retinal artery leaving the main stem in the deep part of the optic nerve head is proximal to the site of the block; (c) when a re-establishment of the circulation by capillary anastomoses occurs between the uveal and retinal circulations in the optic nerve head; or (d) when the obstruction of the circulation is relieved. These events must become effective before irreparable damage to the retinal ganglion cells occurs; unfortunately these cells succumb rapidly, certainly within an hour or so.

Early stages (Fig. 33)

Oedema and necrosis. Oedema and axoplasmic hold-up occur in the retinal nerve fibre layer and necrosis occurs in the retinal ganglion cell layer, so that the retina appears cloudy and white because it interferes with the transmission of the normal redness of the underlying choroid. This is particularly marked in the central part of the retina except at the fovea, an attenuated part of the retina without any nerve fibre or ganglion cell layer, which appears unduly red and prominent, the 'cherry-red spot', against the white background of the surrounding retina.

Attenuation of retinal arteries. The retinal arteries often appear obliterated, but there may be some circulation within the attenuated arteries; the poverty of this is demonstrated by the ready production of fragmentation of the blood column (the *cattle-trucking effect*) on digital pressure of the globe, which embarrasses the circulation by causing a rise in the intraocular pressure.

(a)

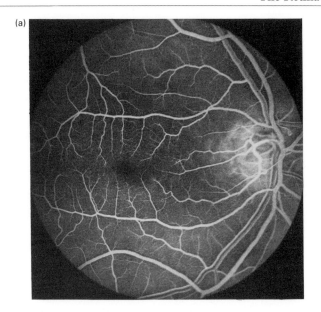

(b)

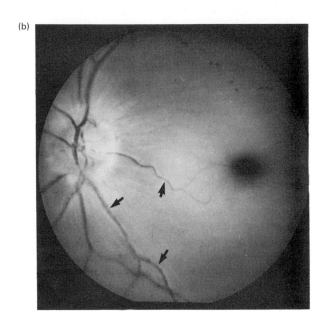

(c)

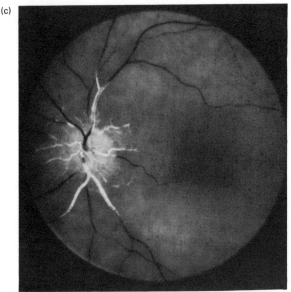

Fig. 33. (a) Fluorescein angiogram of normal retinal circulation. Central retinal artery occlusion: (b) red-free photograph; and (c) fluorescein angiogram. Note (i) retinal oedema obscuring choroidal detail and (ii) segmented blood column (arrows).

The pupillary reflex. The direct pupil reaction to light is affected according to the degree of the visual loss, but the consensual reaction is retained, provided the unaffected eye is functioning adequately.

Later stages

The retinal arteries. These may remain obliterated and appear as white threads, but quite commonly there is a restoration of circulation, although seldom with any restoration of useful vision; there may be a vague awareness of vision in the temporal periphery of the visual field.

Optic atrophy. Pallor of the optic disc becomes evident within four to six weeks of the occlusion following atrophy of the nerve fibres as a result of the degeneration of the retinal ganglion cells and also, to some extent, of the defective blood supply in the optic nerve head.

Macular pigmentation. This usually follows the subsidence of the oedematous changes in the macular area.

Sometimes the early and late changes are limited to certain parts of the retina when the obstruction involves only one or more branches of the artery without involving the main trunk. In such cases only part of the visual field is involved in the form of a sector or quadrant which extends from the region of the fixation spot.

An obstruction of the central retinal artery (or one of its branches) may follow a thrombosis, an embolus or an insufficient circulation.

Thrombosis

A thrombosis may follow arteriosclerotic changes (see above) or inflammatory changes (*arteritis*).

Giant cell arteritis. This is an autoimmune condition affecting the over 60s. It is directed at the internal elastic lamina of arterioles and may therefore affect the ophthalmic or more commonly the posterior ciliary arteries, producing an ischaemic optic neuropathy. A history of malaise and limb-girdle myopathy (*polymyalgia rheumatica*) is usual, and the ocular signs may be preceded by fleeting attacks of blurred vision, severe unilateral headache if there is an accompanying *temporal arteritis*, and pain on chewing. The erythrocyte sedimentation rate (ESR) is almost invariably raised to > 50 mm/h, and biopsy of an involved temporal artery shows an intense round cell infiltration, giant cells and fragmentation of the internal elastic lamina.

The condition demands urgent treatment with systemic steroids to prevent the ocular condition from becoming bilateral; treatment is monitored against the ESR. The majority of cases are self-limiting over six months to two years.

Embolus

A vegetation from a valve of the heart may form an embolus, or portions of blood clot within the left atrium or within a major artery, such as the carotid artery, may form fibrin, platelet or cholesterol emboli which are sometimes multiple and recurrent.

Carotid artery insufficiency

This often starts as a transient blurring or loss of vision. This may spread from above downwards like a blind being lowered from above, or from below upwards like a blind being raised from below, with a restoration of vision within a few seconds or minutes in the reverse direction. These attacks tend to be repeated every few days or weeks, without any precipitating factors or any accompanying features, except occasionally for headache near the affected eye. Rarely the patient is aware of a bruit over the eye. The condition follows a narrowing (and even an occlusion) of the internal carotid artery (involvement of the common or external carotid artery is more rare) which produces a fall in the pressure in the central retinal artery to a level which jeopardises the integrity of the retina. Sometimes the blood supply to the ciliary body is also reduced, causing diminished formation of aqueous humour and ocular hypotension; this may even lead to the development of *anterior segment necrosis* (p.99). A bruit may be detected with a stethoscope over the stenosed carotid artery (or occasionally over the eye), and the site of the stenosis may be demonstrated by a radiograph after the percutaneous injection of a radio-opaque substance into the artery. The diminished pressure in the ophthalmic artery is demonstrated by ophthalmodynamometry; the footpiece of the piston of the dynamometer is applied to the outer surface of the eye after the instillation of a surface anaesthetic, and a gradually increasing pressure is exerted until the retinal arteries show a collapsing pulsation (a measure of the diastolic pressure of the ophthalmic artery), and then until the pulsation just disappears (a measure of the systolic pressure of the ophthalmic artery).

There are sometimes other manifestations of carotid artery insufficiency: transient attacks of hemiparesis of the arm or leg, dysphasia and even acute hemiplegia may result from a unilateral reduction of the cerebral circulation.

Spasm

A hypertonus of the arterial wall occurs in hypertension (see above), but it is unlikely that simple spasm of the central retinal artery is a common cause of obstruction, except in the rare condition called *retinal migraine*. This is transient blindness which may occur in one eye as a result of a vasoconstriction in one or more branches of the central retinal artery in the absence of hypertension. It is suggested that the mechanism of this condition is akin to the changes which occur in the cerebral vessels in migraine. However, retinal migraine, when it occurs repeatedly over a prolonged period of time, may lead eventually to permanent loss of vision.

Treatment

In any obstruction of the retinal arterial circulation it is imperative to improve the circulation as rapidly as possible This may be achieved by the use of vasodilators (amyl nitrite by inhalation, tolazoline or acetylcholine by subconjunctival or retrobulbar injection) or by reducing the intraocular pressure (the removal of aqueous from the anterior chamber by paracentesis is an effective method, but simple massage of the eyeball is also of value). It is also necessary to treat any underlying cause, particularly in cases which give prior warnings of an impending obstruction. The treatment of giant cell arteritis usually involves the use of systemic steroids for a prolonged period. The treatment of carotid artery insufficiency may involve the use of anticoagulants or anti-platelet adhesive agents such as acetylsalicylic acid or dipyrimadole, but a thromboendarterectomy may be necessary. If the thrombus is of long standing, a resection of the affected portion of the carotid artery with an end-to-end anastomosis or with a blood vessel graft may be required. The management of hypertension is discussed on p.121.

Vertebro-basilar artery insufficiency

Vertebro-basilar artery insufficiency may also cause transient episodes of blurred vision of a hemianopic type when one posterior cerebral hemisphere is involved, but if both are involved the blindness is complete (*cortical blindness*, p.342), although unlike peripheral blindness it is not accompanied by a sensation of total darkness. These episodes are often accompanied by sensations of flashing lights, dizziness, vertigo or tinnitus. The ischaemic process may spread to the pons and lower midbrain with involvement of the motor nuclei which are concerned with the extrinsic ocular muscles, so that there may be transient paresis and an awareness of diplopia (see p.255).

Obstruction of the central retinal vein

An occlusion may affect the central retinal vein within the optic nerve head (behind the lamina cribrosa) or may affect one or more of its branches (in front of the lamina cribrosa). The majority of central retinal vein occlusions are associated with systemic hypertension, and one-third have elevated intraocular pressure in the fellow eye. Branch retinal vein occlusions may occur without any dramatic visual symptoms, except when the macular area is involved by haemorrhage or oedema—even then it may not be detected because of the overlap of vision of the two eyes (unless the unaffected eye happens to be closed)—or when the haemorrhage extends into the vitreous. The affected retinal veins are grossly dilated and the disc engorged. If the occlusion is severe, there is secondary closure of the capillary circulation resulting in ischaemia of the retina, manifest as oedema, cottonwool spots and deep retinal haemorrhages.

The majority of branch retinal vein occlusions occur at the arteriovenous crossings, where the vessels lie in a common adventitial sheath, while hemisphere occlusions occur at the disc margins and are associated with chronic simple glaucoma. Peripheral vein occlusions occur in systemic diseases such as sickle cell disease, Eales' disease, sarcoidosis and Behçet's disease, while occlusion of large veins occurs in diabetes. The venous circulation in the retina is restored by pre-existing or collateral channels in or around the optic disc and in areas where normal retina is apposed to diseased retina. The macular area is usually involved by haemorrhage or oedema when the occlusion is complete, but may be spared in branch vein occlusion if away from the macula. The haemorrhages absorb gradually over a period of months, but their presence in the macular area in addition to oedema usually causes permanent impairment of the central vision.

Fluorescein angiography provides a useful guide to prognosis and treatment. The response of the retina to areas of capillary closure is to develop new vessels which are friable and may bleed, producing vitreous haemorrhage, and in cases of complete central vein occlusion new vessel formation may develop on the anterior surface of the iris after an interval of about three months (*rubeosis iridis*). These are prone to cause a gradual obliteration of the filtration angle (*peripheral anterior synechiae*) with the production of an intractable form of secondary glaucoma (*thrombotic glaucoma*) (see p.313).

Treatment There is no specific treatment for the condition, but areas of capillary closure may be photocoagulated to prevent the production of new vessels and their complications and to reverse established new vessels. Attention should be directed to the underlying systemic hypertension and other systemic disease. It is doubtful if anticoagulants are of value once the thrombosis has occurred, but in certain cases they may be used in an attempt to prevent further similar episodes in the same or the other eye; such treatment demands a careful medical assessment as it may lead to other complications because of the increased risk of haemorrhage. The treatment of rubeosis iridis and of thrombotic glaucoma is discussed on p.96 and p.315, respectively.

Renal retinopathy

The retinal changes in renal disease are those of hypertension; the distinguishing features are attributable to the severity and speed of onset of hypertension and the ocular response to it rather than a specific pattern of renal retinopathy. This is due to the different influences on retinal and choroidal blood flow: while the retinal circulation has autoregulation and no sympathetic innervation, the choroidal circulation has a dense sympathetic innervation but no autoregulation. Thus in fulminating hypertension, as in renovascular hypertension (renal artery stenosis) or phaeochromocytoma, the brunt of the damage falls on the choroidal circulation, resulting in choroidal infarcts leading to serous retinal and choroidal detachments. Furthermore a rapid evolution of hypertensive retinopathy occurs: extensive haemorrhages, exudates and cottonwool spots, often with a stellate exudative pattern at the macula, develop with little evidence of chronic vascular changes. These gradually reverse with treatment of the hypertension.

Characteristic retinal appearances in sarcoidosis, connective tissues diseases and amyloid disease will prompt early referral for assessment of the concomitant renal disease.

Uraemia

In severe uraemia there may be total visual loss (*amaurosis*) with headaches, vomiting, convulsions and coma. The amaurosis is not simply the result of the retinal changes (hypertensive and renal retinopathy), but rather the result of a cerebral disturbance (hypertensive encephalopathy) which explains the retention of the pupillary light reflex despite the blindness; this is a form of cortical blindness. (A similar amaurosis may occur in eclampsia and lead poisoning).

Diabetic retinopathy

Diabetic retinopathy occurs in the majority of diabetics. It is not related to the type or severity of diabetes but rather to the duration, through a small proportion of diabetics remain free of retinopathy despite prolonged follow-up. It is always bilateral, though the two eyes may show different degrees of involvement. Microvascular disease is the basis of all diabetic retinopathy and is clearly related to elevated blood sugar concentrations. There is a continuum from background retinopathy through maculopathy to proliferative retinopathy which leads to advanced diabetic eye disease.

There are two pathological sequelae to microvascular disease: first, an abnormal capillary permeability leading to extravasation of the intravascular contents; and, second, an ischaemic response which is consequent upon capillary closure and results in new vessel formation (Figs 34 and 35).

Background retinopathy is the earliest and commonest feature. It presents as a *segmental engorgement* of the retinal veins and *dot* or *punctate haemorrhages* which are often widespread, although they are usually more marked in the central retina between the upper and lower temporal branches of the retinal vessels; these represent saccular *microaneurysms* in the venous side (or sometimes in the arteriolar side) of the capillary bed, particularly in the capillaries which join the superficial and deep retinal capillary networks so that they lie mostly within the inner nuclear layer of the retina. They are the result of sharply localized degeneration in the capillary walls causing the formation of varicose capillary loops, the limbs of which become adherent to one another following the passage of exudates. Later they are the sites of multiple large blot haemorrhages when blood seeps through their walls and also of multiple small glistening yellow-white exudates caused by a seepage of lipoid and mucopolysaccharide material.

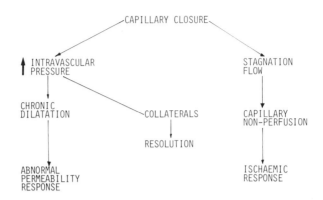

Fig. 34.   Pathogenic mechanisms in diabetic retinopathy.

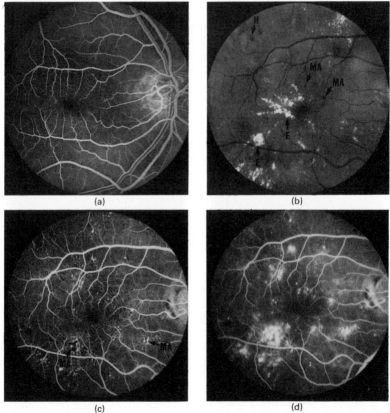

Fig. 35.   (a) Fluorescein angiogram of normal retinal circulation. Diabetic retinopathy:
(b) red-free photograph—note the haemorrhages (H), exudates (E) and microaneurysms
(MA); (c) fluorescein angiogram—early phase; and (d) fluorescein angiogram—late
phase. Note masking by retinal haemorrhages, and vascular leakage.

Background retinopathy may proceed to *diabetic maculopathy*, which is due to oedema as the result of widespread capillary leakage, around which circinate exudates may accumulate. Leaking vessels are delineated by fluorescein angiography and the maculopathy may be reversed by photocoagulation of these vessels or by gentle photocoagulation in the macular region itself. Fluorescein angiography also demonstrates areas of capillary non-perfusion, which tend to occur in the peripheral retina and lead to new vessel formation (*proliferative retinopathy*) on the retina (surface new vessels) or on the disc. New vessels remain on the surface of the retina while the vitreous gel is in position, but once it contracts (an early feature in diabetes) it drags the new vessels off the retina, producing the conditions for advanced diabetic eye disease such as vitreous haemorrhage, retinitis proliferans, traction retinal detachment and thrombotic glaucoma. The now forward new vessels (*rete mirabile*) are prone to recurrent bleeds; retrohyaloid and vitreous haemorrhage produce painless impairment of vision. With time, fibrocytic proliferation into the delicate fronds of new vessels occurs. This in time contracts and exerts a traction upon the retina, leading to a retinal or macular detachment or retinal hole formation. Extensive proliferation on the posterior surface of the vitreous and retina may occur, leading to surface traction. The retinal arteries are seldom involved in the early stages of diabetic retinopathy, but arteriosclerosis is a feature in the later stages and tends to occur earlier and with greater severity than in non-diabetics, so that hypertensive overlay is common in the progress of the disease. Pathologically it is associated with subintimal hyalinization which may be so marked in the precapillary terminal arterioles as to cause their gradual occlusion and disappearance. This may be followed by the development of dilated irregular vessels which extend from the neighbouring venous part of the capillaries into the obliterated arterial portion. Occlusive tendencies in the small branches of the retinal arteries which supply the optic disc tissues probably account for the susceptibility of the optic disc to develop atrophic changes in advanced diabetic retinopathy during the occurrence of any inflammatory condition (e.g. uveitis) or during even limited rises in the intraocular pressure (glaucoma).

Proliferative diabetic retinopathy has histological counterparts in the intercapillary glomerulosclerosis in the kidney (a feature of the Kimmelstiel-Wilson syndrome) and in the peripheral neuropathy.

Rarely in the young diabetic an excessive accumulation of fat in the retinal vessels may be visible, so that the distended vessels appear pale against the light red colour of the fundus background (*retinal lipaemia*). Sometimes diabetic retinopathy is associated with new vessel formation on the anterior surface of the iris (*rubeosis iridis*), particularly when the retinal lesions are severe and long-standing and following cataract extraction; this also occurs in other conditions (see p.96). It is liable to cause secondary glaucoma.

Treatment

Diabetic retinopathy may develop despite adequate control of the diabetes, but a rigid maintenance of control is an important factor in diminishing the progress of the retinal changes. A recent development or a more physiological delivery of insulin by pump in response to the continuous fluctuations in blood sugar has great potential for the future. Undoubtedly careful follow-up of diabetics is essential to observe clinical and angiographic evidence of symptomless proliferative retinopathy. It is treated by photocoagulation either to the new vessels directly or, more logically, to the areas of ischaemic retina. This is known as *panretinal photocoagulation* where numerous burns are delivered to the whole retina excepting the area within the temporal arcades, and it often produces a dramatic regression of the new vessels.

There is little evidence for the efficacy of lipid-lowering agents, but clofibrate, which increases the rate of resolution of hard exudates, may be indicated when the macula is threatened or if there is a marked hyperlipidaemia.

A rapidly progressive proliferative retinopathy , which is rare and usually only occurs in the young diabetic, is probably the only indication for *pituitary ablation*, either by hypophysectomy or by radioactive implant. There are certain criteria which must be verified before considering such drastic treatment: (a) the likely inevitable blindness in the absence of treatment; (b) the presence of reasonable vision in one or both eyes so that there is the possibility of retaining worthwhile visual function if the retinal disease is arrested; and (c) the fitness of the patient to withstand the difficult postoperative period because of the widespread manifestations of endocrine dysfunction requiring careful control by replacement hormone therapy.

Recurrent vitreous haemorrhages are treated by vitrectomy, fibrovascular retinal membranes by intraocular microsurgical dissection, and detachments by releasing the traction. If a retinal hole is present then cryotherapy with external and/or internal tamponade (p.139) is performed. Nevertheless, retinal surgery on diabetics is fraught with difficulty and provided the macular region is intact, peripheral traction detachments are often better left alone.

Diabetic retinopathy produces considerable morbidity, and while those patients with background retinopathy and maculopathy retain their independence, those with proliferative disease are subject to a degree of blindess which entails loss of their independence. Servicing the diabetic community requires particular expertise and liaison with physicians and social service departments.

Toxaemic retinopathy of pregnancy

Toxaemia of pregnancy may occur in the later months of pregnancy (rarely before the sixth month) and the accompanying hypertension leads to a hypertonus of the retinal arteries with the later development of hyperplasia and reactive sclerosis (p.120) if the hypertension persists after the pregnancy. Sometimes, however, the early response of the retinal vessels to the hypertension is followed rapidly by the changes which occur in fulminating hypertension (p.120), but at a much lower level of diastolic pressure than in non-toxaemic hypertension because of the renal element. The oedema and exudate in the retina are usually abundant and sometimes the formation of a subretinal exudate causes a well-marked serous retinal detachment; the affected area shows a characteristic pigmentary disturbance after the subsidence of these oedematous and exudative changes following cessation of the pregnancy.

The connective tissue diseases

In this group of diseases, the connective tissues develop characteristic pathological features of fibrinoid necrosis, granuloma formation and varying degrees of vasculitis, which are probably the result of an autoimmune process whereby host tissues are altered by varying stimuli such as infection or trauma, inducing autoantibody formation. Hence similar clinical features may be present in a range of connective tissue disorders; while some of the ocular manifestations of these diseases may be universal, some are specific and may precede the systemic disorder. Only those connective tissue disorders that have a significant retinal component are discussed.

Systemic lupus erythematosus (SLE)

Also known as *disseminated lupus erythematosus*, this disease represents a widespread autoimmune process involving organ-specific and tissue-specific antibodies to skin, kidneys, spleen, heart, central nervous system and marrow. Various ocular tissues may also be involved, often presenting with keratoconjunctivitis sicca and more rarely with conjunctival scarring with subsequent symblepharon formation, deep keratitis, oedematous changes of the lids, scleritis, and retinopathy characterized by massive fluffy white ('cottonwool') exudates containing cytoid bodies, haemorrhages and sometimes peripapillary oedema. Demonstration of anti-DNA antibodies in the presence of signs of a multisystem disorder is strongly suggestive of SLE.

Polyarteritis nodosa (periarteritis nodosa)

This disease is characterized by widespread necrotizing obliterative lesions of the small arteries and arterioles which assume a nodular appearance as a result of granulomatous or aneurysmal changes. It affects young adults, particularly males, with the occurrence of such general manifestations as pyrexia, haematuria, hypertension, asthma and abdominal pain. There may also be involvement of certain ocular structures: the choroid, with the production of oedematous foci; the retina, with the production of a hypertensive retinopathy in which massive exudates form a characteristic feature; and rarely the extrinsic ocular muscles, with some form of paresis or palsy. A characteristic scleritis with limbal corneal thinning associated with pain may occur in isolation and gives a guide to the systemic diagnosis.

Dermatomyositis

This is an acute or chronic inflammatory condition in which there is involvement of the skin (*dermatitis*) of the face, particularly the eyelids, with spread to the upper extremities and trunk, the mucous membranes of the mouth and pharynx, and the muscles (*myositis*) (see p.263). It is rarely associated with striking retinal changes: distension of the retinal veins and massive oedematous, exudative and haemorrhagic changes, particularly in the macular area. A high percentage of patients with dermatomyositis have occult neoplasms, usually of the gastrointestinal tract.

Toxoplasmosis

The primary involvement of the retina in this inflammatory condition is discussed on p.90.

Cytomegalic inclusion disease

An intrauterine infection of the fetus with the virus of cytomegalic inclusion disease may cause chorioretinitis in the newborn. Multiple foci form in the more peripheral parts of the fundi, sometimes in association with retinal haemorrhage, but the lesions are often less destructive than those in toxoplasmosis. In addition, there are usually cerebral disorders and an X-ray of the skull may show periventricular calcification. Other ocular complications have been described, such as optic atrophy, cataract, destructive membranous conjunctivitis, keratomalacia and uveitis. There may be widespread involvement of the viscera (liver, lungs, heart, kidney and pancreas), providing evidence of its blood-borne nature. Inclusion bodies may be isolated in the urine, in gastric washings, in the saliva, and on liver puncture. This virus has been responsible for bilateral disseminated retinitis in those who are immunosuppressed.

Toxic amblyopia

Certain toxic substances are liable to affect the retinal ganglion cells, particularly those in the macular and paramacular areas, although it is uncertain whether this is a direct effect or an indirect one caused by ischaemia of the retinal capillary vessels. There may also be a toxic effect on the macular and paramacular fibres within the optic nerve.

Tobacco amblyopia

This is usually associated with prolonged smoking of pipe tobacco and follows ingestion (as compared with inhalation) of the smoking products, so that it does not occur in cigarette smoking except rarely when cigarettes are made from pipe tobacco. Characteristically it occurs in elderly men, but it may occur in younger people who are unduly sensitive to pipe tobacco. Tobacco smoke contains large amounts of cyanide, but normally this is detoxicated safely and efficiently following its conversion into thiocyanate. However, in the presence of a metabolic defect (perhaps an inborn error of cyanide detoxification) there is a significantly raised level of cyanocobalamin in the plasma; this is a metabolically inert substance but its presence in excess is an indication of an overwhelming of the body stores of vitamin B_{12} by cyanide. There is gradual failure of the central vision in both eyes; in the early stages this is revealed as a failure of colour perception, particularly in the part of the visual field which lies between the fixation point and the blind spot (*centrocaecal scotoma*), which extends ultimately into the fixation area. Ophthalmoscopic evidence of optic atrophy is only seen in the advanced stages.

Treatment. Total avoidance of tobacco is essential and, if early in the disease, will result in the restoration of central vision. This is facilitated by vitamin B_{12} therapy, provided the disease is recognized before permanent changes occur in the ganglion cells. Vitamin B_{12}, however, is not used simply because of its presumed deficiency. It is given as the hydroxycobalamin form of vitamin B_{12} because this has a strong affinity for cyanide. The diagnosis may be delayed because the visual failure may be regarded simply as the result of 'senile' changes (macular degeneration or cataract), and in any elderly person when the pathological changes within the eyes appear insufficient to account for the visual failure, the coexistence of tobacco amblyopia should be considered with great care.

Alcohol amblyopia

Ethyl alcohol. This seldom produces a toxic amblyopia on its own, but it may be an additional factor which precipitates the effect of pipe smoking and may also foster a nutritional amblyopia (see below).

Methyl alcohol (wood alcohol). This produces widespread and permanent damage to the retinal ganglion cells so that total blindness (or total loss of central vision) is almost invariable; death is also liable to occur because of severe dehydration and prostration.

Quinine amblyopia

The effect of quinine is found particularly when there is sensitivity to the drug. The visual defect follows a retinal ischaemia which is revealed ophthalmoscopically by an attenuation of the retinal arteries. It particularly affects the peripheral vision.

Chloroquine

This drug is liable to bind itself to melanin so that it affects the integrity of the retinal pigment epithelium with a disturbance of function of the rods and cones. Concentric rings of pigmentation occur around the macular area. It also causes characteristic changes in the cornea (see p.65). The retinal changes, unlike the corneal ones, persist even when the drug is discontinued.

Lead retinopathy

Lead intoxication may cause a marked retinal arteriosclerosis and periarteritis with an obliterative type of endarteritis leading to narrowing and sometimes occlusion of the retinal arteries. Similar changes may occur in the cerebral vessels. A lead nephrosis is a cause of uraemia (p.129). Lead may also cause paralysis of the extrinsic ocular muscles.

Nutritional amblyopia

An inadequate diet over a prolonged period, particularly when it is deficient in protein, vitamin B and vitamin A, is liable to cause abnormal changes in the retinal ganglion cells of the macular area. These changes are reversible only when the dietary deficiencies are corrected at a reasonably early stage. It affects the central vision, initially causing an undue fatiguability of the close-reading vision, but eventually leading to a central scotoma. Ophthalmoscopically in the early stages there is oedema of the macular area with occasionally a few small retinal haemorrhages, and in the later stages there is a fine pigmentary disturbance of the affected area. Sometimes there is partial optic atrophy.

Treatment. This should be aimed at speedy correction of the defective diet and of any factors which accentuate this, such as an excessive intake of alcohol or pipe tobacco.

Primary retinal detachment

A primary retinal detachment develops when a break in the integrity of the retina allows fluid from the vitreous to pass into the subretinal space (the space between the neural part of the retina and the pigment epithelium). This break may occur at the site of degenerative changes following previous oedema or haemorrhage (injury or vascular disorder) or following myopic or senile changes, or may be due to an area of abnormal vitreoretinal contact so that retraction of this part of the vitreous pulls on the retina with the formation of a tear; this probably explains the increased incidence of retinal detachment in aphakia, the removal of the lens causing a forward displacement of the vitreous, particularly when the operation is complicated by a loss of vitreous.

There are various forms of retinal breaks—*dialysis, crescentic U-shaped tear,* and *round hole* (Fig. 36).

Dialysis. This is a disinsertion of the peripheral part of the retina at the ora serrata. Characteristically it follows severe contusion of the eye, but it may also follow the rupture of a retinoschisis (p.140), which usually occurs in the lower outer part of the retina.

Crescentic U-shaped tear. This follows traction of the vitreous base and occurs most commonly in the upper temporal or upper nasal quadrant of the retina in the myopic eye. It may be a complication of posterior vitreous detachment leading to dynamic traction at the vitreous base. Its convex border points towards the optic disc. Peripheral to the tear there is a darkened area of retina which represents the site of the vitreoretinal adhesion and forms the *operculum* (or lid) of the tear.

Round hole. This occurs particularly in the peripheral parts of the retina near the ora serrata in areas of retinal degeneration—often in a lattice pattern. There may be more than one hole so that a careful search of the entire retina is essential.

Clinical features

The retina surrounding the tear becomes detached by the spread of subretinal fluid and the detachment gradually extends to involve most of the retina, particularly in the lower part of the eye because the fluid in the subretinal space tracks downwards by the influence of gravity.

(a)

(b)

(c)

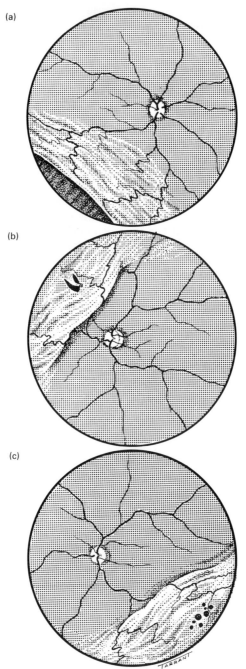

Fig. 36. Retinal detachment in association with (a) a dialysis, (b) a U-shaped tear, or (c) round holes.

The detached area is determined readily on ophthalmoscopic examination as it is seen billowing forward into the vitreous with the formation of retinal folds. Lesser degrees of detachment are detected by the darkening of the vessels in the detached area of retina and by the loss of its normal red appearance. The use of the binocular indirect ophthalmoscope with scleral indentation is essential for careful scrutiny of the peripheral retina, particularly when there is some opacity of the media such as a partial cataract or vitreous haemorrhage. Biomicroscopic examination with a contact lens permits an even more detailed examination of the peripheral retina.

The earliest symptoms may be an awareness of flashes of light caused by the pulling on the retina or disc by a vitreous band, or an awareness of a floating opacity in the field of vision from an opacity of the vitreous, perhaps following a haemorrhage from the retina. Subsequently there is loss of vision in the part of the visual field which corresponds to the affected area; this may be determined accurately using a perimeter (p.343). When the macular area becomes involved in the detachment or in an oedematous process, there is a loss or disturbance of central vision.

Retinal detachment is potentially a bilateral disease, except in cases which follow, for example, trauma or a complicated form of cataract extraction, so that the other eye should be scrutinized carefully at frequent intervals for any early signs of areas of retinal degeneration, such as lattice (a combination of retinal atrophy and degenerative changes in the overlying vitreous), that predispose to detachment, and any such areas treated by cryotherapy or photocoagulation.

Treatment

There are several principles involved, although the techniques differ from case to case.

Rest allows the retinal detachment to subside as far as possible before operation; the particular type of posture adopted depends on the situation of the detachment.

The sealing of the retinal tear or tears may be carried out indirectly by applying cryotherapy to the sclera overlying the area of the tear; the accuracy of this application is verified ophthalmoscopically at operation. This produces a sterile inflammatory reaction of the choroid with the development of an area of choroidoretinal union, so that the tear is obliterated within this area. A similar reaction may be obtained by shining an intense light from a photocoagulator into the eye under direct view with a modified ophthalmoscope, but this photoreaction is effective only when the affected area of the retina is in contact with the underlying pigment epithelium.

Apposition of the detached retina to the retinal pigment epithelium is achieved by internal or external tamponade, the prime objective being to close the retinal hole or holes, following which there is absorption of the subretinal fluid. External tamponade, achieved by suturing a segment of sponge or silicone band on to the sclera, will appose the detached retina to the retinal pigment epithelium. If the area of pathological retina or vitreous is widespread then cryotherapy and a 360° support with an encircling silicone band is used.

The removal of subretinal fluid is frequently required to permit accurate positioning of the scleral explant and is achieved by making one or more small openings in the sclera in the region of the detachment; the evacuation of the subretinal fluid permits the affected area of the retina, including the retinal tear, to become apposed to the underlying choroid so that the process of retinochoroidal coagulation becomes effective.

Removal of vitreous, vitreous haemorrhage or fibrotic retinal membranes (especially in diabetics and post-traumatic cases) by direct closed microsurgical techniques, followed by the insufflation of air, sulphur hexafluoride (SF6) gas, or silicone oil (internal tamponade) to maintain retinochoroidal apposition, has permitted treatment of otherwise inoperable cases, with a restoration of a limited degree of vision. (See also toxic cataract, p.177.)

Secondary retinal detachment

A retinal detachment may occur as a secondary phenomenon in certain conditions in the absence of a retinal tear: an exudative retinal detachment occurs in Coats' disease (p.115), toxaemia of pregnancy (p.132), renal retinopathy (p.128), posterior scleritis, and the Vogt–Koyanagi–Harada syndrome (p.93), in which there is an associated uveitis and inflammatory changes in the cerebrospinal fluid. In these conditions the exudate occurs in the subretinal space between the neural part of the retina and the pigment epithelium. The retina in part or as a whole may also become detached when it is pushed forwards by a mass in the choroid (malignant melanoma), although there is usually also an exudative element in the subretinal space. A traction retinal detachment may occur following contraction of strands of fibrous tissue which pass from the retina into the vitreous and is commonly associated with diabetic proliferative retinopathy or trauma.

Retinoschisis ('retinal cyst')

The development of a cystic space between the layers of the neuroretina is known as *retinoschisis*. It occurs not uncommonly as part of a degeneration of the peripheral retina. However, a retinoschisis with sex-linked recessive inheritance occurs in the periphery of the lower temporal quadrant of one or often both fundi, with a translucent globular detachment which extends to the periphery of the retina without any true hole or dialysis formation, despite the thinness of the retina; there is an associated macular dysplasia. Degenerative retino-schises commonly remain unchanged and are detected only on routine examination because they do not cause any obvious visual symptoms. However, holes may develop in the deeper layers of the retina (outer leaf holes), and should a break occur in the innermost layer (inner leaf hole) then there is a direct communication between the vitreous cavity and the subretinal space and the schisis becomes a retinal detachment and is treated accordingly.

Larval granulomatosis (toxocariasis)

The larva of *Toxocara canis*, a nematode common in dogs and cats throughout the world, may become lodged in the retina with the formation of a unilateral creamy-white umbilicated mass, particularly in the central part of the fundus, which protrudes into the vitreous. This mass is composed of fibrous tissue containing areas of fibrinoid necrosis, and there may be some surrounding retinal haemorrhage or exudative retinal detachment, so that the appearance resembles a retinoblastoma (p.146), a pseudoglioma (endophthalmitis, p.86), or Coats' disease (p.115). The disease is usually acquired in childhood at the 'dirt-eating' stage, when the ova of *Toxocara* from animal faeces may be ingested. The larvae hatch out in the intestine and are liable to become widely disseminated to the liver, lungs and retina by way of the bloodstream and except for the retina, via the lymphatics. The other common manifestations are asthma or urticarial skin eruptions. An eosinophilia is a characteristic feature for several months after the onset. A positive skin test to an intradermal injection of an antigen (1 in 1000) prepared from an adult *Toxocara canis* is of diagnostic value, as are enzyme-linked and immunofluorescent techniques.

Degenerations

Retinal degenerations may be primary or secondary. The primary forms are discussed below. The secondary retinal degenerations may follow any severe disease of the retina (e.g. long-standing retinal detachment, extensive retinal vascular disease) or of the underlying choroid (e.g. malignant melanoma, choroiditis).

Primary retinal degenerations

Macular dystrophy

This is an *'abiotrophy'* of the visual elements in the macular areas of both eyes and becomes evident at any age, hence the terms congenital, infantile, juvenile, adolescent, adult (presenile), or senile, depending on the time of onset. There are often familial and hereditary factors (*heredomacular degeneration*).

In the younger age groups the changes in the macular area are sometimes confined to a slight pigmentary disturbance but in the older person they tend to be more obvious with the appearance of a cyst which leads to partial hole formation, fine haemorrhages, exudates or colloid deposits. The condition may present with distortion of central vision or merely eyestrain following the increasingly greater effort which is required for close work, particularly when this is prolonged to a significant extent. The central vision may remain reasonably good for many years, but eventually it becomes impaired, sometimes unequally in the two eyes. The peripheral vision is retained indefinitely.

Macular dystrophy may occur in different ways according to the site of interference.

Choroid. A degeneration of the choriocapillaris causes a central areolar choroidal dystrophy (p.96).

Bruch's membrane. Colloid bodies form on Bruch's membrane and represent aggregations of outer segment, rod and cone layer debris that have not been processed by the retinal pigment epithelium. When the colloid bodies are profuse the condition may be termed *Tay's choroiditis* or *Doyne's honeycomb choroiditis*—misnomers because the condition is not inflammatory. Large colloid bodies may be termed *drusen*.

Ruptures sometimes occur in the elastic part of Bruch's membrane which appear as radiating dark red lines resembling to some extent blood vessels (*angioid streaks*). These have certain systemic associations, in particular with *pseudoxanthoma elasticum*, a disorder of collagen manifest as lax skin, which is somewhat rugose and particularly noticeable in the neck region, vascular abnormalities, and a predilection for gastrointestinal haemorrhage. Other conditions associated with angioid streaks include sickle cell disease, Paget's disease and Ehlers–Danlos syndrome. Neovascular membranes may develop from the edges of the streaks which may result in bleeding, scarring and impairment of vision (*disciform degeneration*). In some forms of high myopia there may be breaks in Bruch's membrane at the macula which may lead to localized haemorrhage.

Retina. There are various forms of heredomacular dystrophy which predominantly affect the macula associated with more widespread retinal involvement. *Cone dystrophy* with poor visual acuity, photophobia and impaired colour vision is seen ophthalmoscopically as an increase in the pigment of the macular region (*bull's eye maculopathy*) and may be of dominant or recessive inheritance. *Best's vitelline dystrophy*, a dominantly inherited condition primarily affecting the retinal pigment epithelium, is seen as a uniform, well-circumscribed, circular orange lesion in the region of the macula. *Stargardt's disease*, or *fundus flavimaculatus*, is a recessive disorder manifest as a bull's eye maculopathy with multiple reticular yellow flecks distributed mainly in the posterior fundus and located in the retinal pigment epithelium. All these conditions may give rise to electrophysiological abnormalities prior to the development of visible ophthalmoscopic features.

Retinitis pigmentosa (tapetoretinal degeneration)

This primary retinal degeneration is an abiotrophy of the rods, and also of the cones at a later stage, although the earliest changes probably occur in the pigment epithelium. The majority of cases are sporadic, but it is important to determine hereditary patterns if possible because a prognosis and genetic counselling can then be given. Dominantly inherited disease has the best prognosis, retaining good vision (6/12 to 6/18) even into late middle age, while those with recessive disease lose their vision early and seriously. The X-linked group has a visual prognosis which lies between that of the dominant and recessive groups. The condition is almost invariably bilateral. The disease is seldom evident before adolescence and its earliest manifestation may be an awareness of defective vision in dim illumination. At this stage there is commonly an annular scotoma in the mid-peripheral ('equatorial') part of the visual field. This gradually progresses peripherally and centrally, although usually with a sparing of a small island of central vision because of the relative resistance of the cones to the disease; this tubular vision may remain indefinitely, or may be lost in middle age.

There are characteristic changes in the eye. Pigment is deposited in the retina, particularly in its peripheral parts, often with branching processes so that each cluster resembles a bone corpuscular cell; this anomaly determines the clinical designation of 'retinitis pigmentosa'. The pigment sometimes migrates into the perivascular space of the retinal veins so that it forms a zone of sheathing. The retinal arteries become markedly attenuated, and the optic disc becomes gradually atrophic, although the pallor has a waxy quality which differs from the usual whiteness of a primary optic atrophy. Cataract affecting initially the posterior cortical part of the lens is a late feature of the disease.

A peculiar form of the condition occurs in infancy (*Leber's congential amaurosis, retinal aplasia*) or in early childhood, and this is associated usually with a profound disturbance of vision, or even with complete blindness, despite remarkably little abnormality of the fundi on ophthalmoscopic examination. After an interval of months or even years there is a slight attentuation of the retinal arteries and a partial degree of optic atrophy, and eventually these changes become more marked and are associated with scattered retinal pigmentary deposits. By adolescence the appearances resemble to some extent a typical retinitis pigmentosa, but inevitably the visual prognosis of this form is extremely poor from an early age.

Sometimes tapetoretinal degeneration in childhood presents as macular dystrophy with pigmentary changes in the macular areas and a progressive disturbance of central vision, which is in sharp contrast to typical retinitis pigmentosa in which the macular areas are seldom involved until late. The widespread nature of the condition is only evident after an interval of several years when the typical changes occur in other parts of the fundi, but an early diagnosis may be made on the basis of a reduced or absent ERG. This distinction is important because the long-term visual prognosis of macular dystrophy, in which peripheral visual function is retained indefinitely thus permitting some degree of visual independence, is much better than generalized tapetoretinal degeneration.

Occasionally tapetoretinal degeneration in the child is associated with other abnormalities—polydactyly (affecting the hands and feet), hypogenitalism, mental retardation (Laurence–Moon–Biedl syndrome), or with deafness, and when this is congenital also with dumbness (Usher's syndrome), or with external ophthalmoplegia and heart block (Kearns Sayre syndrome). Sometimes an atypical form of retinitis pigmentosa is associated with a chronic polyneuritis leading to an involvement of the peripheral nerves, ataxia and deafness (Refsum's syndrome).

Three conditions are regarded as variants of retinitis pigmentosa:

1. *Retinitis pigmentosa sine pigmento*, in which there is no obvious pigmentary disturbance in the retina. It is unnecessary to regard this as a separate entity because tapetoretinal degeneration may become established in the absence of obvious pigmentary changes.

2. *Retinitis punctata albescens*, in which there is widespread distribution of white spots in the retina. This is a true variant and carries a better visual prognosis than the classical retinitis pigmentosa.

3. Rarely the characteristic features of retinitis pigmentosa may remain confined for an indefinite period to one or more quadrants of the retina.

Treatment. There is no known effective treatment of tapetoretinal degeneration, although many remedies have been suggested. Removal of the cataractous lens is not associated with any unusual complications, but the final visual prognosis is dependent on the extent of the surviving retina.

Degenerations of retinal ganglion cells

Lipoid degenerations of the cerebral and retinal ganglion cells (*cerebromacular degenerations*) produce their effects in three characteristic ways at different ages.

Tay-Sachs disease (Amaurotic familial idiocy). In this condition a widespread lipoid degeneration of the cerebral and retinal ganglion cells occurs which becomes evident between the ages of 6 and 12 months when an apparently healthy baby ceases to make progress. There is a white swelling of the retina caused by the engorgement of ganglion cells with lipoid material, particularly in the central region, except for the fovea which is devoid of ganglion cells so that it stands out in contrast as a well-defined '*cherry-red spot*'. Optic atrophy eventually occurs. Death is inevitable within a year of the onset. The condition is not confined exclusively to Jewish children as commonly stated.

Batten–Mayou disease (Spielmeyer–Vogt disease). This is a lipoid degeneration of the retina, cerebral cortex and cerebellum, which usually occurs about the age of three years, with gradual visual failure and progressive mental deterioration and myoclonus leading to death in adolescence. There is diffuse pigmentary change in the central part of the retina. Optic atrophy is not a conspicuous feature. There are characteristic changes in the lymphocytes in the tail of a thin blood film and on histological examination of a rectal biopsy.

Niemann–Pick disease. In this condition the lipoid changes in the retina are sometimes less marked than the widespread changes which occur in the viscera and the central nervous system; the involvement of the viscera may be determined by a rectal biopsy. It usually occurs about the age of three years and death ensues within a few years.

Treatment. This is limited to the provision of suitable reading glasses in patients who survive, often in the form of telescopic spectacles which are more convenient than a simple hand magnifying lens.

Cystoid degeneration

In cystoid degeneration (*cystoid macular oedema*) cavities form within the retina as the result of disintegration of its neural elements. It may occur in any part of the retina, but has a predilection for the macular area because the avascularity of this region creates difficulties in the resorption of fluid. In fluorescein angiography there is an abnormal fluorescence surrounding the foveal area resulting from a spread of the dye into the retinal tissues in the macular area which assumes a rosette pattern. It occurs in a variety of ways: as a senile degeneration; in any inflammatory condition of the adjacent retina (chorioretinitis) or uvea (posterior uveitis), or sometimes in a remote part of the uvea (pars planitis, p.85); in any vascular disorder of the central part of the retina (central retinal vein thrombosis, central retinal artery occlusion, retinal vasculitis, hypertensive retinopathy, diabetic retinopathy, telangiectasis), following various forms of trauma (commotio retinae and solar retinopathy, p.112) and following cataract operation, usually in an elderly person, even when this is uncomplicated.

Oguchi's disease

Oguchi's disease is a rare congenital and inherited condition affecting both eyes and results from an excessive number of cones with very few rods; there may also be an anomaly of the retinal pigment epithelium. The vision is normal in bright illumination but with extreme night blindness in dim illumination, although dark adaptation may occur gradually over a period of several hours. In normal illumination the fundus appears grey or golden in colour, but it assumes its normal red colour after several hours in the dark (*Mizuo's phenomenon*).

Tumours

Neuroepiblastic tumours

Retinoblastoma

Retinoblastoma is the commonest of the neuroepiblastic tumours of the retina. It may occur spontaneously as a somatic mutation within the retina, by dominant inheritance or in association with chromosomal abnormalities. It develops as proliferations of 'nests' of cells in the retina, particularly in the inner nuclear layer, which fail to become differentiated and assume malignant properties; it is not a glioma but unfortunately this term is frequently used as synonymous with retinoblastoma. The tumour, which develops in the early years of life (usually the third year) is frequently fairly advanced when detected. It is often first noted by the parents as a white mass within the eye, giving the so-called *cat's eye reflex (leucocoria)*, or found by the ophthalmic surgeon during the routine examination of the eyes because of a suspected squint (the squint being the result of loss of vision in the eye). Included in the differential diagnosis of leucocoria are such conditions as Coats' disease (p.115), persistent hyperplastic primary vitreous (p.186), toxocariasis (p.141) and vitreoretinal scarring due to the non-accidental injury syndrome (battered baby syndrome) (p.112).

In the early stages the lesion appears as a localized white elevation of the retina, sometimes with an obvious dilatation of the retinal vessels supplying the affected area but rarely with any associated haemorrhage. This localized lesion is often followed quite rapidly by the development of other small lesions, sometimes regarded simply as seedling deposits from the main tumour but many represent independent foci (evidence of the multicentric nature of the tumour). The proliferating tumour tissue may extend into the subretinal space, causing retinal detachment (*exophytum*) with an associated subretinal exudate, or into the vitreous where it forms large masses (*endophytum*); rarely the tumour spreads extensively within the retina so that involvement of the subretinal space or vitreous is delayed. Particles of tumour tissue may pass forward into the anterior chamber with the formation of deposits on the posterior surface of the cornea (resembling large keratic precipitates), or into the angle of the anterior chamber (resembling inflammatory nodules), leading to a secondary glaucoma, sometimes with enlargement of the eyeball as in infantile glaucoma. A true uveitis may occur in advanced cases. Ultimately the tumour spreads from the eye directly into the orbit by perforating the cornea or sclera or into the brain by passing along the optic nerve with the formation of massive necrotic masses. It rarely forms metastases.

Treatment. Retinoblastoma is a radiosensitive tumour so that irradiation should be the treatment of choice. However, when the tumour is detected in the first eye it is often so far advanced that there is little or no prospect of salvaging any useful vision so that enucleation is the only expedient treatment; it must include as much as possible of the optic nerve. In theory the only indication for enucleation as a primary procedure is when there is involvement of the optic nerve, but it is almost impossible to know the extent of optic nerve involvement preoperatively and thus the likelihood of spread.

There are various methods of dealing directly with a retinoblastoma in a conservative way: (a) external irradiation by a lateral approach to include the whole retina as a primary procedure (the known multicentric nature of the condition means that from the onset the whole retina must be suspect even in the presence of an apparently localized lesion); (b) surface applicators such as a cobalt disc to deal with a localized lesion (particularly a recurrence); (c) photocoagulation or laser treatment to destroy a small lesion and its nutrient vessels; and (d) cryotherapy for a localized lesion.

The role of *chemotherapy* in retinoblastoma has undergone a change in recent years: whereas a few years ago it was reserved for cases which failed to respond to conservative measures and for cases which showed widespread dissemination, it is now regarded as an important part of the primary treatment of any retinoblastoma.

A combination of drugs having different modes and sites of toxicity is frequently effective. The combined use of vincristine (a plant alkaloid) and cyclophosphamide (an alkylating agent) is of value; these drugs are continued over a period of one year. Involvement of the central nervous system inevitably determines a poor prognosis, but systemic lomustine (CCNU) is worth trying because it is an anticancer drug which readily crosses the blood–brain barrier, in contrast to intrathecal methotrexate which has only a limited effect.

Repeated examinations of the second eye or of both eyes in a child with a family history of retinoblastoma are essential and permit the detection of the tumour in its early stages so that conservative treatment may be used. Genetic counselling is an important part of the management of this condition.

Other neuroepiblastic tumours

There are other very rare neuroepiblastic tumours which are only locally invasive.

Astrocytoma. Astrocytoma is a tumour of the retinal glial tissue.

Dictyoma and medulloepithelioma. Both dictyoma and medulloepithelioma are tumours of the ciliary epithelium, which is a prolongation of the neural part of the retina over the ciliary body.

Phakomata

Phakomata are congenital hamartomas which involve different neuroectodermal tissues, often with familial or hereditary features but rarely with malignant propensities.

Tuberous sclerosis (Bourneville's disease)

This tumour is derived from neuroglial tissue or neurilemmal cells. Multiple small nodules occur in the skin (*adenoma sebaceum*), in the cerebral cortex (sometimes causing mental deficiency or epilepsy), in the viscera, and in the heart. Additional skin lesions are depigmented macules (in an *ash leaf* configuration) and shagreen patches of elevated course skin. Rhabdomyosarcoma of the myocardium may occur. Characteristic subungual fibromas occur in the nail beds. The retinal lesions appear as mulberry-like white clusters which project into the vitreous, usually in the region of the optic disc; the active nature of these changes is shown sometimes by the occurrence of haemorrhage in the surrounding retina. Drusen of the optic disc sometimes present a similar appearance (see p.162).

Angiomatosis retinae (von Hippel–Lindau disease).

This tumour is characterized by angioblastomatous formations in the cerebellum, medulla oblongata, spinal cord and viscera (particularly the pancreas and kidney). The retinal lesions appear as isolated dilatations and tortuosities of the retinal arteries and veins, with the production of retinal haemorrhages and exudates which may cause haemorrhage into the vitreous or an exudative type of retinal detachment. Sometimes the affected retinal vessels show an arteriovenous communication. A secondary glaucoma may occur as a terminal event. Less commonly the retina is the site of more solid angioblastomatous formations.

Treatment. The spread of the retinal lesion may be limited by surface diathermy, photocoagulation or irradiation.

Cephalofacial angiomatosis (Sturge–Weber syndrome)

This tumour is characterized by angiomatous formations in the skin of the face (*naevus flammeus*) which are usually limited to the area of distribution of the trigeminal nerve, to the meninges with subsequent calcification, and to the cerebral cortex with the possible production of mental deficiency, epilepsy and hemiplegia. Angiomatous formations may occur in the retina or more commonly in the uveal tract and in the episcleral tissues with the subsequent development of glaucoma. The condition is usually unilateral.

Neurofibromatosis (von Recklinghausen's disease)

This is usually a widespread disease with the occurrence of firm neurofibromatous nodules in the nerves of the subcutaneous tissues (e.g. in the eyelids where, if they are diffuse or *plexiform* they may cause ptosis), in the uveal tract as pale brown iris nodules, in the trabecular meshwork (sometimes leading to glaucoma which may be of the infantile type—*buphthalmos*), in the retina, in the sclera, in the cornea, or in the orbit, producing proptosis. There is a strong association between optic nerve glioma and neurofibromatosis.

8

The Optic Nerve

Structure and function

The optic nerve (the second cranial nerve) is a direct extension of the brain and, unlike a peripheral nerve, resembles the cerebral white matter: its nerve fibres are myelinated (except distal to the lamina cribrosa), its interstices contain neuroglial cells, its external coverings are dura, arachnoid and pia, and there is cerebrospinal fluid in the pia-arachnoid space. The optic nerve fibres arise in the retinal ganglion cells. They pass centripetally within the nerve as the afferent visual fibres which terminate in the lateral geniculate body before being relayed to the visual cortex (p.339), and as the afferent pupillary fibres which are relayed to the parasympathetic parts of the oculomotor nuclei (p.74). The optic nerve may be considered in four parts:

1. The *intraocular part* (Fig.37) begins at the *optic disc* which represents the retinal aspect of the optic nerve as seen with the ophthalmoscope. It marks the exit from the eye of the optic nerve fibres, which are slightly elevated at the disc margin (hence the term *optic papilla*). The optic disc has an average diameter of 1.5 mm and is somewhat oval with the vertical meridian slightly larger than the horizontal one. There is a central depression in the optic disc—the *optic cup* (Fig. 37)—through which the branches of the central retinal artery and of the retinal vein enter and leave the eye, usually along the nasal wall of the cup, but rarely along the temporal wall (*inversion of the disc* or *situs inversus*). The size of the normal optic cup is variable but it seldom occupies more than 70% of the area of the disc. Usually the optic cups in any one individual are similar in size unless there is a marked difference in the refractive error between the eyes (e.g. one eye myopic and the other hypermetropic). It is usual for the cup to lie in the central part of the optic disc. The depth of the optic cup is variable; sometimes it is sufficiently deep to detect the *lamina cribrosa*, a sieve-like connective tissue structure which passes across the optic nerve at the level of the choroid and sclera. The optic cup appears pale because it is devoid of nervous tissue, but the rest of the disc appears pink because the optic nerve fibres contain a capillary network which is supplied by several small arteries. The optic nerve head may be divided into pre- and postlaminar regions on either side of the lamina cribrosa; their blood supply is ultimately derived from the *short posterior ciliary arteries*, the prelaminar region from the peripapillary choroidal

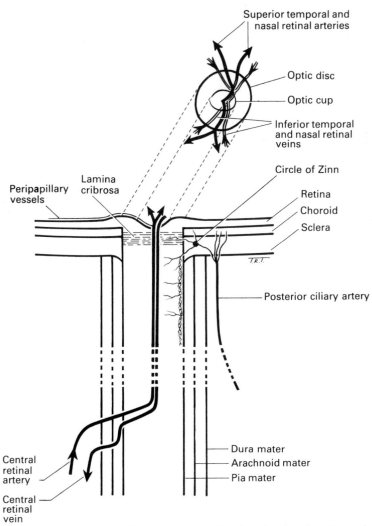

Superior temporal and nasal retinal arteries

Optic disc

Optic cup

Inferior temporal and nasal retinal veins

Circle of Zinn

Peripapillary vessels

Lamina cribrosa

Retina

Choroid

Sclera

T.R.T.

Posterior ciliary artery

Central retinal artery

Central retinal vein

Dura mater

Arachnoid mater

Pia mater

Fig. 37. Longitudinal section of the optic nerve head to show the formation of the optic cup and the lamina cribrosa. The ophthalmoscopic appearance of the optic disc is also illustrated; typical for the right eye, but also for the left in situs inversus.

circulation, the laminar and postlaminar region from the intrascleral circle of vessels (*circle of Zinn*). These and the radial peripapillary network of capillaries derived from the central retinal artery supplying the nerve fibres at the disc surface may be regarded as endarteries, so that occlusion results in irreversible ischaemia because of the lack of anastomoses. Quite frequently the normal disc shows a slight degree of relative temporal pallor, but almost invariably this is present equally in the two eyes.

2.   The *orbital part* lies within the muscle cone formed by the four recti muscles as they pass from the apex of the orbit to the eyeball. Its course is tortuous so that the nerve is not stretched unduly during ocular movement. The *central retinal artery* (a branch of the *ophthalmic artery*) enters the optic nerve a short distance (1.25 cm) behind the eye and travels in the distal part of the nerve before passing to the retina through the optic cup; the *central retinal vein* leaves the eye and the optic nerve in company with the artery. The optic nerve tissue is supplied mainly by small arteries which pass into the nerve from the plexus of vessels in the pia mater, but also to some extent in its axial region by small branches from the central retinal artery.

3.   The *intracanalicular part* lies within the narrow optic canal (formed between the two roots of origin of the lesser wing of the sphenoid and the body of the sphenoid) and is accompanied by the ophthalmic artery. The orbital opening of the optic canal lies at the apex of the orbit.

4.   The *intracranial part* lies between the intracranial opening of the optic canal and the optic chiasm formed by the junction of the right and left optic nerves.

Congenital anomalies

Coloboma of the optic disc

A hole (coloboma) may occur in the optic disc, usually, but not invariably, in association with an inferior coloboma of a sector of the retina and uvea (pp. 78 and 111). More commonly a crescent occurs along the lower border of the optic disc (*Fuch's inferior coloboma*) associated with a 'D'-shaped optic disc head, local retinal hypopigmentation and upper arcuate field defects in a condition known as the *tilted disc*, which should be distinguished from the crescent which occurs in axial myopia as a degenerative change (this most frequently affects the temporal border of the disc, see p. 12).

Other congenital anomalies

Other congenital anomalies include opaque nerve fibres (p.110) and drusen (rarely as a congenital anomaly) (p.162).

Injuries

The optic nerve is liable to become involved in any fracture of the bones in the region of the optic canal—directly by laceration of the nerve or indirectly by interference with its nutrient blood supply or by pressure on the nerve from surrounding oedema or haemorrhage.

Subsequently there is the development of pa
atrophy, but the ophthalmoscopic evidence of th
six weeks after the injury. Sometimes a severe ᴗᵣ
may lead to a partial or complete loss of functior
without any fracture because of haemorrhage withiɩ
the result of its violent concussion against the wall o.
optic canal, or because of a rupture of the nutrient
sudden displacement of the nerve (*contrecoup effect*).

Avulsion of the optic nerve, when the nerve is partiallɣ
torn from the eyeball, occurs in deep penetrating wounɗ
or, rarely, indirectly in a severe contusional injury of the
result of the explosive force which is generated within the
early stages the central fundus is obscured by haemorrɩ
eventually the previous site of the optic disc is apparent as a 'hɩ
a mass of proliferative scar tissue. The retinal vessels are m
attenuated. The eye is blind unless the avulsion is only partial,
part of the visual field is retained.

Optic neuritis

Optic neuritis is an inflammatory condition of the optic nerve in which
a process of demyelination is associated with oedematous changes in the
surrounding tissues. It is usual to distinguish between two forms—
papillitis, in which the disease occurs in the optic nerve within or near
the eyeball, and *retrobulbar neuritis*, in which it occurs in some part of
the optic nerve away from the eyeball. The condition commonly
presents dramatically with sudden loss of vision of the affected eye,
although sometimes it is preceded by a vague awareness of discomfort
in the eye or by a slight defect of the vision during the previous day or
so. The visual loss is usually severe so that there may be merely an
appreciation of movement or light (rarely even an absence of light
perception), but sometimes the visual loss is limited to the central or
paracentral part of the visual field with, characteristically, a loss of
colour perception. It is evident that, although some optic nerve fibres
are affected directly, many other fibres are involved only indirectly by
the oedema which surrounds the focus of demyelination; this accounts
for the relatively good visual prognosis of certain cases. There is a
relative afferent pupillary defect of the affected eye; this is simply an
expression of the conduction defect of the afferent visual pathway. In
the early stages there may be pain in the affected eye, particularly on
movement of the eye, and pressure on the upper surface of the eyeball
near the insertion of the superior rectus tendon may elicit obvious
tenderness.

The optic disc in the acute phase may reveal no obvious abnormality
or sometimes only a slight oedema, but when the lesion is adjacent to
the optic nerve head (*papillitis*), the disc oedema may be marked, with

w haemorrhages in the peripapillary part of the retina; when the
nal changes are widespread it is termed a *neuroretinitis.*

The subsequent changes which occur in the affected optic nerve
bend to a large extent on the nature of the demyelinating process.
btic neuritis is a feature of several different conditions.

Disseminated sclerosis (multiple sclerosis)

In disseminated sclerosis, scattered foci of demyelination occur in the
central nervous system, usually in young adults who are otherwise
healthy, with a characteristically variable periodicity. It tends to run a
fluctuating course with acute exacerbations at irregular intervals and
with intervening periods of improvement and quiescence; it may
eventually enter a more chronic and persistent phase. Optic neuritis
occurs in nearly half of all cases, typically but not invariably as the first
manifestation of the disease. Many years may elapse (five to ten years or
even much longer) before the next manifestations of the disease occur
(e.g. paraesthesiae, ataxia, disturbances of bladder control). Indeed it is
reasonable to consider optic neuritis as the only manifestation of the
disease, so that the absence of subsequent manifestations does not
preclude the diagnosis of disseminated sclerosis. The optic neuritis is
usually confined to one eye initially, but the other eye may be involved
similarly some months or years later; sometimes both eyes are involved
simultaneously. Some patients are aware of impaired vision after
exercise or a hot bath (*Utoff phenomenon*), and others are aware of
upper limb paraesthesiae induced by neck flexion (*Lhermitte's sign*).
As a general rule there is gradual restoration of vision within a few
weeks of the onset of the optic neuritis, with only a small paracentral
scotoma or a localized, more peripheral field defect as the remaining
legacy of the disorder, but sometimes the central vision is permanently
affected by a residual central scotoma. Colour vision tends to be
permanently affected, but the changes may be subtle and only
detectable using the Farnsworth Munsell test. Pupillary abnormalities
often persist, again as subtle variations from the normal. The majority
of cases show the development of some pallor of the optic disc,
particularly in the temporal region because of the predilection for the
papillomacular bundle to be involved in the process. Red-free light
ophthalmoscopy may demonstrate nerve fibre bundle defects in the
peripapillary retina. Visual, auditory or spinal evoked responses, which
demonstrate a delay in conduction along myelinated fibres, give added
evidence for demyelination of other nerves, thus supporting a diagnosis
of disseminated sclerosis. It is important to record the pattern of
recovery of vision; if there is no recovery after two months, a further
search must be made for other lesions of the anterior visual pathway.
There is no known treatment for this disease, but systemic and orbital
steroids have been used in an attempt to reduce the recovery time.

Encephalomyelitis

Optic neuritis, usually affecting both eyes, may occur as part of an encephalomyelitis in association with one of the exanthemata—measles, chicken pox, herpes zoster, mumps, whooping cough, infectious mononucleosis, or one of the virus diseases—or following an undue sensitivity to certain substances (diphtheria, tetanus and pertussis immunization, sulphanilamide, isoniazid, DDT) or the toxic encephalopathic state which occurs in hydrocephalus (p.161). Sometimes blindness may ensue as the result of an encephalopathy in the absence of optic neuritis, so that it is a form of cortical blindess (p.342); this has followed triple antigen immunization.

Neuromyelitis optica (Devic's disease)

In this condition a bilateral optic neuritis occurs in association with a myelitis, usually in young children; similar cases which do not show myelitis may be considered as modified forms or as manifestations of encephalomyelitis. The prognosis for restoration of useful central vision is sometimes remarkably good considering the obvious uniform pallor of the optic disc which characterizes the later stages of the condition, but there is inevitably some degree of permanent defect.

Encephalitis periaxialis diffusa (Schilder's disease)

Optic neuritis is a rare feature of this condition (p.342).

Toxic and metabolic disorders

Toxic or metabolic disorders that produce bilateral optic neuritis include Leber's hereditary optic atrophy, tobacco and methyl alcohol amblyopia, pernicious anaemia, tropical neuropathy and occasionally diabetic neuropathy.

Ischaemic optic neuropathy

This condition affects the elderly with sudden impairment of vision due to occlusion of part or all of the vascular supply to the optic disc, resulting in an acute ischaemia with disc swelling and haemorrhages. It is usually caused by giant cell arteritis or arteriosclerosis. Vision does not recover and the disc develops a segmental or total pallor. If the investigations confirm giant cell arteritis and immediate intensive steroid treatment (intravenously then orally) at an initial dose of 80 to 100mg/day is instituted, there is less likelihood of a similar involvement in the other eye.

Optic disc oedema

It is generally accepted that the term *papilloedema* is restricted to optic disc swelling due to raised intracranial pressure (*plerocephalic oedema*), but optic disc oedema may occur in other ways.

Increased intracranial pressure (papilloedema). This is the classical form of disc swelling and may be produced by obstruction of the normal flow of cerebrospinal fluid, for example in aqueduct stenosis, or more commonly as the result of some intracranial space-occupying lesion; this is usually a tumour, particularly in the posterior cranial fossa (mid-brain, cerebellum), but more rarely it may be an inflammatory focus (abscess, gumma or tuberculoma) or sometimes an extensive extradural haemorrhage or severe meningitis. It is essentially bilateral but is sometimes unequal and is occasionally unilateral, but in the latter case has no localizing value; if associated with anosmia and optic atrophy in the other eye, it is known as the *Foster Kennedy syndrome*.

It is important to realize that raised intracranial pressure may be present without papilloedema. The mechanism of papilloedema is not clearly established but it is suggested that it is related to an obstruction to the normal flow of axonal particles (axoplasmic hold-up) or to failure of absorption of cerebrospinal fluid, or that it may be the result of compression of the retinal vein as it passes obliquely through the subarachnoid space of the optic nerve because of the raised pressure of the cerebrospinal fluid. It seems likely, however, that an overloading of the optic disc with blood from the arterial circle of Zinn is also of importance in its genesis as the increased resistance to blood flow in the pial plexus causes a diversion of blood from the arterial circle to the tissues of the optic disc. It may occur also because of the high diastolic pressure in the cerebral arteries following the increased capillary resistance of the cerebral tissues subjected to a raised intracranial pressure. These theories explain the absence of papilloedema in an atrophic optic disc (which is devoid of an adequate arterial circulation), despite obvious oedema of the otherwise healthy optic disc of the other eye.

Obstruction of the venous outflow from the eye (in the absence of an increased intracranial pressure). This may occur in central retinal vein thrombosis, in retinal vasculitis, in any form of increased blood viscosity such as polycythaemia and macroglobulinaemia, in cavernous sinus thrombosis, in carotico–cavernous anastomosis, or in any orbital lesion which causes a marked rise in the intraorbital tension (orbital tumour, orbital cellulitis, dysthyroid disease, orbital granulomas).

Uveitis. Optic disc swelling may occur when there is a patch of active choroiditis in the central part of the fundus, particularly in a juxtapapillary situation, and is also a feature of panuveitis in association with a generalized retinal oedema.

Optic neuritis. Optic neuritis in the anterior part of the optic nerve (*papillitis*, p.153) may cause optic disc swelling.

Hypertensive retinopathy. Papilloedema is a feature of the malignant form of hypertensive retinopathy (p.119), with involvement of both eyes.

Ischaemic optic neuropathy. Ischaemic optic neuropathy (p.155) produces acute swelling of the optic disc and is the commonest cause of optic disc swelling on one side and optic atrophy on the other, the latter representing a resolution of a previous ischaemic episode.

Collagen disorders. The retinopathy which occurs in collagen disorders (p.133) is usually associated with disc oedema.

Infiltration of the optic nerve head. This may occur in leukaemia, lymphomas, carcinoma and sarcoidosis. The mass of abnormal tissue interrupts either the normal circulation or the axoplasmic flow at the optic nerve head, causing optic disc oedema.

Lead poisoning. Disc oedema may be produced in various ways—as part of a retinopathy, as a plerocephalic oedema in association with an encephalopathy, or as part of an optic neuritis (papillitis).

Metabolic disorders. Hypercapnia, usually associated with chronic obstructive airways disease and hypocalcaemia can cause optic disc oedema.

Benign intracranial hypertension. This usually affects apparently healthy young people, particularly females, often following antibiotic treatment or following withdrawal of systemic corticosteroids. There is raised intracranial pressure and well-marked bilateral papilloedema. Ventriculography shows a decreased size ('*squeezing*') of the ventricles, which is the result of oedema of the brain. Headaches are common, and sometimes giddiness and vomiting may occur; in the female these symptoms may be most marked shortly before menstruation. There may be transient disturbances of the vision, rarely the vision may become permanently impaired as the result of a compressive (consecutive) optic atrophy. A paresis of the sixth cranial nerve may also occur. Some cases appear to be the result of thrombosis of a major cerebral venous sinus, but in many cases there is no known aetiology, although it has been suggested that there is some electrolyte imbalance in certain cases.

Where there is evidence of imminent visual impairment, surgical decompression of the optic nerve sheath is indicated.

Hypotony of the eyeball. Rarely a persistently low intraocular pressure, such as may occur after a glaucoma 'drainage' operation in which the operation area is draining excessively, is associated with some disc oedema.

Note: A false appearance of disc oedema may be found in high degrees of axial hypermetropia because of 'crowding' of the optic nerve fibres at the disc margin (*pseudopapilloedema*). Rarely the optic disc margins are markedly elevated as a congenital anomaly.

In papilloedema the dilatation of the vessels on the optic disc surface with extensions on to the surrounding retina causes a hyperaemia; the increased permeability of these vessels accounts for the oedema which elevates the disc margins—initially on the nasal side, subsequently on the superior and inferior margins and finally on the temporal margin—with a reduction in the size or even an obliteration of the physiological cup. The dilatation of the retinal veins and the retinal oedema are limited to the peripapillary region, with spread into the macular region in severe cases; these changes are followed by the production of varying amounts of retinal haemorrhage. Fluorescein angiography illustrates the presence of the dilated vessels, with an early filling of the disc capillaries, and there is leakage of fluorescein in the oedematous areas of the disc, with spread of the dye into the surrounding retina, particularly in relation to the retinal vessels. In chronic papilloedema the well-marked vascular network on the surface of the disc is strikingly evident. There is usually no awareness of any visual impairment, unless the macula is affected, but careful examination of the visual field shows enlargement of the blind spot. In the later stages the oedema may subside without leaving any obvious ophthalmoscopic signs, but usually there is some permanent blurring of the disc margins; in severe or persistent cases there is some degree of secondary atrophy with a corresponding visual impairment and sometimes even total blindness.

Treatment. This depends entirely on the cause of the optic disc swelling.

Optic atrophy

It is convenient to distinguish between two forms of optic nerve atrophy—primary and secondary.

Primary optic atrophy

The term *primary optic atrophy* is applied to optic atrophy which is the result of a disease process affecting the optic nerve fibres directly within the optic nerve or indirectly because of involvement of their parent cells (the ganglion cells) in the retina.

Involvement of the optic nerve

Congenital causes. A *coloboma* of the optic disc (p.152) appears as an atrophic area because of the absence of optic nerve fibres in that region. *Optic disc (optic nerve) hypoplasia* is a developmental anomaly in which there is poverty or absence of optic nerve fibres in the optic nerve head and usually also in the adjacent part of the optic nerve, although the framework and blood vessels of the nerve are present. It may be unilateral or bilateral, and it is associated almost invariably with profound visual impairment or even complete blindness. It is apparent ophthalmoscopically as a small excavated optic disc which is grey or white in colour and usually there is some attenuation of the retinal arteries; the significance of the small size of the disc may be overlooked because this is also a feature of the hypermetropic disc in early childhood, but on careful observation a faint line is apparent around the hypoplastic disc which represents what would have been the extent of the disc in the absence of the hypoplasia. Hypoplasia may be an isolated event, but sometimes there is an associated neurological disorder with anomalies of midline structures, particularly an absence of the septum pellucidum (*septo-optic dysplasia*). There may also be associated endocrine dysfunction with a deficiency of growth hormone; this requires early replacement therapy otherwise there will be permanent short stature.

Inherited causes. Optic atrophy may present in early life as the result of a dominant or autosomal recessive inherited disorder. In addition, in *Leber's hereditary optic atrophy* there is a fairly rapid loss of vision in both eyes in the late teenage period or in early adult life. It is usually transmitted by the female with a recessive, sex-linked mode of inheritance; at one time it appeared almost exclusively in males but more recently has also been found in females. The initial loss of vision may be profound (as in bilateral optic neuritis), but subsequently there is usually a restoration of peripheral vision, although seldom of central vision. The optic discs frequently show a uniform pallor, but sometimes this is limited to the temporal parts of the discs. The condition may be related to an inherent metabolic defect in the conversion of cyanide to thiocyanate (i.e. in the detoxification of cyanide). The sex distribution, which has undergone a change in recent years (at one time exclusively male but now with a significant number of female cases), and the relatively late onset (despite the inherited nature of the condition) may be an indication that environmental factors, especially those related to smoking, precipitate the disorder. This is illustrated by the lower thiocyanate concentration in the plasma of smokers with Leber's disease as compared with normal smokers.

Traumatic causes. Trauma may cause various degrees of optic atrophy following severence of part or all of the optic nerve fibres, either directly or more commonly indirectly following a disruption of the nutrient blood vessels (p.152).

Optic atrophy may be found in infancy as the result of brain damage from some obstetric complication, such as a premature separation of the placenta or a slow moulding and compression of the head during labour leading to rupture of some of the small veins draining into the longitudinal sinus or to tears in the tentorium cerebelli and falx cerebri with the production of rupture of the straight sinus or its tributaries. In such cases the optic atrophy is part of the brain damage which follows a disruption of vital structures by haemorrhage. Sometimes optic atrophy is the result essentially of a state of anoxia in the neonatal period, so that it may form part of the respiratory distress syndrome of the newborn.

Inflammatory causes. Optic neuritis (p.153) leads to an atrophy of the optic nerve fibres in the affected part of the nerve, but a primary form of optic atrophy may occur without any preceding optic neuritis in neurosyphilitic conditions, particularly in association with tabes dorsalis or general paralysis of the insane; in these conditions the peripheral vision is affected first but later the central vision is involved, sometimes with total blindness.

Neoplastic causes. A glioma of the optic nerve (p.162) causes a progressive destruction of the optic nerve fibres.

Involvement of the retinal ganglion cells

Certain retinal diseases are associated characteristically with some degree of primary optic atrophy, such as toxic amblyopia (p.135) or tapetoretinal degeneration (p.143). In addition, any advanced form of retinal disease, such as long-standing retinal detachment or retrolental fibroplasia, is likely to eventually be associated with some degree of optic atrophy.

Secondary optic atrophy

The term *secondary optic atrophy* is applied to optic atrophy which is the result of an indirect involvement of the optic nerve fibres by a disease process which causes pressure on the optic nerve. It is liable to occur, therefore, in any disorder which increases the intraorbital tension—for example, orbital tumour, orbital cellulitis, thyrotrophic exophthalmos (which exerts localized pressure on the optic nerve in the orbit), meningioma (which restricts the passage of the optic nerve through the optic canal), carcinomatous deposits, Paget's disease of the surrounding bone or oxycephaly—or which causes pressure on the optic nerve in its intracranial course—for example, pituitary tumours extending into the region of the anterior chiasmal angle or optochiasmal arachnoiditis. It is likely, of course, that these forms of secondary optic atrophy are the result of the effect of pressure on the nutrient vessels of the nerve fibres rather than of direct pressure on the nerve fibres. The optic atrophy which is associated with cupping of the optic disc in chronic simple glaucoma and with papilloedema is of a similar secondary nature.

Optic atrophy may also occur in *hydrocephalus*, when it may be produced in different ways. It may follow a shift in the position of the brain stem so that there is a stretching of the optic nerves or chiasm, with a consequent disruption of their nutrient vessels. It may follow meningitis, (which is prone to occur when the hydrocephalus is associated with a meningomyelocele—a form of spinal dysraphism), which occurs as a result of spread of infection or blood-borne spread from a urinary tract infection. It may also occur when the meningitis causes a toxic encephalopathic state with a secondary rise in the intracranial pressure (see above), or when it causes a toxic cardiopathy with the production of a right-sided cardiac failure which leads to a further increase in the intracranial pressure, even in the presence of a Spitz–Holter valve because of interference with the ventriculo-atrial shunt. It may follow a precipitous dilatation of the third ventricle which causes severe pressure on the optic chiasm, leading sometimes to a sudden blindness which is permanent unless the pressure is relieved as a matter of urgency; this condition is sometimes associated with a persistent turning down of the eyes (the so-called *'setting-sun' phenomenon)*. Furthermore, optic atrophy may occur in hydrocephalus simply as the result of long-standing papilloedema (*consecutive optic atrophy*, see below). Sometimes a severe disturbance of vision or even blindness may ensue in hydrocephalus in the absence of optic atrophy as the result of encephalopathy causing a water-logging of the brain; this represents a form of cortical blindness.

In primary and secondary optic atrophy, there is a gradual loss of the normal pink colour of the disc as a result of loss of the integrity of the arterioles which supply the capillaries of the optic nerve head; the margins of the optic disc retain their normal clear-cut outlines. If, however, optic atrophy follows optic disc swelling the margins of the disc appear blurred. Such atrophy should not necessarily be termed secondary atrophy as it may be primary atrophy (as in papillitis) or secondary atrophy (as in papilloedema); the term *consecutive optic atrophy* may be used clinically.

The patient's awareness of developing optic atrophy depends to a large extent on the nature of the field defect; a peripheral restriction of the visual field is detected often only in the late stages, but a central or para-central scotoma is more likely to become apparent in the early stages.

Drusen

This term is applied to translucent glistening bodies composed of concentric laminations of hyaline material which develop on the optic disc as an inherited degenerative condition with involvement usually of both eyes; rarely they occur as a congenital anomaly. They sometimes proliferate and project into the vitreous, but occasionally they lie buried within the disc so that there may be an ophthalmoscopic appearance suggestive of optic disc swelling. They are often associated with abnormal retinal vessel crossings and branchings; on fluorescein angiography the absence of any increase in the normal fluorescence of the optic disc and of any extension of the fluorescence into the surrounding retina confirms the diagnosis of buried drusen. The drusen autofluoresce. They are liable to affect the optic nerve fibres with the production of visual field defects such as an enlarged blind spot or a nerve bundle defect. Tuberous sclerosis (p.148) of the optic disc may present with a similar appearance.

Tumours

The different forms of optic nerve tumour are classified according to their tissue of origin in the nerve or in its surrounding sheaths.

Glioma

This is the commonest form of optic nerve tumour. It occurs usually in early childhood, sometimes in association with neurofibromatosis. It arises from the neuroglial framework of the optic nerve, usually in its orbital part, with possible spread forwards to the region of the optic nerve head or backwards to the optic chiasm (with consequent enlargement of the optic canal which is demonstrated radiographically). The main features of the condition are marked visual loss and optic atrophy of the affected eye; not infrequently some degree of visual loss occurs in the other eye when there is involvement of the optic chiasm. Proptosis is not a common feature in the earlier stages of the condition.

Meningioma

This tumour, which usually occurs in adult life before middle age, arises in the arachnoid sheath. A large growth occurs causing proptosis and diplopia because of displacement and impaired mobility of the eyeball. Visual defects are seldom evident until the later stages of the condition because the optic nerve tissue is not invaded directly by the tumour. Optic disc swelling is a characteristic feature and may be associated with shunt vessels at the disc head; if severe it may lead to some degree of optic atrophy.

Fibroma

This is a relatively benign tumour which arises in the dural sheath in childhood, with the production of a slowly increasing proptosis and impaired mobility of the eye; visual impairment does not occur except in the later stages.

Treatment

This consists of local excision of the tumour by a lateral approach (lateral orbitotomy—*Krönlein's operation*) or by a transfrontal approach, depending on the site and extent of the tumour. In a glioma this entails removal of the optic nerve but in a sheath tumour it may be possible to retain part of the nerve.

9

The Lens

Structure and function

The lens is a biconvex structure which lies behind the iris (from which it is separated by the narrow posterior chamber) and in front of the vitreous (from which it is separated by the narrow retrolental space). The central part of its anterior surface lies immediately behind the pupil where it forms part of the posterior boundary of the anterior chamber, and the most prominent part of this surface (the anterior pole of the lens) lies about 3 mm behind the posterior surface of the cornea. The lens is composed of three main structures: capsule, epithelium and fibres.

Capsule

This surrounds the lens and is concerned with the alterations which occur in the shape of the lens during accommodation (Fig. 7, p.10). It is thicker peripherally than centrally (Fig. 8, p.10) and is attached to the ciliary body through the *zonule (suspensory ligament)*. It is also concerned with fluid transference between the lens and the aqueous humour; the lens is dependent on this fluid for its nutrition because it is avascular; the capsule is also concerned with maintaining the correct amount of fluid in the lens.

Epithelium

The lens is developed from ectoderm and appears at an early stage as a small vesicle. The anterior part of the vesicle forms the lens epithelium; the posterior part is concerned with the formation of the earliest lens fibres (the embryonic fibres) so that the epithelium is present only over the anterior part of the lens. In the equatorial region the epithelial cells become elongated and are concerned thereafter in the formation of the lens fibres.

Fibres

These comprise the bulk of the lens and are distributed according to their time of formation in different zones; the embryonic fibres which lie in the centre of the lens are surrounded in succession by the fetal fibres, infantile fibres, adolescent fibres and adult fibres (Fig. 38).

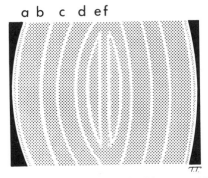

Fig. 38. Optical section of the lens: (a) capsule; (b) cortex; (c) adult nucleus; (d) infantile nucleus; (e) fetal nucleus; (f) embryonic nucleus.

The embryonic fibres form a homogeneous mass, but the other fibres form characteristic suture lines (e.g. the Y-shaped sutures of the fetal fibres) which represent the lines of junction between the terminals of the fibres. It follows that the oldest fibres pass towards the centre of the lens where they remain indefinitely, in contrast to the old cells of the skin, also an ectodermal structure, which are shed from its outer surface throughout life. In later life the older fibres form a solid mass of 'dead' fibres—the *nucleus*—which may be differentiated into its embryonic, fetal, infantile, adolescent and adult components, and the newer fibres form a surrounding mass of 'living' fibres—the *cortex.*

The lens is concerned with the transmission and refraction of light rays. Its normal transparency is achieved by the clear nature of its structures, by the absence of any blood vessels, and by a correct fluid balance within the lens.

Congenital anomalies

Ectopia lentis

In this condition, which is usually bilateral, there is partial dislocation of the lens resulting from defective formation of part of the zonule, so that the lens is displaced by the remaining intact zonule. The limited action of the zonule causes the lens to become more spherical (thus almost invariably producing myopia) and there is usually also a considerable degree of astigmatism because of a tilting of the lens. The rim of the lens is visible in the defective area on dilatation of the pupil, but in more advanced cases it may encroach also on the undilated pupil so that the patient is aware of two blurred images in each eye—one through the dislocated lens (a phakic image) and the other through the space produced by the dislocation (an aphakic image). The lack of support of the iris by the dislocated lens produces a tremulous wobbling of the iris (*iridodonesis*).

Sometimes ectopia lentis is associated with other developmental anomalies, either of an ocular nature such as ectopic pupil, aniridia or megalocornea, or of a more general nature such as Marfan's syndrome, homocystinuria or Marchesani's syndrome. Marfan's syndrome (a dominantly inherited condition) and homocystinuria (due to deficiency of an enzyme cystathione synthetase and inherited recessively) have similar skeletal features of arachnodactyly (long spidery hands and feet), kyphosis and osteoporosis, but the former has hypermobile joints while the latter does not. Whereas the subluxation in Marfan's syndrome is present from birth and non-progressive, that of homocystinuria is progressive and may be complicated by total dislocation either anteriorly or posteriorly. Furthermore, homocystinuria is associated with a tendency to thromboembolic episodes, which makes general anaesthetics hazardous. The abnormal amino acid is demonstrated by chromatography of urine or blood.

The complications of ectopia lentis are poor visual acuity and the risk of amblyopia, cataract formation and glaucoma, which may be due to pupil block or dislocation of the lens into the anterior chamber, or may be of a phacolytic nature (p. 176 and 314).

Treatment. As far as possible every attempt should be made to achieve some form of vision by the use of correcting lenses through the phakic (or sometimes through the aphakic) part of the pupil. Treatment is usually conservative, maintaining a close watch on the visual acuity. Lens extraction is only indicated in cataract formation, pupil-block glaucoma or uncorrectable poor acuity, and is attended by an increased complication rate of vitreous loss and retinal detachment.

Coloboma of the lens

This is a localized indentation of the lens, usually of the lower part, in association with defective formation of a small portion of the zonule.

Anterior or posterior lenticonus

This is a condition of excessive curvature of the anterior or posterior poles of the lens. It causes a marked increase in the effectivity of the axial part of the lens with the production of high myopia, but there is usually considerable distortion of vision, even after optical correction, because of its localized nature.

Spherophakia

In this condition there is an excessive curvature of both the anterior and posterior surfaces of the lens. It is liable to be associated with cataractous changes and may also lead to a secondary glaucoma because the spherical shape of the lens is liable to block the passage of aqueous through the pupil (pupil-block glaucoma).

Persistent vascular sheath

Remnants of the vascular network that surrounds the lens are commonly present, but rarely interfere with vision. They include persistent pupillary membrane and epicapsular stars (pp. 77 and 78).

Cataract

Congenital cataract is considered on p.168.

Injuries

Cataract may be the result of an injury to the lens. It may be caused by a break in the integrity of the lens capsule (perforating injury) or the result of concussional effects without such a break (blunt trauma), sometimes in association with a ring-shaped deposit of pigment on the anterior capsule of the lens following the imprint of the pigmented posterior layers of the iris on its anterior surface. *Dislocation* may also follow trauma.

Exfoliation of the lens capsule may follow exposure to infrared rays, as in the glass-blowing industry. Parts of the capsule become detached so that they project into the anterior chamber or become rolled up like parchment on the surface of the lens; this should not be confused with *pseudoexfoliation of the lens capsule* (p.314).

Cataract

A cataract represents a loss of transparency of the lens following changes in the physical and chemical characteristics of its fibres—for example, because of a denaturation of the lens proteins or an alteration in the hydration of the lens following some abnormality of the lens capsule or of the constituents of the lens.

Cataractous changes may be detected directly by focal illumination, when they appear as white opacities within an otherwise clear lens; these opacities may occur in the cortex—*anterior cortical cataract, posterior cortical cataract* or *peripheral cortical cataract*—or they may occur in the nucleus—*nuclear cataract.* They may also be detected indirectly on ophthalmoscopic examination, when they appear as black opacities against the background of the red reflex of the fundus. In advanced cases the whole lens becomes opaque so that it prevents the appearance of any red reflex; this absence of a red reflex does not necessarily imply that the cataract is *mature*, a term which is reserved for a cataract which is so complete that the iris fails to cast any shadow on its anterior surface.

Cataract may be considered according to the time of its onset— *congenital* (or *developmental*) or *senile* (sometimes *presenile*)—or according to its association with some other condition such as ocular disease, ocular trauma, endocrine dysfunction, skin disorders, myotonic dystrophy, Down's syndrome, and inborn errors of metabolism such as cystine storage disease (cystinosis) and galactosaemia.

Congenital (or developmental) cataract

The term *congenital cataract* is applied to various forms of cataract which are present at birth (thus correctly termed *congenital cataract*) or which appear in the earlier (or even in the later) years of life as a result of some defect which is congenitally determined (thus probably more accurately termed *developmental cataract*). These forms of cataract are the result of hereditary, toxic, nutritional or inflammatory influences. Fifty per cent of congenital cataracts are idiopathic and an isolated finding; those that are hereditary are usually dominantly inherited. Of those caused by congenital infections, rubella has accounted for the majority in the past, but toxoplasmosis, cytomegalovirus and herpes simplex may all be implicated. Some cataracts are associated with chromosomal abnormalities such as Down's and Turner's syndromes.

Anterior polar cataract

This is an isolated form of cataract in the region of the anterior pole of the lens following a developmental anomaly in association with strands of persistent pupillary membrane. It may also follow damage to the anterior part of the lens as the result of contact of the lens with the cornea following perforation of the eye. The opacity usually remains localized and, in the absence of corneal scarring, has little or no effect on the vision.

Anterior pyramidal cataract

This is a more obvious anterior polar cataract with a projection of the opaque area into the anterior chamber.

Posterior polar cataract

This is an isolated form of cataract in the region of the posterior pole. It is usually the result of contact of the lens with the hyaloid artery during

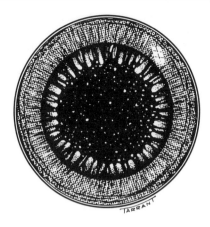

Fig. 39. Dot and flake (coronary) cataract.

development. Sometimes a remnant of the artery projects from the affected area into the retrolental space and vitreous.

Nuclear cataract (cataracta centralis pulverulenta)

This is the result of the formation of fine dots, often of a yellow colour, in the central part of the lens (the embryonic and fetal parts). It seldom interferes significantly with vision.

Sutural cataract

This is an accumulation of fine white dots in the sutures of the lens fibres, particularly in the Y (or fetal) sutures. They do not affect vision.

Dot and flake cataract (Fig. 39)

Fine dot opacities which appear blue (*blue-dot cataract*) or larger flake opacities which appear white (*coronary cataract*) are common features in the more peripheral parts of the lens. They lie between normal lens fibres and represent areas of degeneration of isolated fibres. They are often present in youth and may increase in number with age, but seldom interfere significantly with vision until later life when they become associated with senile lens changes.

Lamellar (or zonular) cataract (Fig. 40)

This cataract affects only a particular zonule of the lens. It consists of a concentric layer of opacity, sometimes narrow but often very extensive, within an otherwise clear lens except for fine lines of opacity which pass

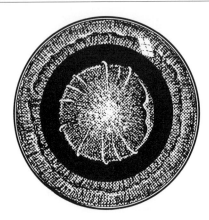

Fig. 40.   Lamellar cataract.

from the circumference of this layer towards its centre like the spokes of a wheel. The congenital form is sometimes due to an inherited trait, usually of a dominant type, and is frequently bilateral, but it may be associated with the rubella syndrome or it may occur as an acquired form after injury, in association with some other ocular disease, or as a result of parathyroid deficiency (p.178).

Coralliform cataract

This appears as a collection of opacities in the nuclear part of the lens resembling a mass of coral.

Axial fusiform cataract

This appears as a narrow spindle-like cataract extending from the anterior pole to the posterior pole.

Cataract in galactosaemia

This type of cataract may first become apparent in the early weeks of life as a refractive ring ('drop of oil' as seen with the ophthalmoscope) in the centre of the lens, leading to complete opacification of the lens. It is due to the accumulation of dulcitol, an abnormal product of the deranged galactose metabolism which has strong osmotic properties and occurs because of an enzyme deficiency. A transferase deficiency leads to the more severe form of galactosaemia, with hepatomegaly jaundice, haemolysis and eventually mental retardation, while a deficiency of galactokinase leads to the formation of cataract later in childhood, usually without other signs. The diagnosis is readily made biochemically and the condition is reversible with a galactose-free diet if implemented in the early stages, and which must be continued for life; if the cataract is well established then surgery is required.

Rubella cataract

Rubella cataract is essentially of a congenital nature because it is the result of maternal rubella (German measles) during pregnancy, particularly during the first eight weeks. The cataract is frequently complete but is sometimes of the lamellar type. It commonly affects both eyes, but may be strictly unilateral. Live rubella virus may persist in the cataractous lens for two or more years after birth and this is an important factor in the management of such cases (see below).

Maternal rubella may be responsible for other abnormalities of the eyes: microphthalmos, buphthalmos, diffuse corneal oedema, embryopathic pigmentary retinopathy (p.111), and defective development of the dilator muscle of the iris so that there is a persistent miosis. It may cause other general abnormalities such as congenital heart defects and perceptive deafness; their association with cataract constitutes the *rubella syndrome*. The recent introduction of rubella immunization has reduced the incidence of this condition.

Investigation of congenital cataract

A careful family history, examination of urine and blood for electrolyte or amino acid anomalies and serum for evidence of intrauterine infection are the basic requirements, but it is also important to perform a detailed examination of the eye for evidence of co-existing ocular disorders which may affect the prognosis.

Treatment of congenital cataract

Complete bilateral congenital cataracts require early surgical treatment because a failure to use the eyes in the early weeks or months of life causes *stimulus deprivation amblyopia* (p.231) and a loss of central fixation which make responses to later treatment negligible. These complications are still more prone to occur in unilateral complete (or even partial) cataract and the prognosis for restoration of central vision is invariably poor unless the operation is performed in the first few weeks of life and followed by occlusion of the unaffected eye and the provision of a contact lens to correct the aniseikonia which is inevitable in uniocular aphakia. Partial bilateral cataracts, particularly of the lamellar type, are often best left alone because they may be compatible with adequate vision in the distance and remarkably good close reading vision. In such cases the optical disadvantages of aphakia and the long-term risks of an ocular complication like retinal detachment, uveitis or secondary glaucoma outweigh the advantages of an improved level of distant vision following a cataract operation.

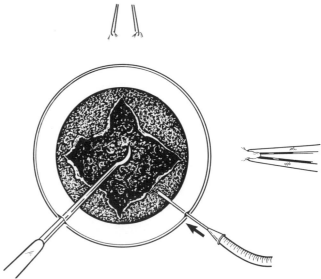

Fig. 41. Discission of the anterior lens capsule with a Ziegler's knife. Note the preplaced needle which is attached to a saline reservoir so that the anterior chamber is maintained throughout the operation.

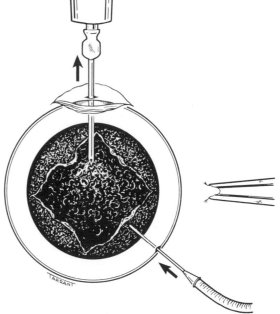

Fig. 42. Aspiration of lens material by a Scheie needle which is inserted into the anterior chamber by an *ab externo* approach at the upper part of the limbus. Note the preplaced needle which is attached to a saline reservoir so that the anterior chamber is maintained throughout the operation.

A congenital cataract is removed most readily by *aspiration* after *discission*. The anterior chamber is maintained throughout the operation with saline by means of a preplaced needle, and, after an adequate opening of the anterior lens capsule (*discission*) with a Ziegler's needle (Fig. 41), the lens material is aspirated through a large bore needle (such as the Scheie needle) which enters the anterior chamber by a subconjunctival approach at the limbus (*ab externo* approach) (Fig. 42).

Alternatively a lensectomy may be performed with the recently developed microsurgical suction-cutting instruments, which permit a more complete removal of the lens matter with less distortion of the globe. Certainly there is no indication to confine the operation to a simple discission with a reliance on subsequent spontaneous absorption of the lens material because this is liable to create the need for multiple discission operations and the liberated lens material is prone to cause uveitis; this applies particularly in the rubella cases when an intense endophthalmitis may destroy the eye despite intensive anti-inflammatory measures. It follows that the surgical treatment of a complete rubella cataract, which must be early to avoid intractable stimulus deprivation amblyopia, demands the removal of all lens material (because it contains live virus); if however, a destructive endophthalmitis occurs in the first eye, removal of the cataract from the second eye should be delayed until at least the age of two years.

It is essential in the surgical treatment of congenital cataract to avoid any interference with the posterior capsule of the lens because of the frequency of attachment of the vitreous to this part of the capsule, and because perforation of the posterior capsule is associated with an increased incidence of macular oedema. It follows that intracapsular extraction is contraindicated because it is prone to cause a loss of vitreous which greatly increases the risk of subsequent retinal detachment. In bilateral congenital cataracts which are confined to the more central parts of the lenses, an adequate level of vision may be obtained by securing some degree of mydriasis (e.g. by the use of atropine 1/16% drops once daily), or sometimes by carrying out an optical iridectomy in the upper or lower outer segment of the eye.

There are many variables in assessing the prognosis for good vision—for example, whether the condition is unilateral or bilateral, the age of onset of visual impairment and the degree of amblyopia, the presence of other ocular or systemic disorders, and the understanding and commitment by the parents to numerous hospital attendances to correct, ideally with contact lenses, the sometimes variable refractive error.

Senile cataract

The term senile is applied to all forms of cataract which develop spontaneously in the absence of any congenital disorder, ocular disease,

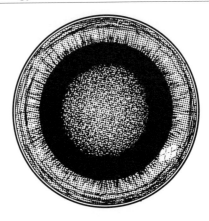

Fig. 43. Nuclear senile cataract.

ocular trauma, or associated systemic disorder, and, although it is prone to occur in the elderly, it may occur at an earlier age so that it is sometimes termed *presenile*. Presenile cataract may occur in certain families as an isolated event, sometimes showing a certain degree of 'anticipation' so that the cataract occurs slightly earlier in each succeeding generation. It occurs classically in *Werner's syndrome* which is a heredofamilial condition with posterior cortical cataract which usually affects one eye more than the other, premature greying of the hair, premature baldness, scleroderma affecting particularly the face and extremities, chronic ulceration of the legs and feet, hypogonadism, and sometimes osteoporosis, blue sclerotics and peripheral arterial calcification. There are various forms of senile and presenile cataract.

Nuclear sclerosis

Changes in the nucleus of the lens are to some extent natural because some gradual hardening and loss of elasticity is inevitable, but when marked it causes distortion of the vision, particularly for distant objects, and increases the refractive power of the lens, causing an increased myopia (or decreased hypermetropia). This accounts for the myopia which develops in some elderly people who are then often able to read small print without glasses—a surprising event to an elderly person who has required reading glasses for many years.

Nuclear cataract (Fig. 43)

It is usual for nuclear sclerosis to progress to true cataract formation so that the central part of the lens becomes opaque. This type of cataract is not particularly noticeable on straightforward examination because

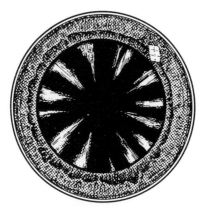

Fig. 44.   Cuneiform senile cortical cataract.

the pupil remains 'black' owing to the clarity of the surrounding cortical parts of the lens, but it may be detected readily by focal illumination or by ophthalmoscopic examination.

Cortical cataract

Incipient cataract. In the early stages of cortical cataract there is an abnormal accumulation of fluid between the lens fibres (perhaps as a result of an increased permeability of the lens capsule) so that, although the lens appears somewhat cloudy, there is no true opacification.

Immature cataract. Changes occur in the lens fibres which produce irregular white opacities. These are usually distributed within the periphery of the cortex in a radial manner (*cuneiform cataract*) (Fig. 44), but sometimes they assume a more uniform distribution in the posterior cortex (*cupuliform cataract*). Occasionally these changes are associated with a marked increase of fluid within the lens which may even cause swelling of the lens (*intumescent cataract*) with a consequent embarrassment of the filtration angle which may lead to secondary glaucoma.

Maturity. The whole lens becomes opaque with disappearance of the iris shadow which is normally apparent on the anterior surface of the lens and with absence of any red reflex. The vision becomes reduced to a vague awareness of hand movements (HM) or even to a mere perception of light (PL) but with retention of the ability to discern the direction from which the light is coming; this normal projection of light is tested by shining a bright light from different areas of the visual field into the eye and asking the patient to point to the various sources of the light. Failure of perception of light (no PL) is evidence of some additional lesion within the eye, such as vitreous haemorrhage, retinal detachment or optic atrophy. Defective projection of light in a particular direction is evidence of some more localized lesion within the eye, a finding which necessitates a guarded prognosis for restoration of useful vision after the cataract operation. Diagnostic ultrasound is a useful technique for assessing the integrity of the posterior segment in the presence of a dense cataract and will identify retinal detachments, choroidal tumours, some foreign bodies and some macular diseases.

Hypermaturity. This should be avoided by the treatment of a cataract before it becomes completely mature, because hypermaturity is liable to cause various complications:

1. *Morgagnian cataract.* The cortical cataract becomes liquefied and the hard nucleus sinks to the lower part of the capsule. This is frequently associated with a tremulousness of the iris on movement of the eye (*iridodonesis*).

2. *Dislocation of the lens.* The cataractous lens becomes dislocated into the vitreous (or more rarely into the anterior chamber) because of an associated degeneration of the suspensory ligament of the lens. This is also associated with iridodonesis.

3. *Phacolytic glaucoma.* This follows a leakage of lens material through the defective capsule into the anterior chamber where it accumulates within phagocytic cells; these cells may block the filtration angle causing secondary glaucoma (p.314).

4. *Lens-induced uveitis.* This follows a leakage of lens material through the capsule causing uveitis in an eye previously sensitized to lens protein (see p.95).

Complicated cataract

Complicated cataract is the result of various forms of long-standing ocular disease, such as recurrent severe uveitis or a retinal detachment which has failed to respond to treatment, and it is likely that it is the result of a general metabolic disorder of the diseased eye. It forms characteristically in the posterior cortical part of the lens, sometimes with striking colour changes in the affected region as a result of the diffraction of the light rays by the tiny opacities (*polychromatic lustre*).

Traumatic cataract

Any break in the integrity of the lens capsule following a perforating injury (e.g. the all-too-frequent perforation in the young child caused by scissors or some sharp-pointed toy, or the entry of a metallic fragment in the industrial worker) or following inexpert instrumentation during an intraocular operation (e.g. a penetrating keratoplasty or certain glaucoma operations) is followed by cataractous changes. These may remain localized if the opening in the capsule becomes sealed rapidly, but otherwise the whole lens becomes cataractous. If the opening in the capsule is large, the persistent permeation of aqueous into the lens results in the gradual dissolution and eventual absorption of the lens material, but sometimes the liberation of lens material into the anterior chamber causes an anterior uveitis or a secondary glaucoma by an impairment of the drainage of aqueous through the filtration angle.

Cataract may also follow injury of the eye in the absence of any perforation of the lens capsule—for example in severe contusion of the eye (*concussion cataract*) or exposure to irradiation, radar waves or to infrared rays; this usually takes the form of small opacities in the anterior or posterior subcapsular parts of the cortex, but sometimes larger leaf-life zones of opacity radiate out from the centres of these areas (the so-called *rosette cataract*).

Toxic cataract

Cataract may follow the systemic administration of various drugs, such as chlorpromazine, ergot and the corticosteroids, or even the topical administration of drugs of the anticholinesterase group (DFP and Phospholine Iodide) and steroids. The opacities usually start in the anterior or posterior subcapsular regions. Some metals given for therapeutic reasons (topically or systemically) or absorbed by frequent contact in certain industrial processes may lead to a pigmentation of the anterior lens capsule, with the eventual development of anterior subcapsular opacities, including silver (argyrosis), mercury (mercurialentis), copper (chalcosis) and iron (siderosis). Posterior subcapsular vacuoles may occur following retinal detachment surgery in which sulphur hexafluoride (SF6) gas or silicone oil have been used for internal retinal tamponade—those due to SF6 tend to reverse spontaneously with absorption of the gas, but silicone-induced opacities persist.

Endocrine cataract

Diabetes mellitus

True diabetic cataract is rare because of the early diagnosis and treatment of diabetes. It is more likely to occur in adolescents and progresses rapidly in both eyes with the formation of subcapsular opacities, particularly posteriorly, and then with complete opacification and intumescence. Sometimes this is reversible, provided the diabetes is controlled before the oedematous lens changes are followed by an irreversible denaturation of the lens proteins. Senile cataract in diabetics is similar to that which occurs in non-diabetics, although there is some evidence that it may occur more frequently and earlier and that it may progress more rapidly in diabetics. An increased tendency to haemorrhage and a more marked liberation of pigment from the posterior surface of the iris are two features often noted during a cataract extraction in diabetics, but the greater liability to postoperative infection is not now common because of the improved control of the disease and the use of antibiotics.

Transient changes in the refraction of the eye are a common feature in diabetes during periods of faulty control of the disease. Hyperglycaemia causes a decrease in hypermetropia (or an increase in myopia) and hypoglycaemia causes an increase in hypermetropia (or a decrease in myopia), changes which are caused by alterations in the relative water content of the cortical and nuclear parts of the lens leading, respectively, to an increased or decreased effectivity of the lens.

Parathyroid deficiency

Hypoparathyroidism, which is characterized by an increased excitability of the neuromuscular system (tetany) as a result of hypocalcaemia, may be occasionally associated with a localized subcapsular cataract late in the disease. This may remain localized so that some years later it appears as a lamellar cataract. Spasmodic movements of the eyelids may occur in tetany.

Hypothyroidism

Cataract in the form of subcapsular opacities may rarely occur in cretinism.

Other types of cataract

Atopic cataract

Certain severe skin conditions, such as generalized eczema in children or scleroderma, are rarely associated with cataract formation, following a disturbance of the lens epithelium which is akin to that occurring within the skin. In *Rothmund's syndrome* the development of cataract in early childhood is associated with poikiloderma and with various forms of vascular disturbance.

Cataract in myotonic dystrophy

Anterior and posterior subcapsular flaky opacities may occur in myotonic dystrophy—a condition of generalized muscular disturbance affecting particularly the hands, arms and legs, with the production of a peculiar form of weakness in which the affected muscles, after a delayed and relatively weak contraction, exhibit an inability to achieve a spontaneous relaxation (this is detected readily in the handshake of such patients). These subcapsular changes gradually extend to involve the whole lens in a presenile type of cataract. Ptosis (p.199) may occur in this condition. These patients may have respiratory and pharyngeal weakness, and associated cardiac defects which make general anaesthesia, particularly with muscle relaxants, hazardous.

Cataract in Down's syndrome

Fine opacities within the fetal (Y) sutures and blue-dot and coronary opacities within the peripheral parts of the lens are commonly found to a much greater degree in Down's syndrome than in the normal population. A localized arcuate opacity within the lens is also a feature in some patients; this is a distinctive change.

Uniocular cataract

A uniocular cataract may simply represent asymmetrical development of bilateral cataract, but it may indicate underlying ocular disease such as previous trauma (whether blunt or perforating), an intraocular neoplasm or retinal detachment, or may complicate the condition of heterochromia iridis. When the fundus cannot be seen in these cases, radiological and ultrasonic investigations should be performed prior to surgery.

Treatment of cataract

The absence of any accepted medical method of preventing or treating cataract, despite innumerable claims over the years, determines the necessity for surgical treatment, but each case must be assessed carefully and the following estimations made before advising operation:

Estimation of the corrected distant and near visual acuities of the affected (or more affected) eye. Certain forms of cataract, such as a nuclear cataract, may be compatible with quite reasonable vision, although the interpretation of 'reasonable' varies with the intellectual capacity and occupation of the individual. For example, an elderly person may be content with poor distant vision if the near vision is reasonably good, whereas a younger person may have entirely different requirements. Sometimes in cataract the vision may be improved for a time simply by a change of spectacle lenses (e.g. as a compensation for the increasing myopia in a nuclear lens sclerosis) or by preventing a too marked constriction of the pupil by the use of dark glasses or a mydriatic sufficiently weak to allow the retention of some accommodation (e.g. atropine 1/16% drops once daily).

Estimation of the corrected distant and near visual acuities of the unaffected (or less affected) eye. It is not possible with conventional spectacle lenses to obtain the use of the two eyes together (binocular vision) after a cataract operation on one eye owing to the marked size difference (aniseikonia) of the two retinal images. This difficulty may be overcome by a contact lens or by an acrylic lens implant in the anterior or posterior chamber, the latter being maintained in the most physiological position by retaining the posterior capsule (*extracapsular extraction*—see below). Implant displacement, chronic iritis, and biodegradation may occur, but the principle complication is damage to the endothelium, which particularly occurs during insertion of the lens. Peroperative and postoperative endothelial contact may lead to corneal endothelial decompensation and bullous keratopathy. However, attention to careful microsurgical techniques, the use of correct intraocular irrigating solutions and the use of air or a viscous aqueous substitute to protect the endothelium during implantation have led to the present popularity of implants. They permit an earlier return to binocularity, and avoid the disturbing optical aberrations and field defects inherent in aphakic spectacle wear.

Estimation of the potential visual function of the affected eye after operation. This entails a determination of any coexisting ocular disease, such as vitreous haemorrhage, retinal detachment, senile macular degeneration, diabetic retinopathy or optic atrophy. When the cataract is immature this is possible after the instillation of a mydriatic. If, however, the cataract is extensive, reliance must be placed on indirect methods:

1.   The relation of the corrected visual acuity to the degree of cataract. A reduction in acuity which is greater than would be expected from the cataract is suggestive of some coexistent lesion, and, as discussed above, even a mature cataract never reduces the vision beyond the level of 'perception of light with accurate projection'.
2.   Examination of the visual field using simple confrontation or the perimeter (p.343) may indicate some other abnormality.
3.   Examination of the less affected eye. The recognition of a condition which tends to affect both eyes, such as macular degeneration, makes it possible that it is present also in the cataractous eye.
4.   Determination of any childhood squint which may have caused an amblyopia and sometimes a loss of central fixation with or without an eccentric retinal fixation (see p.231). In such a case the central

vision would be improved to only a limited extent after a cataract operation. This is excluded best by a careful history; the presence of a squint of the cataractous eye is not necessarily an indication of a childhood squint as it may have followed simply the dissociation of the two eyes by the defective vision of one eye. In a congenital (or developmental) cataract which is confined solely or largely to one eye, the affected eye is usually amblyopic following its disuse (stimulus deprivation amblyopia), often with a loss of central fixation, and any associated squint is incidental.

5.   Detection of any abnormality of the eye which might progress after the operation, thereby affecting the visual prognosis. For example, an early corneal dystrophy, particularly affecting the corneal endothelium as in Fuchs' dystrophy (p.67) tends to advance rapidly following the inevitable trauma to the cornea during the removal of the lens. In addition, evidence of a previous uveitis is an indication of an increased likelihood of a postoperative uveitis, particularly if soft lens material is liberated at the operation. Evidence of an active uveitis is usually a contraindication to operation, except when the uveitis is of the lens-induced type (p.95) or in a child with uveitis of the form which occurs in Still's disease (p.93) when persistence of some degree of uveitis is inevitable.

6.   Assessment of retinal function by electrodiagnostic tests (p. 109).

7.   The use of diagnostic ultrasound for the detection of lesions in the posterior segment.

Estimation of the maturity of the lens. A mature cataract usually demands early treatment, irrespective of other considerations because of the complications which tend to follow hypermaturity (see p.176).

Cataract surgery

Preparation of the patient. It is important to exclude or treat before operation any general conditions which might cause adverse complications such as haemorrhage, infection or iris prolapse. These include diabetes, cardiovascular disease, renal disorders and bronchitis.

Preparation of the eye. It is essential to eliminate any surface infection, especially of the lids. When a routine culture of the conjunctival sacs determines the presence of pathogenic organisms, even in the absence of any obvious infection, an appropriate antibiotic should be given. However, most surgeons rely on topical antibiotics (e.g. chloramphenicol drops) without recourse to culture. A source of organisms which might give rise to postoperative intraocular infection and its devastating sequelae is an obstructed nasolacrimal system, so that any history of a persistently watering eye necessitates syringing of the nasolacrimal duct to ensure its patency.

The operation. This depends on the particular form of cataract. The surgical treatment of congenital cataract which occurs in early life is discussed on p.171.

In *extracapsular extraction* the anterior capsule of the lens is removed by a capsulotomy needle, so that the solid nucleus and as much as possible of the soft cortical lens fibres are expressed from the eye through the upper limbal incision; a simultaneous irrigation aspiration cannula is used to remove the remaining cortical lens material. The technique of phacoemulsification has recently been developed whereby ultrasonic fragmentation of the lens tissue is followed by aspiration, the procedure requiring only a small incision (1 to 2 mm). This operation does not interfere with the integrity of the posterior lens capsule; sometimes it is necessary to cut a small hole in this capsule (a needling or capsulotomy) some weeks or months later to provide clear vision. Recently, the neodymium: YAG laser photodisruptor has been used to create this hole.

In *intracapsular extraction* the lens is removed intact within its capsule by grasping the capsule with special non-cutting forceps (intracapsular forceps), by the use of suction apparatus (erysiphake), or by cryosurgery, whereby the tip of the cryoprobe is securely attached to the capsule and the underlying lens fibres by the formation of a blob of ice. The difficulty of dislocating the lens from its zonular attachments to the ciliary body without rupturing the capsule, particularly when unduly resistant as in the younger patient or in an immature cataract, may be overcome by a partial digestion of the zonule with a solution of alpha-chymotrypsin (Zonulysin) behind the iris a few minutes before the removal of the lens. An intraocular lens may be inserted following intracapsular or extracapsular cataract extraction. Recently there has been a trend towards posterior chamber implants because of their more physiological position, facility of dilatation of the pupil postoperatively, and less risk of damaging the endothelium; they necessarily require an extracapsular technique so that the implant may rest in the capsular bag.

Complications. Disturbance of the vitreous is one of the main complicating features of a cataract extraction and is more likely in the intracapsular extraction. Vitreous loss is serious because it predisposes to the development of uveitis or a retinal detachment, but a forwards displacement of vitreous into the anterior chamber, even in the absence of vitreous loss, may also be serious as it may lead to glaucoma by obstructing the flow of aqueous (*pupil block*). Several procedures help to maintain the vitreous in its correct place during and after the operation: (a) the prevention of spasm of the orbicularis oculi muscle of the eyelids during the extraction by facial akinesia; (b) the prevention of spasm of the extrinsic ocular muscles during the extraction by retrobulbar anaesthesia (these two procedures only apply when the operation is performed under local anaesthesia—as a rule general anaesthesia is preferred unless there is some contraindication); (c) the restoration of the anterior chamber after the extraction by the insertion of air or saline, which is retained because of adequate direct suturing of the limbal incision; and (d) the facilitation of the circulation of aqueous within the eye after the operation by providing one or two small holes in the peripheral parts of the iris (*peripheral iridotomies* or *iridectomies*).

Haemorrhage into the anterior chamber (*hyphaema*) after the operation usually absorbs within a few days, but rarely it has to be removed by irrigation because of the development of secondary glaucoma. Rarely severe haemorrhage occurs within the eye during the extraction (*expulsive choroidal haemorrhage*), particularly in an elderly person with defective choroidal vessels, because of the sudden reduction in the intraocular pressure which follows opening the eye. Massage of the eye before commencing the operation lowers the intraocular pressure and diminishes this risk, but lowering of the intraocular pressure by an osmotic agent like oral gycerol, or intravenous mannitol is more certain and may be adopted as a routine if there is doubt about the intraocular pressure or in the presence of a high degree of myopia, which increases the risk of vitreous loss. During general anaesthesia, muscle relaxants and hyperventilation further reduce the risk.

Prolapse of iris into or through the limbal incision may occur in a restless patient, sometimes after severe coughing, but its incidence is reduced by the adequate closure of the limbal incision with direct sutures. It may occcur after spontaneous resolution of aphakic pupil-block glaucoma. An iris prolapse usually should be abscissed, but sometimes it may be replaced, provided the prolapse is only within the wound without any true exposure and is of recent onset so that a uveitis (which might lead to a sympathetic ophthalmitis, p.94) is unlikely.

Sometimes *cystoid degeneration of the macula* may occur spontaneously after a cataract operation, even when this is uncomplicated. It usually occurs in an elderly person, so that there may have been a predisposition to its development, but vitreous traction is often an important factor.

Postoperative intraocular infection (endophthalmitis) may occur within days of the operation or even as long as years later, particularly if there is imperfect wound closure. The patient complains of pain, while the eye is chemosed, inflamed and shows the signs of an aggressive intraocular inflammation manifested as a hypopyon with a fibrinous exudative response in the anterior chamber and a vitritis precluding a satisfactory view of the retina. Immediate treatment is with intensive topical and subconjunctival antibiotics, which can be modified following identification and sensitivity of the organism by gram stain and culture of fluid obtained from the anterior chamber and the vitreous. When there are signs of resolution, topical steroids are added to the regimen to minimize the toxic effects of acute inflammation upon the retina, uvea and corneal endothelium.

Dislocation of the lens

This follows a defect in the zonule which may be due to (a) a congenital anomaly (p.165); (b) trauma (p.167); or (c) degenerative conditions, such as a mature cataract secondary to a long-standing retinal detachment or in advanced infantile glaucoma (buphthalmos), when there is an enlargement of the eye but not of the lens.

The dislocation may be incomplete (as in ectopia lentis, p.165) or complete when the lens becomes dislocated anteriorly into the anterior chamber or posteriorly into the vitreous.

Anterior dislocation

This is almost invariably followed by such complications as secondary glaucoma (due to obstruction of aqueous flow through the pupil by the lens), corneal degeneration (due to contact of the lens with the posterior corneal surface), or anterior uveitis. The only effective treatment is usually removal of the lens, although sometimes the lens may be restored to its normal position after pupillary dilatation (by the instillation of a mydriatic) where it is maintained thereafter by pupillary constriction (by the instillation of a miotic).

Posterior dislocation

This has little effect initially except visually because of the aphakia, so that a correcting lens is necessary in the interests of clear vision. There are, however, many later complications including adhesion of the lens to the lower peripheral part of the retina by an inflammatory exudate, intense uveitis, secondary glaucoma, and retinal detachment. It is usually advisable therefore to remove such a lens, although this involves the loss of some of the vitreous during the opening of the eye at the corneoscleral junction (because of the vitreous which surrounds the lens), so that the results of the operation are sometimes poor, and in certain circumstances it is expedient to adopt a 'wait-and-see' policy. Closed intraocular microsurgery has reduced the complications of this operation, and a conservative policy is now less common.

10

The Vitreous Body

Structure and function

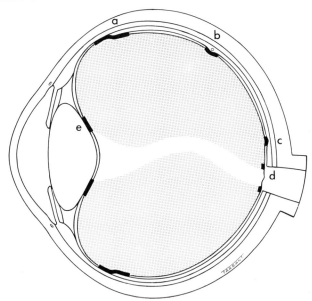

Fig. 45. Attachments of the vitreous: (a) at the vitreous base: ora serrata and pars plana; (b) to retinal vessels; (c) at the fovea; (d) at the margins of the optic disc; and (e) to the posterior lens capsule. The unshaded area is Cloquet's canal.

The vitreous body is a transparent gel-like substance which fills the space between the posterior surface of the lens and its zonule, the internal limiting membrane of the retina, the ciliary body, and the optic disc. It is formed by a combination of fine fibrillar micellae of non-branching collagen, which is stabilized by a mucopolysaccharide, *hyaluronic acid*, with 99% of the structure being made up of water. At the periphery, or the *cortex*, the concentration of collagen and hyaluronic acid is higher and the fibrillary arrangement is more compact, imparting greater rigidity. Cellular elements with phagocytic and possibly secretory potential reside in the cortex.

The outer cortex has a firm fibrillar union with the internal limiting lamina of the retina, which is derived from the retinal neuroglial cells (*Müller's cells*). This union is especially strong over the *pars plana* and *ora serrata* (vitreous base), at the disc and adjacent to the retinal vessels (Fig. 45). The anterior surface of the vitreous appears on slit-lamp microscopy to be separated from the posterior surface of the lens by a narrow capillary space (the *retrolental space*), but in fact this contains a homogeneous type of vitreous which has a narrow circular zone of tenuous attachment to the posterior lens capsule. A narrow 'canal' (*Cloquet's canal*) passes through the vitreous from the central part of the posterior lens capsule to the optic disc (Fig. 45), but it is not a true space because it contains modified vitreous; it represents the site of the hyaloid artery which is present in the developing eye but disappears before birth.

Examination of the vitreous requires a fully dilated pupil in order to observe both the static and dynamic (during and immediately after eye movement) appearances with the slit-lamp, mirrored contact lens and the indirect ophthalmoscope.

Congenital anomalies

Persistent hyaloid remnants

Small persistent remnants of the hyaloid artery or its branches constitute vitreous 'floaters' (*muscae volitantes*) (see below). Sometimes a persistent hyaloid artery may ramify in a remnant of the posterior fibrovascular sheath which lies behind the developing lens in intrauterine life with the formation of a *persistent tunica vasculosa lentis*.

Persistent hyperplastic primary vitreous

In this condition active hyperplastic changes originate in the anterior part of the vitreous after birth in association with a persistent tunica vasculosa lentis. A mass of vascularized tissue forms behind the lens either in a localized area or over the whole posterior surface; it sometimes passes round the equator of the lens to its anterior surface. This tissue varies in thickness from a thin membrane to a thick mass extending into the anterior part of the vitreous. The anterior chamber usually becomes shallow with a consequent narrowing of the filtration angle. Characteristically the ciliary processes become elongated, atrophic and drawn out to become incorporated in the mass; zonular fibres may also extend into the mass. Usually the peripheral retina is involved in these changes so that it becomes disorganized and detached. The development of uveitis or secondary glaucoma is a likely terminal event. The condition may be unilateral or rarely bilateral. There is no effective treatment; an attempt may be made to incise the mass of tissue but there is unlikely to be any significant visual improvement because of the other changes in the eye. In addition, an intense stimulus deprivation amblyopia will be present, even in the relative absence of other changes.

Injuries

Damage to the vitreous occurs in perforating injuries where the vitreous may become incarcerated into the wound, stimulating glial and retinal pigment epithelial proliferation. Where a foreign body has penetrated the eye, traversed the vitreous and become impacted on the retina, there is a fibrocytic proliferative response at the entry site, impaction site and along its intravitreal route. When the fibrous tissue contracts, vitreous traction (*static traction*) along the length of the fibrosis (*transgel traction*) results in retinal traction and possibly retinal detachment. Foreign body removal is ideally an intraocular procedure accompanied by vitrectomy to pre-empt the fibrosis.

Loss of vitreous during surgery may induce transgel traction if the gel is incarcerated in the wound, and may lead to retinal traction and possible retinal detachment or macular oedema.

Vitreous haemorrhage

Haemorrhage may occur from abnormal vessels such as the new vessels formed in response to ischaemia in conditions such as branch retinal vein occlusion, diabetes, sickle cell retinopathy, as part of a haematological disorder such as leukaemia or thrombocytopaenia, or following posterior vitreous detachment.

An *intragel haemorrhage*, which disperses rapidly through the gel producing painless impairment of vision, takes longer to clear than a *retrohyaloid haemorrhage* which does not clot and forms fluid levels. Concentration of degenerating red blood cells on the posterior hyaloid face produces a yellow/orange uniform appearance known as an *ochre membrane*.

Inflammation

Inflammatory cells may invade the vitreous secondary to uveitis, choroidoretinitis (e.g. due to toxoplasmosis), retinal vasculitis or candidiasis and may be pronounced in the anterior vitreous with toxocaral infestation. A typical feature of pars planitis (p.85) is the confluent exudate that lies on the posterior hyaloid face in association with white globular opacities.

The vitreous may also be invaded by inflammatory cells during an acute meningitis, producing a globular white opacity known as a *pseudoglioma*, or may be the site of amyloid deposition. It is rarely the site for deposition of reticulum cell sarcoma masses.

Vitreous in diabetes mellitus

Vitreous involvement in diabetes contributes greatly to the morbidity of the disease. Detachment of the vitreous occurs earlier in diabetics but not in those with background retinopathy alone. It usually occurs (a) following neovascularization and fibrocellular proliferation on the retina and posterior hyaloid face, so that solid retraction of the vitreous (without collapse of the gel) results in avulsion of the new vessels, and retrohyaloid haemorrhage; (b) following contraction of the fibrotic proliferating tissue leading to static traction on the retinal surface (*epiretinal membrane*); or (c) between points of abnormal vitreoretinal adhesion, with the development of retinoschisis, retinal detachment or macular oedema. These cases, hitherto virtually untreatable, have a potential for vision following the development of the microsurgical intraocular techniques of vitrectomy, removal of fibrocellular traction bands, endophotocoagulation of the retinal new vessels and internal tamponade to retinal breaks (see p.132).

Opacities in the vitreous

Small particles may occur in the vitreous gel (the *muscae volitantes*) as the result of congenital remnants or of coagulations of protein material, usually in association with an increased fluidity of the vitreous. Sometimes they remain undetected by the patient unless they are viewed against a bright background, but they are visible particularly when they lie in the central part of the vitreous and are more clearly defined when they lie near the retina; to some extent they are most troublesome in the introspective type of person. The opacities, which appear subjectively as black spots or threads, shift on movement of the eye, but this change in position is not precise so that on attempting to view them against a particular part of the background they flit rapidly away; this is in contrast to the scotoma which follows a retinal lesion, such as a macular haemorrhage, which may be viewed precisely in any desired direction. The opacities may be observed with the ophthalmoscope or, when anteriorly placed, with the slit-lamp miscroscope, but sometimes they are too small to be readily visible.

There are other primary opacities in the vitreous which are seldom associated with any subjective awareness: peculiar small white particles which are composed of calcium soaps—the so-called *asteroid bodies*—occur rarely in old age, even sometimes in the absence of any obvious ocular disease and usually as a unilateral phenomenon, and numerous clusters of glittering golden cholesterol crystals—*synchisis scintillans*—occur in long-standing uveitis or vitreous haemorrhage and cascade through the degenerate fluid vitreous.

Degenerations

Syneresis

In myopia and advancing age or adjacent to local chorioretinal disease there is an aggregation of the collagen fibrils which leaves optically empty cavities (*lacunae*) within the vitreous gel, which is then therefore more mobile. The aggregated collagen fibrils, if sufficiently posterior, may induce the sensation of floaters (see above).

Posterior vitreous detachment

Cleavage of the cortex from the internal limiting membrane of the retina, or more likely along a plane within the cortical gel, resulting in a separation from the retina constitutes a *posterior vitreous detachment*. This is a common occurrence with age and in myopia and also following vitreous haemorrhage or retrohyaloid haemorrhage, which may occur in various retinal disorders or in subarachnoid haemorrhage.

There are two types of posterior vitreous detachment:

1. Posterior vitreous detachment without collapse of the gel, where there is a retraction of the vitreous from the retina without syneresis; this is a common accompaniment of diabetes where neovascular membranes grow on to the posterior hyaloid face and are avulsed, with the retraction inducing retrogel haemorrhage.

2. Posterior vitreous detachment with collapse of the gel occurs in a degenerate vitreous, where the syneretic lacunae discharge their contents through a rupture in the cortical layers into the retrohyaloid space. The vitreous remains attached at the vitreous base and at any site of anomalous vitreoretinal adhesion, and the increased mobility of the gel will exert dynamic traction at these sites. Anomalous vitreoretinal adhesion occurs over areas of degenerate retina such as lattice degeneration, over retinal vessels (particularly areas of retinal neovascularization, for example, in branch vein occlusion or diabetes) and over areas of focal choroidoretinal inflammation. This dynamic traction may result in avulsion of vessels leading to retrohyaloid haemorrhage, or creation of retinal tears that predispose to retinal detachment. If there is a break in the retina, the pigment epithelium is exposed and the presence of pigment cells on the posterior vitreous face or in the remaining gel is striking evidence of retinal hole or detachment formation.

11

The Eyelids

Structure and function

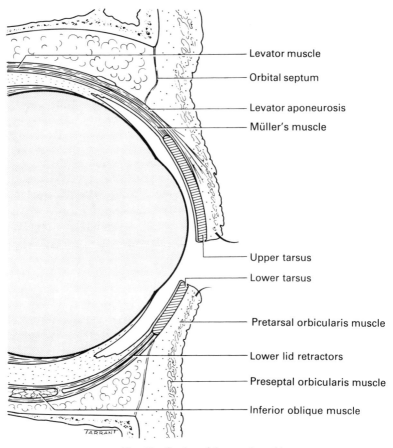

Levator muscle

Orbital septum

Levator aponeurosis

Müller's muscle

Upper tarsus

Lower tarsus

Pretarsal orbicularis muscle

Lower lid retractors

Preseptal orbicularis muscle

Inferior oblique muscle

Fig. 46. Section of the anterior orbit.

The upper and lower eyelids are modified folds of skin consisting of orbital and palpebral portions; in the upper eyelid the orbital portion extends down from the eyebrow to cover the upper part of the orbit and the palpebral portion covers the upper part of the eyeball. In the lower eyelid the orbital portion extends up from the cheek to cover the lower part of the orbit and the palpebral portion covers the lower part of the eyeball. The subcutaneous layer of the eyelids contains the *orbicularis oculi muscle* which is innervated from its deep surface by the facial (seventh cranial) nerve and forms an oval sheet of concentric muscle fibres surrounding the eyelids (Fig. 46). The palpebral parts of this muscle, particularly of the upper lid, are used in gentle lid closure, and the orbital parts are also brought into play in forcible lid closure. Closure of the lids is associated reflexly with an upwards movement of the eye which is effective before the lids are fully closed (*Bell's phenomenon*). The orbicularis muscle is concerned also in the drainage of the tears (see p.210). Deep to the orbicularis muscle is the tissue plane that contains the vascular and nervous supply to the lids.

Closure of the upper lid by the orbicularis muscle is opposed by the combined actions of the striated *levator palpebrae superioris muscle* and its associated smooth *superior palpebral muscle (of Müller)* which retract the lid (Fig. 46). The levator is a voluntary muscle which is innervated by the oculomotor (third cranial) nerve and extends into the upper lid from its origin in the apex of the orbit. It becomes aponeurotic and has a widespread insertion into the anterior surface of the tarsal plate and into the orbital septum, which passes from the upper margin of the tarsal plate to the orbital rim. From its origin on the inferior surface of the levator muscle, the involuntary smooth muscle, supplied by the cervical sympathetic nerve, passes forwards to be inserted into the upper margin of the tarsal plate.

The palpebral opening is the entrance into the conjunctival sac which is bounded by the upper and lower lid margins; these margins terminate laterally in an acute angle (the *lateral canthus*), which is attached to the bony orbit by the *lateral palpebral ligament*, and terminate medially in an elliptical junction (the *medial canthus*) which is attached to the bony orbit by the *medial palpebral ligament*. When the eyelids are opened in the normal way with the eyes directed straight ahead, it is usual for the upper margin of the cornea to be covered slightly by the upper lid margin and for the lower margin of the cornea to be at the same level as the lower lid margin. In the infant the upper lid margin is often above the cornea (with the appearance of an *upper scleral rim*) and in the older adult there is a tendency for the lower lid margin to lie below the cornea (with the appearance of a *lower scleral rim*).

The lid margin is a narrow zone (about 2 mm in width) which separates the outer (skin) surface of the eyelid from its inner (palpebral conjunctiva) surface; the junction of the medial one-sixth and lateral five-sixths of the lid margin is represented by a papilla which contains the lacrimal punctum (see p.290). There are also other structures on the lid margin:

1.   Two or three irregularly placed rows of short stout hairs (the *eyelashes* or *cilia*), which are more numerous in the upper than in the

lower lids, are placed anteriorly on the lid margin. The eyelashes are renewed rapidly after epilation, reaching their normal size within about ten weeks. They provide some degree of protection to the eyes and are associated directly with *sebaceous glands (of Zeis)* and indirectly with *sweat glands (of Moll)*.

2. The *intermarginal sulcus* lies behind the lashes and is visible clinically as a 'grey line'. It is important surgically because it represents the line of division of the lid into its anterior portion (skin and orbicularis muscle) and its posterior portion (tarsal plate and conjunctiva).

3. The openings of the ducts of the *Meibomian (tarsal) glands*, 30 to 40 in the upper lid and 20 to 30 in the lower lid, lie immediately behind the grey line. These large sebaceous glands lie within the *tarsal plate*, a dense formation of connective tissue within each lid which provides the palpebral portion of the lid with some degree of rigidity. Their sebaceous secretions on the lid margins prevent an overspilling of the normal tear flow from the conjunctival sac. The secretions also form the surface layer of the precorneal fluid, thus preventing an undue evaporation of the tears from the surface of the cornea.

Congenital anomalies

Epicanthus

This is a semilunar fold of skin which passes from the medial part of the eyebrow in a crescentic manner towards the lower lid, so that it tends to obscure the medial canthus and to increase the apparent breadth of the nose. It occurs to a minor degree in most young children, but usually disappears spontaneously as the bridge of the nose becomes formed in the early years of life except in certain races, such as the Chinese and Japanese, and in Down's syndrome, when it remains as a permanent feature. It is usually bilateral, although not always symmetrical. Epicanthic folds tend to give a false appearance of a convergent squint (see p.236). A more severe form of epicanthus occurs in association with congenital ptosis and inevitably also with marked narrowing of the palpebral fissure *(blepharophimosis)*; this condition requires correction by a plastic operation to deal with the epicanthus and some months later by a further operation to deal with the blepharophimosis.

Coloboma of the eyelid

A notch in the lid margin, usually at the junction of the middle and inner thirds of the upper eyelid, may occur as a developmental anomaly. It may be corrected by a plastic operation for cosmetic reasons and for protective reasons if the notch is sufficiently large to cause undue exposure of the cornea, which may occur even during closure of the lids.

Ankyloblepharon

Rarely a small area of adhesion between the upper and lower lid margins may occur as a congenital anomaly, evidence of the fact that the lids are adherent to one another at an early stage of development. Such an adhesion is treated by simple division.

Congenital ptosis

Drooping of the upper lid may occur as a congenital anomaly of the levator muscle; it may be unilateral or bilateral and is sometimes associated with a weakness of the extrinsic ocular muscles, particularly those concerned with elevation of the eye. Most of these defects are caused by a failure in the development of the affected muscle or muscles so that they are myogenic in origin, but a few cases are neurogenic in origin. The degree of ptosis is variable; usually it is largely a cosmetic defect because it is not sufficiently marked to prevent the eye from functioning visually. In severe cases the affected eye is likely to develop stimulus deprivation amblyopia as a result of its disuse, although this is avoided in bilateral cases because of the necessity to tilt the head backwards to achieve any form of vision.

In the *Marcus Gunn jaw-winking phenomenon*, unilateral congenital ptosis is replaced by a marked retraction of the affected lid during the opening of the jaw (so that it is recognized by the mother at an early stage of life during the act of sucking). This retraction increases on deviating the jaw away from the affected eye and decreases on deviating the jaw towards the affected side. The condition is probably the result of an abnormal nervous connection between the oculomotor nerve serving the levator muscle and the motor part of the trigeminal nerve. As a general rule the phenomenon becomes less obvious when the child becomes older, and operative treatment is seldom if ever indicated because it would necessitate the elimination of levator function by a myectomy (to avoid the retraction of the lid) and subsequent correction of the persistent ptosis using the frontalis muscle in a brow suspension procedure; this tends to give an asymmetrical appearance to the upper eyelids and logically would necessitate similar surgical procedures on the unaffected upper lid.

The detection of ptosis is obvious on simple inspection of the eyelids. Assessment of the degree of levator function demands the prevention of any upwards movement of the eyebrow by pressing on it with the finger so that the frontalis muscle is not allowed to exert an indirect elevating influence on the lid.

Treatment. The surgical correction of congenital ptosis is seldom carried out before the age of four years unless the ptosis is sufficient to prevent the development of central vision; after that age it is easier to assess the extent of the operation because in the early years of life there may be some degree of spontaneous improvement.

The choice of operation depends on the severity of the ptosis and the degree of levator function. For a mild ptosis (2 mm) with good levator function (more than 10 mm excursion from extreme down gaze to extreme up gaze), a posterior approach to remove the upper border of the tarsal plate and part of Müller's muscle and the adjacent conjunctiva is satisfactory (*Fasanella–Servat operation*). Moderate and severe ptosis require some form of levator muscle resection, a posterior approach (*Blaskovic operation*) through the conjunctiva if the levator function is fair (6 to 10 mm) thus preserving the skin crease, or an anterior approach (*Everbusch operation*) through the skin if the levator function is poor, with the creation of an artificial skin crease. If the levator function is less than 3 mm, a brow suspension technique is employed where strips of fascia lata provide a link between the frontalis muscle and the upper tarsus so that the patient raises the eyebrow to reduce ptosis.

Distichiasis

Rarely the Meibomian glands fail to develop and are replaced by extra rows of eyelashes which turn inwards so that they rub on the cornea. They should be removed by electrolysis puncture or by cryotherapy which destroys the follicles of the aberrant eyelashes.

Injuries

Lacerations

A laceration requires immediate suturing to ensure healing of the lid without subsequent structural deformity; this applies particularly when the lid margin is involved , because unless great care is exercised in suturing the cut ends into perfect apposition the lid margin becomes notched, which may subsequently interfere with the tear film.

Burns

A superficial burn is treated simply by eliminating any infective agent with an application of cetrimide 1% lotion to the affected area and then applying some form of antibiotic cream until healing is complete. A severe burn involving a large area of the lid or its whole thickness demands urgent and effective treatment because the exposure of the eye which follows the failure of the lid to protect the eye may result in

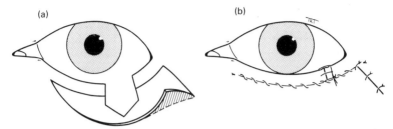

Fig. 47. Correction of lid laxity. (a) Pentagonal excision of full-thickness lid. (b) Wound closure.

serious damage to the eye. A tarsorrhaphy may provide sufficient protection, but an early plastic repair is the most satisfactory procedure.

Abnormal positions of the lid margins

The integrity of the eye is dependent to some extent on a correct positional relationship between the margins of the eyelid, particularly the upper one, and the eyeball. This is upset in two conditions— *ectropion* and *entropion*.

Ectropion

In this condition the lid margin is everted so that it fails to be in contact with the surface of the eye, with exposure of the palpebral conjunctiva and persistent epiphora. It may be produced in two main different ways.

Atonic conditions

A marked weakness of the orbicularis oculi muscle occurs in facial palsy, with a sagging and ectropion of the lower lid, usually termed *lagophthalmos* because of the inability to close the eyelids properly. An atonic condition of the skin and the underlying pretarsal orbicularis muscle in the elderly, leading to horizontal lid lengthening, also predisposes to the development of ectropion, which is increased by the tendency for the patient to wipe the lower lid persistently in a lateral direction because of an associated epiphora. The treatment of this type of ectropion depends on its severity. A true lagophthalmos may be lessened by realigning and reapposing the lower lid to the globe by shortening the lateral and medial canthal ligaments, by decreasing the extent of the palpebral aperture by a lateral tarsorrhaphy (a union of the lateral part of the upper and lower eyelid margins) or by supporting the lower lid with a fascial sling. A senile ectropion may be relieved by a full-thickness resection of part of the lid to reduce the horizontal laxity (Fig.47). When the ectropion is of small degree and confined to its medial part so that epiphora is the main symptom, it is relieved simply by opening the punctum and the adjacent part of the canaliculus (three-snip operation), usually in conjunction with a cauterization of the adjacent palpebral conjunctiva to try and appose the lid to the eyeball. Marked medial ectropion demands a lid-shortening procedure with a diamond-shaped excision of the tarsus immediately below the inferior punctum.

Cicatricial conditions

The occurrence of scarring in the eyelids following trauma (e.g. gunshot wounds, burns), severe inflammation or previously treated neoplastic disease may cause an ectropion of the upper or lower lids. Treatment involves excision of the scar tissue and restoration of the defective area by a skin graft, deriving maximum benefit from the remaining skin by the use of a Z-plasty.

Entropion

In this condition either the upper or lower lid margin is inverted so that the lashes rub against the eyeball, causing irritation and discharge and sometimes fine abrasions of the cornea which may lead to ulceration.

Lower lid entropion

Congenital. A simulated form of entropion may occur in early childhood when the fold of skin which is present immediately below the lower eyelid margin is unduly prominent (*epiblepharon*) so that on a downward movement of the eye the lid margin becomes inverted and the lashes rub on the cornea causing discomfort. The condition usually resolves spontaneously, but in severe cases the fold of skin may be excised (without any removal of the underlying orbicularis oculi muscle) and the edges of the wound united with fine silk sutures.

Spastic entropion. Spasm of the orbicularis oculi, which accompanies the irritation of any inflammatory condition of the surface of the eye or follows a simple bandaging of the eye, may cause an entropion of the lower lid, particularly in an elderly person who has a loss of the normal elasticity of the connective tissues of the lower lid. The entropion is often relieved simply by removing the cause of the irritation, or as a temporary measure by applying a strip of adhesive tape from the lid margin towards the cheek, or by inserting everting sutures through the conjunctiva below the tarsal plate which are made to emerge and tied just beneath the lash line.

Involutional or senile entropion. With age a number of degenerative changes take place in the orbit, eyelid muscles, and tendons and tarsal plate. Atrophy of the retro-ocular fat leads to enophthalmos, the lower lid retractor muscle (inferior palpebral muscle of Müller) lengthens allowing freer movement of a less rigid tarsal plate, while the orbicularis muscle and tarsal plate become stretched. All these combine to produce a relative increase in the horizontal length of the lid margin which therefore lacks stability.

Everting sutures correct minor cases, but a more logical approach is to reverse the lid laxity by performing a lid-shortening procedure which entails a full-thickness removal of a section of lid appropriate for good apposition of the remaining lid margin (Fig. 47). This may be combined with everting sutures. However, if failure of the lid retractor is the fault, as judged by no deepening of the inferior fornix on downward gaze, a tarsal fracturing technique is used, whereby a full-thickness incision is made through the lid 4 to 5 mm from and parallel to the lid margin; the combination of everting sutures and dense scar tissue formation maintains correct lid position. When there is lid laxity and a failure of the retractor, a horizontal lid-shortening procedure and a tarsal fracture are performed simultaneously.

Cicatricial entropion. An entropion may follow any form of scarring of the lid (traumatic, inflammatory or neoplastic) and as there is less tissue to manipulate, special plastic surgical techniques using skin, mucous membrane and tarsal grafts are employed.

Upper lid entropion

This follows cicatrizing disease of the conjunctiva and tarsus, whether infective—such as trachoma, adenovirus or staphylococcal disease—or immunological—such as mucous membrane pemphigoid or the ocular sequelae of erythema multiforme— or from injuries, particularly chemical. It is potentially more serious than lower lid entropion because of the great excursion of the lid margin, which may have metaplastic lashes or keratinization of the conjunctival epithelium, with adverse effects on the corneal surface. In a worldwide context, entropion is a major factor in the pathway to blindness because the associated ocular discharge attracts eye-seeking flies which transmit both the agent of trachoma (*Chlamydia*) and also bacteria responsible for acute corneal infection. The entropion must be carefully assessed prior to surgery, with particular attention to severity, the degree of lid margin keratinization, the bulk of the tarsal plate and the presence of deep tarsal disease inducing lid retraction.

Treatment by rotation of the lashes and the keratinized conjunctiva away from the globe may be done through the skin or through the

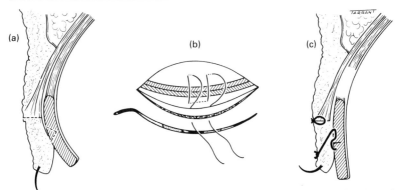

Fig. 48. Correction of upper lid entropion. (a) Lid margin split; excision of horizontal wedge from tarsal plate. (b) Position of everting sutures. (c) Disinsertion of Müller's muscle to advance the posterior lamella; tractional tarsal suture everts the anterior lamella.

conjunctiva, usually with a splitting of the lid into anterior and posterior lamellae at the grey line to facilitate rotation, with special care to avoid lid retraction which may lead to exposure, by disinserting Müller's muscle from the upper border of the tarsal plate (Fig. 48).

Abnormal movements of the eyelids

Blepharospasm

Spasm of the eyelids may occur in any inflammatory condition of the eye, particularly when there is photophobia, so that it is an exaggeration of the normal protective mechanism of the eye. It occurs sometimes on attempting to examine the eye in children and may then be associated with an eversion of the lids so that the conjunctival surfaces of the lids become exposed, thus preventing any view of the eyeball; in babies it is sometimes necessary to open the lids with a special retractor. The condition of *essential blepharospasm*, a progressive and bilateral disorder of involuntary repetitive firm closure of the lids, is an uncommon but cosmetically and socially disabling disorder (occasionally unilateral), for which avulsion of the branch of the facial nerve supplying the orbicularis muscle is the only reasonable means of achieving a long-term remission, although such a procedure has no influence on the underlying cause of the blepharospasm which is probably a disorder of the basal ganglia. Blepharospasm is also a feature of other extrapyramidal disorders, particularly Parkinson's disease.

Myokymia

This refers to fine rhythmical contractions of an involuntary nature which occur from time to time within a small portion of the orbicularis muscle of either lid. There is a marked subjective awareness of this phenomenon, but the contractions are scarcely visible on inspection. It is essentially a functional condition which is produced by fatigue and eyestrain. Rarely these involuntary movements are more marked and widespread, as in a tic, which is sometimes associated with trigeminal neuralgia (tic doloureux).

Ptosis and lid retraction

Acquired ptosis

Ptosis (drooping of the upper lid) is commonly a congenital anomaly (p.193), but it may also be an acquired condition.

Myasthenia gravis

Ptosis is often a presenting feature of this autoimmune disorder of voluntary muscle in which acetylcholine receptor antibodies block the normal transmission of efferent motor impulses across the myoneural junction. Presenting in young adults and more often in females, the condition has strong associations with disorders of the thymus—10% have a thymoma, while 70% have thymic hyperplasia. Other muscles may also be involved, for example the extrinsic ocular muscles, the pharyngeal muscles, and more rarely the skeletal muscles. The disease runs a progressive course, often with apparent remissions and characteristically with an increase of the condition at times of fatigue, so that it is more obvious towards the end of the day. Ocular myasthenia occurs in the majority of patients at some time. It affects the levator and extrinsic ocular muscles, occasionally with signs that may mimic disorders of the brain stem, and is brought out by fatiguing the affected muscles. It is invariably associated with orbicularis muscle weakness and over-excursion of the upper lid following rapid vertical movement from down gaze to the primary position (Cogan's sign) is usually present. Myasthenia is a clinical diagnosis; the administration of the short-acting anticholinesterase edrophonium chloride (Tensilon)—which produces a temporary amelioration of the paresis—is only rarely required, and must only be done in the presence of resuscitation facilities.

A myasthenic syndrome may occur with carcinoma, usually of the bronchus, as part of autoimmune thyroid disorders or related to drugs such as penicillamine and the aminoglycoside antibiotics. Such cases rarely present with ocular signs, do not have acetylcholine receptor antibodies and rarely respond to edrophonium.

Treatment. Anticholinesterases, such as neostigmine or the longer acting pyridostigmine, are the mainstay of treatment and are usually sufficient for the purely ocular form of the disease. More widespread muscular involvement benefits from thymectomy, steroids and immunosuppression, but the effects of plasmapheresis tend to be short-lived.

Horner's syndrome

A small degree of ptosis follows paresis of the smooth muscle of the upper lid as the result of involvement of the cervical sympathetic nerve in any part of its long course from hypothalamus, through the dorsolateral brain stem, synapsing in the upper thoracic spinal cord and then passing in close relation to the apex of the lung to the superior cervical ganglion, where it makes a final synapse before being distributed to the face and orbit in company with the branches of the internal carotid artery. The ptosis is associated with a slight narrowing of the palpebral aperture. This accounts for the suggestion of some degree of enophthalmos, but this is a false impression. There is also some constriction of the pupil (*miosis*) because of loss of tone in the dilator muscle of the pupil, and decreased sweating of the affected side of the face. The site of the lesion is usually determined by the associated clinical features; lesions may be due to syringomyelia, poliomyelitis, multiple sclerosis, vascular or neoplastic diseases of the brain stem, tumours of the apex of the lung, or trauma to the side of the neck.

Pharmacological tests of denervation hypersenitivity can distinguish between pre- and postganglionic sympathetic lesions. Classically, the lack of monoaminoxidase in postganglionic lesions allows weak sympathomimetic drugs such as adrenaline 1/1000 to dilate the pupil (with no effect on the normally innervated pupil), and conversely prevents the dilator action of cocaine which requires mono-aminoxidase for its action. Sometimes, however, the responses are equivocal and more accurate information is gained by using phenylephrine 1% or hydroxyamphetamine.

Neurogenic lesions

Any lesion of the oculomotor nerve (third cranial nerve) (p.255) may be associated with ptosis. Rarely the Marcus Gunn phenomenon (p.193) may occur as an acquired condition.

Myopathic lesions

Ptosis is a characteristic feature of an ocular myopathy (*progressive external ophthalmoplegia*, p.262), and it may occur in myotonic dystrophy, although cataract (p.178) is the more usual ocular complication. The ptosis which occurs in thyrotrophic exophthalmos (*exophthalmic ophthalmoplegia*) may be the result of changes within the levator muscle, but it is also mechanical because of swelling of the upper eyelid (p.291).

Mechanical lesions

Any abnormal tissue within the upper lid which increases its bulk (e.g. haemorrhage, oedema, trachomatous scarring, neoplastic deposits) may cause ptosis.

Traumatic lesions

Ptosis which follows trauma is usually the result of involvement of the oculomotor nerve or of the cervical sympathetic nerve, but the levator muscle may be affected directly by a traumatic lesion of the upper lid, for example following the surgical exploration of the upper part of the orbit.

Treatment

This is essentially treatment of the condition which is causing the ptosis; correction of the ptosis by operation (p.194) is less frequent than in the congenital form of the condition. Sometimes spectacles with a metal crutch which presses backwards against the junction of the palpebral and orbital parts of the upper lid are of value, but they tend to cause discomfort. A special form of haptic contact lens which supports the upper eyelid is more effective.

Lid retraction

Lid retraction is discussed on p.289 in relation to endocrine exophthalmos.

Inflammatory conditions

Blepharitis

It is customary to consider two types of blepharitis, squamous or non-ulcerative and ulcerative, but the marked decrease in ulcerative cases in recent years is an indication that to a large extent they merely represent cases of non-ulcerative blepharitis in which there is a secondary infection; this is usually avoided by the use of topical antibiotics. The squamous type is characterized by hyperaemia of the lid margins, some swelling and redness of the eyelids, fine powdery deposits or scales on the eyelashes, and sometimes by a tendency for increased loss of the eyelashes. It is usually chronic and the abnormal changes are accentuated by a tendency to rub the eyelids. It is essentially a seborrhoeic condition, hence its increased incidence in childhood, particularly in early adolescence, but it may also be induced by constant exposure to an irritant such as smoke or cosmetics. The occurrence of secondary infection, usually of a staphylococcal nature, increases the severity of the condition with obvious sepsis in the region of the eyelashes; in the later stages permanent distortions (*trichiasis*) of the eyelashes may cause some of them to rub on the cornea with increased irritation of the eyes and the development of corneal ulceration. It is obvious that the ulcerative form of blepharitis is prone to occur in dirty surroundings and in conditions of malnutrition, or in association with other diseases, such as the exanthemata, when there is a lowered resistance to infection so that its incidence is greatest in childhood. A hypersensitivity response to *Staphylococcus* probably accounts for much of the chronic low-grade inflammatory conjunctival response in these patients.

Blepharitis may sometimes be associated with dermatitis (eczema) of the eyelids; this may be of an infective or allergic nature. Acne rosacea is invariably associated with blepharitis.

Treatment. The immediate treatment consists of maintaining the eyelid margins as free as possible from discharge, powdery deposits or scales by the application of cottonwool soaked in a bland lotion like saline, and the elimination of any secondary infection by the use of an appropriate antibiotic ointment; the isolation of the infective agent and an assessment of its sensitivity to various antibiotics determines the particular drug used. The elimination of any associated dermatitis or seborrhoeic condition of the face and scalp is also of value. Weak topical steroids help to reduce the hypersensitivity response. The long-term treatment is aimed at eliminating conditions of poor hygiene and malnutrition which foster its continuance. Ingrowing eyelashes may be removed with epilation forceps, but they almost invariably regrow within a few weeks and it may be necessary to destroy the follicles of the offending lashes by electrolysis puncture or cryotherapy.

Infective dermatitis

The lids may be affected by a variety of infective agents: bacterial conditions such as furunculosis, sycosis barbae and impetigo contagiosum; fungal conditions such as tinea (ringworm) and actinomycosis; parasitic conditions such as the crab louse, scabies and myiasis (fly maggots); and viral conditions such as herpes simplex, herpes zoster ophthalmicus, verruca, and molluscum contagiosum can all affect the eyelids. Dermatitis of the eyelids is a feature of dermatomyositis (see p.134).

Herpes simplex. This is discussed on p.54.

Herpes zoster ophthalmicus. This unilateral condition causes a swelling of the eyelids, particularly the upper one, with a characteristic vesiculation of the skin and with similar involvement of the skin of the affected side of the face and scalp within the distribution of the ophthalmic division of the trigeminal nerve (fifth cranial nerve).

The other ocular complications are keratitis (p.56), uveitis (p.89), secondary glaucoma (p.314), internal ophthalmoplegia (p.103) and external ophthalmoplegia (p.254).

Verruca . This is an infective type of simple wart; it may be single or multiple on the eyelid, and particularly occurs near the lid margin.

Molluscum contagiosum. This viral condition forms a raised globular mass on the lid, which is usually single, but may be multiple, and occurs in the region of the lid margin where it may be obscured to some extent by the lashes. It has a characteristically umbilicated centre. This appearance may be suggestive of a basal cell carcinoma (rodent ulcer), but it lacks the nodularity which is evident on palpation of such a lesion. It is commonly associated with a mild but chronic follicular conjunctivitis with superficial punctate keratitis which does not respond to antibiotic treatment. Incision of the lesion with curettage of the contents, which show numerous eosinophilic inclusion bodies, cures the condition.

Allergic dermatitis

The lids are prone to be affected by external agents which produce an allergic response resulting in a moist eczema and oedematous swelling. There are many such irritants, for example drugs such as atropine, cosmetics such as mascara and nail varnish (which is transferred to the eyelids from the fingernails by rubbing the eyes), various chemicals used in industry, various metallic substances such as nickel (which characteristically causes the 'spectacle' form of dermatitis because of its use in some spectacle frames), and plants such as *Primula*. The lids may also show an allergic response in certain systemic conditions such as the ingestion of shellfish in hypersensitive individuals.

Treatment. The main aim of treatment is to eliminate the offending agent. The local reaction may be relieved by the administration of topical steroids, but sometimes antihistamine drugs are necessary to combat the condition.

Stye (external hordeolum)

This is an infective condition of the follicle of the eyelash or its associated sebaceous glands of Zeis. It is usually acute, with considerable pain and tenderness of the eyelid. The affected part of the lid margin becomes swollen, red and tense with the production of a yellow 'head' which points along the line of an eyelash before finally discharging its purulent contents, and there is a surrounding oedematous reaction. Sometimes a stye may be chronic; recurrent styes may be associated with blepharitis as part of a seborrhoeic diathesis.

Treatment. The most effective treatment is to hasten its discharge by the application of heat, usually in the form of hot spoon bathings; this involves the use of a large wooden spoon (wooden simply because the handle of a metal spoon becomes too hot to hold) to which a large wad of cottonwool is attached by a bandage and, after dipping it into a bowl of boiling water, the pad is gradually brought near the eye (which is kept closed) so that the steam from the pad circulates around the eye; when the pad is sufficiently cool, it is held against the eye. This process is repeated several times over a period of 10 to 15 minutes. Rarely it is necessary to incise the stye at the lid margin to facilitate the discharge of the pus.

Chalazion (internal hordeolum or meibomian cyst)

This is an enlarged tarsal gland resulting from an accumulation of its sebaceous products because of a failure of their expulsion through the tarsal duct owing to some obstruction by foreign material such as a particle of dirt. The affected gland ceases to enlarge after a few days or weeks because the accumulated material obliterates the formative basal cells of the gland. The cyst usually forms a round painless projection on the conjunctival surface of the lid or a pouting of the blocked duct on the lid margin. Subsequently the cyst becomes organized with the formation of a relatively solid mass. Sometimes a carcinoma may show a similar appearance. More rarely there is secondary infection of the cyst with the production of pain and oedema of the surrounding parts of the lid. This oedema is particularly marked when the infected tarsal cyst lies near the lateral or medial canthus; in this situation the cyst may be difficult to palpate, although its presence is determined by an area of tenderness on gentle prodding with a glass rod. A generalized infective condition of the tarsal glands *(meibomianitis)* is sometimes associated with blepharitis and acne rosacea.

Treatment. Sometimes a chalazion subsides spontaneously within a few weeks, but usually it is necessary to evacuate its contents by curettage after making a vertical incision over the conjunctival surface of the cyst,which is secured by a special clamp. In long-standing cases it is also necessary to excise part of the thickened wall, but care should be taken to retain the overlying conjunctiva so that a mass of scar tissue on the inner surface of the lid is avoided. The excised tissue should be examined histologically if there is any suggestion of malignancy; this certainly should be carried out when the lesion recurs after a short interval.

Cysts

Cyst of Moll

A cyst of Moll is a small translucent cyst at the lid margin which protrudes in the region of an eyelash. Simple puncture is usually followed by recurrence and the cyst should be excised.

Sebaceous cyst

Sebaceous cysts may assume different forms in the eyelid; a simple cyst of one of the sebaceous glands of the skin is excised in the usual way if sufficiently large and the multiple small white spots which are slightly elevated above the surface level (milia) may be shelled out if necessary. The conditions which may arise in the specialized sebaceous glands (glands of Zeis and tarsal glands) are discussed above.

Tumours

Papilloma

This is a benign wart which may assume various forms: usually it appears as a raised vascular mass, but it may remain relatively flat, particularly in the elderly person. Rarely it becomes pigmented. Sometimes a cutaneous horn may form on its surface. It may be treated by simple excision.

Angioma

This is a benign malformation of the blood vessels of the skin. It may appear as a bright red area owing to a proliferation of capillary vessels (*capillary angioma* or *telangiectasis*) or as a blue-coloured area due to the formation of abnormal venous channels (*cavernous angioma*). An angioma of the eyelid may be associated with a similar condition of the face (*'port-wine' stain*) or with angiomas elsewhere (as in the Sturge–Weber syndrome, p.149). An angioma of the lid in a baby is often noticed first when the child cries, because it then becomes larger.

Treatment is seldom indicated in the young child, unless the angioma is sufficiently large to prevent adequate opening of the eye so that stimulus deprivation amblyopia is likely to occur, because an angioma almost invariably becomes less obvious as the child grows older; the extent of spontaneous regression can be assessed simply in the young child by the degree of blanching which occurs on gentle pressure over the lesion with a glass lens. Surgical treatment using the cutting diathermy is the treatment of choice to reduce the excessive bulk and secondary ptosis of the lid.

Xanthelasma

This is a benign disorder of lipid deposition which develops in the unicellular sebaceous glands present in the medial parts of the upper and lower eyelids with the formation of several yellowish, slightly raised masses. They may be removed by simple excision for cosmetic reasons. It is commonly a familial condition, but onset in early adult life merits investigation of lipid and cholesterol metabolism.

Molluscum sebaceum (keratoacanthoma)

This is a benign condition but develops with alarming rapidity and may simulate a squamous cell carcinoma clinically because of its destructive nature and also sometimes histologically. The centre of the lesion is characteristically excavated and filled with keratin. Treatment is by excisional biopsy.

Carcinoma

Malignant tumours of the eyelids assume different forms:

Squamous cell carcinoma (epithelioma). This may arise spontaneously or rarely as a result of malignant change in a papilloma. It causes a localized nodular tumour which eventually breaks down centrally to form an area of ulceration with destruction of the affected tissues of the lid. It is liable occasionally to form metastases. It may masquerade as squamous blepharitis or a recurrent chalazion.

Basal cell carcinoma (rodent ulcer). This is the commonest form of carcinoma of the eyelid and occurs characteristically at the lid margin, particularly of the lower lid, or in the skin around the medial canthus. It forms a nodular lesion which readily and repeatedly breaks down, with crust formations in its central ulcerated zone. The surrounding nodular part of the lesion gradually spreads with extensive involvement and destruction of the neighbouring tissues, but without any tendency to form metastases.

Basosquamous carcinoma. Clinically it is sometimes difficult to distinguish between the squamous cell and basal cell types of carcinoma, and it is not surprising, therefore, that an intermediate form exists which shows features of both types.

Intraepithelial carcinoma (Bowen's disease). This is a rare form of carcinoma of the lid and is discussed in relation to the conjunctiva on p.40.

Treatment of carcinoma. In all cases of suspected carcinoma the histological examination of a biopsy specimen is essential; this routine procedure avoids the erroneous identification of some of these lesions as, for example, chalazion or molluscum sebaceum. The surgical excision of a lid carcinoma involves removal of sufficient surrounding healthy tissue to ensure complete removal of the lesion. This is a difficult task when the carcinoma involves the whole thickness of the lid or the region of the lid margin and it may be necessary to carry out elaborate plastic procedures to repair the defect in the lid after the removal of the tumour. In some of these cases, irradiation may provide a more satisfactory result.

Melanoma

The various forms of melanomas which involve the lid are discussed in relation to the conjunctiva on p.40.

Other conditions of the eyelids

Syphilitic conditions

A primary chancre of the eyelid presents as an acute inflammatory swelling with an associated preauricular and submaxillary adenitis in the primary stage of the disease. A skin rash may involve the eyelids in the secondary stage of the disease, and a gumma may involve the deeper tissues of the lid, particularly the tarsal plate (so that it mimics a chalazion), in the tertiary stage of the disease.

Oedematous conditions

Oedema of the eyelids is a common feature in a wide variety of conditions of the lids or of their adjacent structures, for example traumatic, inflammatory or allergic disorders. It is also a feature of any condition which causes an increased pressure within the orbit (such as endocrine exophthalmos or proptosis resulting from an orbital tumour), and of certain systemic conditions such as renal dysfunction or cardiac failure.

Blepharochalasis

Blepharochalasis is the term applied to the redundant folds of skin which occur sometimes in the upper lid and also, more rarely, in the lower lid, of the elderly person. It may be treated in certain cases by simple excision but usually its correction requires treatment of the whole skin of the face (the plastic operation of 'face-lift').

12

The Lacrimal Apparatus

Structure and function

The lacrimal apparatus consists of the structures concerned in the production and drainage of the tears.

The production of tears

Tear production occurs in the lacrimal gland, which lies in the upper and outer corner of the orbit in a recess immediately behind the orbital margin so that it is seldom possible to palpate the normal lacrimal gland. The main (or orbital) part of the gland (the *superior lobe*) is continuous behind with the smaller (or palpebral) part (the *inferior lobe*) which curves forwards to end in the region of the superior fornix. The tears, which are secreted in both parts of the lacrimal gland, pass into the eye via openings from the inferior lobe in the superior fornix; this secretion is regulated by the secreto-motor fibres of the greater superficial petrosal nerve which is derived from the facial nerve, and ultimately from the superior salivatory nucleus. There are also scattered nodules of lacrimal gland tissue (the *accessory lacrimal glands*) in various parts of the conjunctiva. It should be noted that tear formation is very scanty in the first few weeks of life and becomes reduced in advanced age. The lacrimal and accessory lacrimal glands produce the aqueous phase of the tear film, whilst the goblet cells of the conjunctiva produce the deep or mucous layer and the meibomian glands the superficial or oily layer.

Measurement of tear production

A rough guide to tear production is obtained using *Schirmer's test*— one end of a strip of filter paper (4 mm in width) is inserted into the lateral part of the inferior fornix of each eye with the main part of the paper projecting over the lid margin and down the cheek. The extent of the passage of tears down the paper is measured over a short period (up to five minutes). In normal eyes the rate of formation is very variable— sometimes it is most profuse because of the mechanical stimulus of the filter paper—but when it is less than 5 mm over a period of five minutes the flow may be regarded as subnormal.

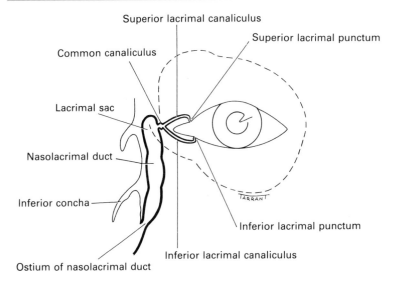

Fig. 49. The structures concerned with the drainage of tears.

The drainage of tears

This takes place along the lacrimal passages (Fig. 49), which are lined by a mucous membrane and are in continuity with the nasal mucous membrane so that they are liable to catarrhal affections.

The lacrimal puncta. There are two *puncta* (*superior* and *inferior*), one for each eyelid, which represent small circular openings on the lid margins near their medial ends. The upper punctum functions much less efficiently than the lower one for purely mechanical reasons.

The lacrimal canaliculi. Each punctum opens into a *canaliculus* which runs for a short distance vertically before passing horizontally in a medial direction to the region of the medial canthus, where the two canaliculi (*superior* and *inferior*) join to form the *common canaliculus*.

The lacrimal sac. The common canaliculus opens into the *lacrimal sac* which lies in a recess (the *lacrimal fossa*) between the most medial part of the lower orbital margin (the *anterior lacrimal crest*) and the *posterior lacrimal crest*.

The nasolacrimal duct. The lower part of the lacrimal sac is continuous with the *nasolacrimal duct* which passes downwards (and very slightly backwards and outwards) to open into the inferior meatus of the nose with a valvular mechanism at its opening. In the fetus the duct is initially a solid cord of cells which becomes canalized later; sometimes in the newborn there is a failure of this canalization or failure of the valvular mechanism at the opening of the duct to become effective, but usually these defects are only temporary.

The drainage of tears is an active process involving the lacrimal pump which is dependent on the integrity of the orbicularis oculi muscle of the eyelids: closure of the lids draws the lacrimal fluid from the puncta and canaliculi into the sac by a suction effect, and opening of the lids forces the lacrimal fluid from the sac into the nasolacrimal duct and then into the nose through the lower end of the duct, the valvular mechanism of which opens during this movement.

The main function of the tears is to maintain a normal degree of moisture of the eyes which is essential for the health of the surface tissues, particularly the cornea; lacrimal fluid is one of the constituents of the precorneal film (p.45). The tears also contain an enzyme (lysozyme) which has an important antibacterial effect so that, in the absence of any active inflammation, a culture of the conjunctival sac is often negative. There are several other antibacterial substances in the tear film, such as lactoferrin, immunoglobulins, and non-lysozymal enzymes. The presence of these enzymes determines the fact that repeated irrigations of the eye, which dilute their influence, are unwise procedures in any inflammatory condition, except to remove a copious discharge from behind the eyelids.

The patency of the lacrimal passage

The patency of the lacrimal passage is assessed by the following methods:

Syringing. This consists of irrigating the tear sac with saline after passing a cannula into the lower canaliculus through the lower punctum; the process is then repeated, passing a cannula through the upper punctum into the upper canaliculus. The entry of the cannula is facilitated by dilating the punctum and the early part of the canaliculus with a dilator (Nettleship's dilator). Free entry of the fluid into the nose (and into the throat when the patient is lying flat) implies patency of all the passages. No entry of fluid into the nose and regurgitation of fluid from both canaliculi implies some obstruction beyond the point of formation of the common canaliculus (i.e. in the lacrimal sac or nasolacrimal duct). No entry of fluid into the nose and regurgitation of fluid only from the canaliculus which is being syringed usually implies some obstruction in the canaliculus before the formation of the common canaliculus.

Radiographic examination. Irrigation of the lacrimal passages with a radiopaque substance such as Lipiodal provides a radiograph which gives an accurate picture of the site of obstruction.

Fluorescein test. The detection of fluorescein in the nasal secretions after instillation of the dye into the conjunctival sac is of diagnostic value provided the result is positive; a negative result is not conclusive evidence of an obstruction because the dye may fail to pass into the nose in sufficient quantities to be detected readily.

Excessive watering of the eyes

Excessive watering of the eyes may be the result of overabundant production of tears (lacrimation) or of failure of adequate drainage of the tears (epiphora).

Excessive lacrimation

This may be induced by any noxious stimulus of the eye such as inflammatory conditions (e.g. conjunctivitis, keratitis, uveitis), traumatic conditions (e.g. foreign bodies, chemical agents, ingrowing eyelashes) or closed-angle glaucoma, which all exert their effects by a reflex action relayed by afferent stimuli through the trigeminal nerve and then by efferent stimuli through the greater superficial petrosal nerve. It is also induced by excessive exposure to bright light, when the afferent part of the reflex is the afferent visual pathway. Excessive lacrimation also follows various emotional stimuli.

Epiphora

This occurs because of some failure of the adequate drainage of tears:

1. Failure of the punctum of the lower lid to lie in correct apposition to the eyeball, caused by ectropion or entropion of the lid; treatment involves rectification of the eyelid defect (see Chapter 11).
2. Failure of the patency of the punctum or canaliculus of the lower lid. This may be simply due to a small foreign particle or an eyelash, so that the epiphora is relieved by removal of the obstruction. It may also be the result of an accumulation of infective material, usually in the form of fungi (actinomyces) which proliferate to form a thick yellowish-white cheese-like material; the epiphora is relieved by removing the infective material, if necessary after opening the punctum and the associated part of the canaliculus (the *'three-snip' operation*), and by

treating the affected epithelium with silver nitrate 1% or weak iodine. Canalicular stenosis may follow infection with herpes simplex virus or *Chlamydia trachomatis*. It also follows injury of the medial part of the lower lid which involves the punctum or canaliculus directly or sometimes indirectly as the result of a later reparative fibrosis; fibrosis of the punctum may respond to a 'three-snip' operation, but fibrosis of the canaliculus requires more elaborate surgical treatment (see below). Sometimes, however, it is possible to prevent this fibrosis by a plastic repair performed shortly after the injury; for example, severance of the lower canaliculus may be repaired by inserting a nylon thread into the cut ends of the canaliculus, if it is possible to identify them, before suturing the torn lid. The thread is subsequently removed once healing is complete and this necessitates leaving the free end of the thread beyond the punctum at the time of the operation. Damage to the punctum is usually easier to repair.

3. Failure of the lacrimal sac and nasolacrimal duct to drain the tears as a result of some form of obstruction.

Congenital stenosis of the nasolacrimal duct

Failure of the nasolacrimal duct to become canalized or failure of the valvular mecahnism at the lower end of the duct to become effective results in an accumulation of the lacrimal and conjunctival secretions within the sac; this stenosis is liable to foster the occurrence of infection (*dacryocystitis*). Sometimes the infective element is the primary and not the secondary event so that a narrow but patent duct may become blocked by the occurrence of inflammatory changes in its mucous membrane. The regurgitation of the contents (mucous, mucopurulent or purulent) of the lacrimal sac into the conjunctival sac is associated with conjunctivitis. The condition is sometimes unilateral.

Treatment. The control of any infective element by local antibiotics (as for conjunctivitis, see p.31) is the first essential, and this may relieve the obstruction in the duct permitting its final canalization. This process may be aided by instructing the mother to press on the lacrimal sac (pressure on the skin of the most medial part of the lower lid immediately behind the anterior lacrimal crest) in the hope of expressing the contents of the sac down the nasolacrimal duct. If the obstruction persists, it is necessary to relieve the obstruction. This may be achieved by simple syringing with saline through the punctum of the lower eyelid, particularly if the cannula is inserted just beyond the common canaliculus to achieve a more forcible entry of the fluid into the duct; this manoeuvre also serves to verify that the lower canaliculus is not the site of the obstruction. If the syringing fails to relieve the obstruction, a fine lacrimal probe should be passed down the length of the nasolacrimal duct, approaching it by way of the upper punctum and upper canaliculus; this route is favoured because the probe may damage the epithelial lining of the canaliculus leading to the development of an obstruction, an unfortunate complication in the lower canaliculus but of much less importance in the upper one. The majority of cases recanalize spontaneously by the age of six months, so that intervention prior to this time is seldom necessary. If the obstruction persists after six months, syringing and usually also probing is carried out under a short general anaesthetic.

Dacryocystitis

This may occur in the infant, as described above, but is usually a disease of adults, particularly after middle age and in the female. Infection of the tear sac may arise from direct spread of infective material from the conjunctiva into the sac or from retrograde spread of infective material from the nasopharynx, but it is usually the result of infection following stagnation of tears within the lacrimal sac as the result of an obstruction of the lower end of the lacrimal sac where it joins the nasolacrimal duct or within the duct, particularly in an area of narrowing in conjunction with some catarrhal swelling of the mucous lining of the duct. This causes an accumulation of pus or mucopus within the tear sac which regurgitates into the conjunctival sac through the canaliculi and puncta, particularly after pressure over the lacrimal sac. Rapid control of the infection by local and systemic antibiotics may relieve the obstruction, although it may be necessary after the resolution of the acute stage to obtain proper patency by syringing of the sac. Sometimes the obstruction at the lower end of the sac persists, with the development of a distended sac (a *mucocele*) which contains a mucous type of fluid, often without any infective constituent.

If the lacrimal sac is extensively involved in the infection, and particularly if the infection is prolonged (so-called *chronic dacryocystitis*), the sac becomes shrunken because of fibrosis. In other cases chronic infection of the sac is followed by acute dacryocystitis. This presents suddenly with a tense swelling which projects from the lacrimal fossa with redness and oedema of the overlying and surrounding skin. It may respond to intensive treatment with systemic antibiotics, but sometimes there is abscess formation with subsequent discharge of pus spontaneously of after incision; in either event the obstruction at the lower end of the sac is unrelieved and the sac remains infected. Chronic dacryocystitis is usually associated with recurrent conjunctivitis and even sometimes with a septic type of keratitis; it may be of particular danger in an intraocular operation because it predisposes to purulent endophthalmitis, but this is a less likely complication in the antibiotic era.

Treatment. The obstruction of the nasolacrimal duct is very seldom relieved by a probing, except as discussed above in the early months of life, and any occasional success is usually only short-lived. The removal of the tear sac (*dacryocystectomy*) may be advised after acute dacryocystitis to prevent further infection, but this does not relieve the epiphora; the main indication for such an operation is in the elderly patient who is not fit for general anaesthesia; sometimes the subsequent epiphora is not unduly troublesome because of the natural reduction of tear production in old age. The most effective treatment is to perform an anastomosis between the medial half of the lacrimal sac and the nasal mucosa which lines the middle meatus of the nose (*dacryocystorhinostomy*). Stenosis of the lower canaliculus is difficult to relieve surgically, but an effective method is to break down the obstruction by a probe during the conduct of a dacryocystorhinostomy and then to pass one end of a thin plastic tube from the opened tear sac into the lower canaliculus, out of the lower punctum, into the upper punctum and along the upper canaliculus to the sac where it is then passed, with the other end of the tube, through the opening in the nasal mucosa to the lower part of the nose just behind the nostril; if possible this tube is retained for several weeks or even months to ensure the patency of the previously obstructed canaliculus, with subsequent repeated syringings for a few weeks. Canalicular stenosis near the entrance to the lacrimal sac requires open dissection under microscopic control.

Carcinoma of the lacrimal sac

This may occur as a primary event or due to spread of a carcinoma from the neighbouring nasopharynx. It causes epiphora because it results in obstruction of the sac or duct. The extent of the lesion may be determined by radiographic examinations and by surgical exposure (which will also provide material for a biopsy examination), but postoperative irradiation is necessary because the diffuse nature of the lesion usually prevents its complete removal.

Diminished watering of the eyes

A diminished supply of tears is the result of two main conditions: (a) a reduction in the formation of tears; or (b) a decreased ability of the tears to reach the eye. A reduction in the formation of tears occurs in any destructive process of the lacrimal gland, such as tumour formations, inflammatory conditions, atrophic conditions such as Sjogren's disease—although sometimes this reduction is preceded by a short period of increased tear formation—or in any defect of the afferent part of the lacrimation reflex because of impairment of the trigeminal nerve. A decreased ability of the tears to reach the eye occurs in any severe chronic inflammation of the conjunctiva that causes obstruction of the channels which are concerned in the passage of tears into the conjunctival sac from the lacrimal gland, such as trachoma, mucous membrane pemphigoid or Stevens-Johnson syndrome, or sometimes as a result of trauma such as a lime burn, which particularly affects the accessory lacrimal glands. Impairment of tear secretion may be an early sign of cerebello-pontine angle tumours, which interefere with the secreto-motor supply to the lacrimal gland.

Riley-Day syndrome (familial dysautonomia)

This condition becomes evident in infancy, usually occurring in the Jewish child, with difficulty in swallowing, recurrent respiratory infections and failure to thrive. There is a marked tendency to dehydration with excessive perspiration, but characteristically with an absence of tears which may lead to corneal ulceration. There is impaired corneal sensation and hypersensitivity of the pupil to cholinergic drops such as pilocarpine.

Treatment. The eyes should be kept moist with artificial tears (methylcellulose drops); recently hydrogel contact lenses have also proved to be of value in protecting the cornea.

Disorders of the lacrimal gland

Dacryoadenitis

Acute dacryoadenitis

This causes a painful swelling of the lacrimal gland which becomes easily palpable and is associated with considerable oedema of the overlying part of the upper lid. Abscess formation is rare. Rarely it is the result of a local ocular infection. Sometimes it is a feature of mumps, infectious mononucleosis, sarcoidosis or gonococcal disease.

Chronic dacryoadenitis

This causes a painless swelling of the lacrimal gland and usually has a granulomatous origin (e.g. tuberculosis, sarcoidosis). Sometimes both lacrimal glands are involved together with the salivary glands and this symptom complex is termed *Mikulicz's syndrome* (p.92). Ultimately the condition may regress spontaneously, but sometimes a granulomatous response may mask a malignant condition of the gland.

Tumours

These are not common. Benign mixed tumour and adenoid cystic carcinoma constitute the majority of such tumours, and metastatic deposits may occur.

Benign mixed tumour

Known as mixed because it often contains mesenchymal as well as epithelial elements, this tumour affects middle-aged persons. They present with a long history, usually more than 12 months, of a painless swelling of the upper lid with displacement of the globe (*proptosis*) in a forwards and downwards direction, often showing a limitation of movement, particularly on elevation, with consequent diplopia. There is usually radiological evidence of enlargement or destruction of bone in the lacrimal fossa. Because incomplete removal of such a neoplasm often leads to recurrences with definite potential for malignant change, biopsy is not performed and the tumour is removed in its capsule in toto.

Adenoid cystic carcinoma

This is an aggressive epithelial carcinoma presenting, again in middle age, but with a short history of swelling and proptosis accompanied by boring pain, which probably testifies to its propensity for periosteal and neural invasion. Because of the short history, radiological signs may be absent, but local bony sclerosis or destruction in the region of the gland may be evident. Some of these tumours have areas of calcification. The decision to carry out a biopsy therefore depends on the length and pattern of the history, associated signs and radiological findings. Confirmation of adenoid cystic carcinoma demands local excision via a lateral orbitotomy, with exenteration of the orbital contents if there is failure to respond to irradiation. The prognosis is poor but those with intracranial extension may benefit from chemotherapy.

The reticuloses

More rarely the lacrimal gland may be involved in one of the reticuloses (such as lymphoma, lymphosarcoma and leukaemia), sometimes as an isolated event (particularly in the elderly), but at other times in association with general manifestations of the disorder. The localized lesions usually respond to irradiation, but if the lesions become widespread some form of general anticancer therapy (cytotoxic drugs, chemotherapy) is necessary to try and control the disease.

Cysts

These are essentially retention cysts of the lacrimal gland fluid and occur most often in the palpebral part of the gland so that they are visible in the superior fornix after eversion of the upper lid. Simple incision usually only gives a temporary effect, and excision of the whole cyst is necessary to avoid recurrence.

13

The Extrinsic Ocular Muscles

Structure and function

There are six extrinsic ocular muscles concerned with the rotatory movements of each eye (*uniocular movements*). These movements take place around a variable centre of rotation and are distinct from *translatory movements*, which represent movements of the eye from side to side, up and down, and backwards and forwards in the absence of any rotation.

Lateral rectus

This arises near the apex of the orbit and passes forwards on the lateral side of the eye to be inserted on the lateral surface of the sclera in front of the equator of the eyeball. It runs in the horizontal meridian of the eye and rotates the eye outwards (abduction) (Fig. 50).

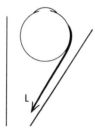

Fig. 50. The action of the right lateral rectus muscle (L) in the primary position (abduction).

Medial rectus

This arises near the apex of the orbit and passes forwards on the medial side of the eye to be inserted on the medial surface of the sclera in front of the equator. It runs in the horizontal meridian of the eye and rotates the eye inwards (adduction) (Fig. 51).

Superior rectus

This arises near the apex of the orbit and passes forwards and outwards above the eye to be inserted on the upper surface of the sclera in front

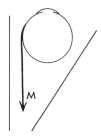

Fig. 51.   The action of the right medial rectus (M) in the primary position (adduction).

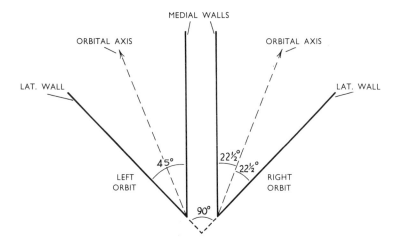

Fig. 52.   The direction of the orbital axes.

of the equator. It runs in the line of the orbital axis (Fig. 52) thus forming an angle (usually regarded as 23°) with the vertical meridian of the eye in the primary position. (The primary position is the position of the eye when it is directed straight ahead, so that there is an absence of any horizontal or vertical deviation, with an absence also of any torsional deviation and with the head held vertically erect.) In that position, the superior rectus muscle rotates the eye upwards (elevation), rotates the eye inwards (adduction) and twists the eye inwards (intorsion); when the eye is in a position of 23° abduction it causes only elevation becauses it runs then in the vertical meridian; when the eye is in a position of 67° adduction it causes only adduction and intorsion because it then runs at 90° to the vertical meridian; and when the eye is abducted beyond 23° it continues to cause elevation, but also causes abduction and extorsion (twisting outwards) (Fig. 53).

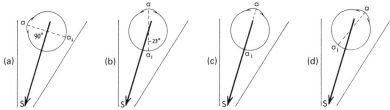

Fig. 53. The actions of the superior rectus (S): (a) in 67° of adduction (adduction and intorsion); (b) in the primary position (elevation, adduction and intorsion); (c) in 23° of abduction (elevation); and (d) beyond 23° of abduction (elevation, abduction and extorsion). $a-a_1$ = vertical meridian of the eye.

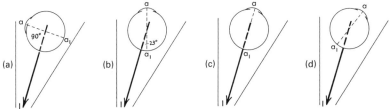

Fig. 54. The actions of the inferior rectus (I): (a) in 67° of adduction (adduction and extorsion); (b) in the primary position (depression, adduction and extorsion); (c) in 23° of abduction (depression); and (d) beyond 23° of abduction (depression, abduction and intorsion). $a-a_1$ = vertical meridian of the eye.

Inferior rectus

This arises near the apex of the orbit and passes forwards and outwards below the eye to be inserted on the lower surface of the sclera in front of the equator. It runs in the line of the orbital axis (Fig. 52). With the eye in the primary position it rotates the eye downwards (depression), rotates the eye inwards (adduction) and twists the eye outwards (extorsion); when the eye is in a position of 23° abduction it causes only depression because it then runs in the vertical meridian; when the eye is in a position of 67°adduction the muscle causes only adduction and extorsion because it runs then at 90° to the vertical meridian; and when the eye is abducted beyond 23° it continues to cause depression but also causes abduction and intorsion (Fig. 54).

Superior oblique

This arises near the apex of the orbit and passes forwards on the upper and medial surface of the eye to the anterior part of the roof of the orbit where it hooks round a pulley (the *trochlea*) before passing backwards and outwards above the eye, at an angle of 54° with the vertical meridian in the primary position, to be inserted on the upper and outer surface of the sclera behind the equator. This partial reversal of its line of pull causes it to rotate the eye downwards (depression) despite its situation above the eye; it also rotates the eye outwards (abduction) and

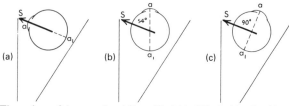

Fig. 55. The actions of the superior oblique (S): (a) in 54° of adduction (depression); (b) in the primary position (depression, abduction and intorsion); and (c) in 36° of abduction (abduction and intorsion). a–a_1 = vertical meridian of the eye.

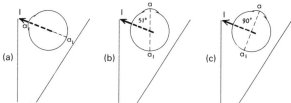

Fig. 56. The actions of the inferior oblique (I): (a) in 51° of adduction (elevation); (b) in the primary position (elevation, abduction and extorsion); and (c) in 39° of abduction (abduction and extorsion). a–a_1 = vertical meridian of the eye.

twists the eye inwards (intorsion). When the eye is in a position of 54° adduction it causes only depression because it then runs in the vertical meridian, and when the eye is in a position of 36° abduction the muscle causes only abduction and intorsion (Fig. 55).

Inferior oblique

This arises from the anteromedial part of the floor of the orbit and passes backwards and outwards below the eye, at an angle of 51° with the vertical meridian in the primary position, to be inserted on the lower and outer surface of the sclera behind the equator. Pull of the muscle from in front causes it to rotate the eye upwards (elevation) despite its situation below the eye; it also rotates the eye outwards (abduction) and twists the eye outwards (extorsion). When the eye is in a position of 51° adduction it causes only elevation because it then runs in the vertical meridian, and when the eye is in a position of 39° abduction it causes only abduction and extorsion (Fig. 56).

It should be noted that the angles given above for the vertical muscles represent average figures and that there are frequently wide variations—this is discussed later on p.249 in the context of the A and V phenomena.

It should also be noted that the vertical muscles are able to carry out isolated movements because the other effects cancel each other out. A movement of elevation by the superior rectus and inferior oblique does not induce any torsion because the intorsion of the superior rectus is cancelled by the extorsion of the inferior oblique. A movement of depression by the inferior rectus and superior oblique does not induce any torsion because the extorsion of the inferior rectus is cancelled by the intorsion of the superior oblique. Similarly, a movement of intorsion by the superior rectus and superior oblique does not induce any vertical movement because the elevation of the superior rectus is cancelled by the depression of the superior oblique, and a movement of extorsion by the inferior rectus and inferior oblique does not induce any vertical movement because the depression of the inferior rectus is cancelled by the elevation of the inferior oblique.

Binocular movements

The movements of the two eyes together may be of a conjugate or disjunctive nature.

Conjugate movements

These are co-ordinated movements of the two eyes in the same direction *(version movements)* which occur in the following six main directions (the *cardinal positions* of the eyes), with one muscle in each eye concerned primarily in each movement:

1. *Dextroelevation* (up and to the right)   Right superior rectus
                                                 Left inferior oblique
2. *Dextroversion* (to the right)   Right lateral rectus
                                                 Left medial rectus
3. *Dextrodepression* (down and to the right)   Right inferior rectus
                                                 Left superior oblique
4. *Laevoelevation* (up and to the left)   Right inferior oblique
                                                 Left superior rectus
5. *Laevoversion* (to the left)   Right medial rectus
                                                 Left lateral rectus
6. *Laevodepression* (down and to the left)   Right superior oblique
                                                 Left inferior rectus

This illustrates that in any movement of the eyes, paired muscles which are *synergists* (*agonists*) contract together, and it should be noted also that paired muscles which are *antagonists* simultaneously relax (in an active way) by the phenomenon of *reciprocal innervation*; for example, in a movement of dextroelevation the right inferior rectus and left superior oblique act as antagonists with the right superior rectus and left inferior oblique acting as agonists.

The range over which conjugate movement is possible is termed the *binocular field of fixation*, and it forms a circle of about 45 to 50° from the primary position, except below when it is restricted on both sides to about 35° by the nose (Fig. 57), but its full extent is seldom used because head movements are usually brought into play when there is

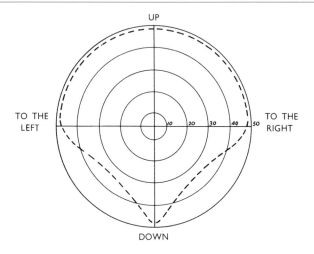

Fig. 57. The binocular field of fixation.

more than about 20° rotation. It is measured using the perimeter after removing the central fixation target (p.343). Both eyes follow the moving target along the arc of the perimeter at 15° intervals over the 360°, until there is an appreciation of diplopia of the target; this marks the limit of the binocular field of fixation in that particular meridian. This appreciation is facilitated by the use of a red goggle over one eye and a green goggle over the other, so that at the limit of the binocular field of fixation the target becomes red or green and not a mixture of the two colours as in binocular viewing. However this provides a slightly reduced field of fixation in the presence of a paresis because of the dissociating effect of the coloured goggles.

Disjunctive movements

These are co-ordinated movements of the two eyes in opposite directions (*vergence movements*) which occur in two directions; *convergence* (or *positive convergence*) when each eye is turned inwards, and *divergence* (or *negative convergence*) when each eye is turned outwards from a convergent position.

The nervous control of ocular movement

The extrinsic ocular muscles are influenced by three main systems: the afferent system, the efferent system and the extra-pyramidal motor system.

The afferent system

The afferent system has several components:

1. *Visual stimuli* travel in the afferent visual pathway; the visual awareness of an object may induce a particular form of ocular movement. This is part of the *psycho-optical reflex.*
2. *Proprioceptive stimuli* arise in the labyrinth (the semicircular canals provide information about movements of acceleration or deceleration of the head, and the utricle and saccule provide information about the position of the head in space), in the neck muscles and in the extrinsic ocular muscles. These are part of the *postural reflexes.*
3. *Auditory stimuli* arise in the inner ear.

The efferent system

The efferent part of the motor system has several components:

1. *Cortical centres,* or *frontal centres,* are concerned with the production of binocular movements as a result of a voluntary desire or in response to a command. The *occipital centres* are concerned with the production of binocular movements in response to a visual stimulus, and are part of the *psycho-optical reflex* pathways. The right cerebral hemisphere is concerned with movements to the left, and the left hemisphere with movements to the right. (The term centre may be incorrect because experimental evidence indicates that wide areas of the cerebral cortex may exert such motor effects).

2. *Intermediary centres,* or *supranuclear centres,* are described in the tectal part of the midbrain in the region of the superior colliculi for vertical movement, in the pretectal region for convergence, and near the sixth cranial nerve nuclei for lateral movement, but the evidence for these is essentially clinical and is at variance with experimental evidence based on precise stereotaxic methods and sensitive recording devices; these show several reactive areas in the brainstem near the midline or within the median plane for vertical movements, and also several reactive areas in the brainstem (the tegmentum of the midbrain and pons, the central grey matter, the vestibular nuclei, the paramedian zone and the reticular activating system), which represent a vast mass of interrelated neurons in the segmental part of the central core of the brainstem, for lateral movements. It is evident, therefore that, the true location of the intermediary centres is at present ill-understood.

3. *The third, fourth and sixth cranial nuclei* and their *cranial nerves* are also included. The third cranial nucleus, which lies on each side of the midbrain, controls four extrinsic ocular muscles—the medial rectus, superior rectus, inferior rectus and inferior oblique. The fourth cranial nucleus, which lies on each side of the midbrain, controls one extrinsic ocular muscle—the superior oblique. The sixth cranial nucleus, which lies on each side of the pons, controls one extrinsic ocular muscle—the lateral rectus. The *medial (posterior) longitudinal bundle (fasciculus),* which runs through the brainstem, forms a nervous link between these three paired cranial nuclei (Fig. 66, p.257).

The extrapyramidal motor system

The motor system of the eye is also controlled by the extrapyramidal motor system, which is a complex nervous mechanism (comprising cortical centres, basal ganglia, nuclear masses in the midbrain and the reticular formation, and the cerebellum). These are concerned in the maintenance of proper degrees of muscle tone and rhythm which are essential for the conduct of precise ocular movement; the reticular formation appears to function as a master control mechanism because of its ability to modify and integrate the vast assortment of conflicting sensory impulses.

The movements of the eyes are influenced also by the fascial tissues of the orbit.

The development of binocular vision

Binocular vision is achieved by using both eyes together so that the separate images arising in each eye are appreciated as a single image by a process of fusion. This achievement is an acquired ability, not simply an inborn one, and is built up gradually during the early weeks and months of life, provided there is a proper co-ordination of various abilities:

1.   The ability of each retina to function properly from a visual point of view, particularly the central part of the retina (the fovea). This necessitates a reasonably intact retina and an absence of any significant defects in the transparent structures of the eye (the cornea, the anterior and posterior chambers, the lens and the vitreous).

2.   The ability of the visual areas of the brain to promote fusion (bifoveal fixation) of the two separate images transmitted to them from each eye, so that a single mental impression is achieved of the object. This is made possible by the forwards direction of the eyes in man, so that the visual field of one eye almost completely overlaps the visual field of the other eye (the *binocular field of vision*) (see Fig. 76, p.318), and within the parts of the retina of one eye which are concerned with this binocular field are several visual elements which correspond with similar visual elements in identical parts of the retina of the other eye. In this way any small object in the binocular field of vision may be regarded as producing a stimulation of corresponding retinal points, although this has a physiological rather than an anatomical significance. The association of the visual fibres from corresponding retinal points is achieved in the brain by the rearrangement of these fibres from each eye at the optic chiasm (see p. 324).

3.   The ability of each eye to lie correctly in its bony orbit, so that the visual axis (the line which passes from the object of fixation to the fovea) of each eye is directed to the same object at rest and during movement (central fixation). The control of the position of the eye

demands carefully integrated controlling mechanisms which may be considered in three groups—mechanisms which give information to the brain (the *fixation reflexes*), mechanisms which produce the movement (the *motor responses*) and mechanisms which steady the movement (the *steadying influences*).

The *fixation reflexes* are concerned with informing the brain about the positions of the eyes and may be of two types—visual or postural. Visual information is the result of each retinal receptor possessing a projection in a particular direction in space, so that stimulation of a receptor by an object gives information on the position of that object, quite apart from the visual detail of the object. The central point of the retina (the fovea) has a straight-ahead type of projection (the *principal visual direction of the fovea*) so that it is concerned with direct fixation of an object, whereas the other retinal receptors are concerned with objects in the paracentral and peripheral parts of the field of vision. The *psycho-optical reflex* is composed of the *fixation reflex* (the fixation of an object by one or both eyes), the *refixation reflex* (the change in fixation from one object to another object or the maintenance of fixation on a moving object by one or both eyes), the *conjugate fixation reflex* (the fixation of an object which involves a conjugate movement of both eyes), the *disjunctive fixation reflex* (the fixation of an object which involves a disjunctive movement of both eyes), and the *corrective fusion reflex* (the maintenance of fusion in the primary position and during conjugate and disjunctive movements by the strength of the fusional influences—*fusional vergence reflex*—despite a tendency to develop a squint (*heterophoria*).

Postural information is of a more primitive kind and is the result of the existence within the muscles of the eye, head and neck of specialized structures (muscle spindles and tendon organs) which record the amount of contraction and relaxation of each muscle so that the position of the eyes in relation to one another and in relation to the position of the head is known. It is also the result of impulses from the labyrinthine mechanisms (see above). These postural reflexes are responsible for the fact that the eyes continue to move together even when one eye is totally blind, although there is usually an eventual deviation of the blind eye.

The influence of the complex efferent motor systems—the *motor responses*—and the influence of the extrapyramidal motor system—the *steadying influences*—are discussed above (p.222).

4. The ability of the mechanism which turns the eyes inwards to a near object (*convergence*) or outwards from a convergent position to a distant object (*divergence* or *negative convergence*) and the focusing mechanisms of the eye *(accommodation)* to achieve an adequate degree of harmony. The mechanism of accommodation has been discussed on pp.9 and 77. The mechanism of convergence is essentially a reflex, with three components in addition to reflex accommodative convergence: *tonic reflex convergence*, which implies the existence of some inherent

tonus of the medial recti; *proximal reflex convergence*, which is induced simply by the presence of a near object; and *fusional reflex convergence*, which is exerted to maintain fusion of an object of fixation.

There is a close relationship between the mechanisms of accommodation and reflex convergence: a unit of accommodation (A)— one dioptre (1D)–is inevitably accompanied by the stimulus to induce an appropriate degree of accommodative convergence (AC) (measured in prism dioptres—Δ); this is the accommodative convergence and accommodation relationship (the AC/A ratio). During the binocular fixation of an object 1m from the eyes, so that each eye exercises 1 D of accommodation, there is a total convergence of the two eyes of 6Δ in the presence of an average interpupillary distance of 60mm. Thus in emmetropia and orthophoria the theoretical AC/A ratio is 6 (i.e 6Δ/1D), but in practice the normal ratio is about 4. A lower than normal ratio is necessary in uncorrected hypermetropia (because accommodation must exceed convergence) and a higher ratio is necessary in uncorrected myopia (because convergence must exceed accommodation) if binocular vision is to be maintained at different distances of fixation by the influences of the fusional vergence reflex. The AC/A ratio may be measured in different ways; the *heterophoria method*, which compares the differences in the latent deviation of the eyes (the *phoria*) at distant and at near fixation; the *gradient method*, which compares the change in the phoria at a fixed point of fixation during the application of convex spherical lenses (which reduce accommodation) and concave spherical lenses (which increase accommodation); the *graphic method*, which measures the convergence response of the eyes to different concave spherical lenses on the synoptophore and compares these with the normal responses graphically; and the complicated *fixation disparity method*, which is concerned with the disparity (*retinal slip*) which may occur within Panum's areas (areas of retinal correspondence, i.e. the retinal areas in which slightly dissimilar images from an object must project to be perceived in depth) in a phoria under certain circumstances.

Orthophoria

The development of binocular vision permits the visual axes of the two eyes to be directed to a particular object in the primary (straight ahead) position, during all forms of conjugate and disjunctive movement, and at all distances of fixation (near and far); this ideal state is termed *orthophoria* and it should be maintained rigidly even when the eyes are dissociated from one another by occlusion of one eye which prevents the normal controlling influences of the fusion mechanism, but this is often an unrealized ideal even in normal persons.

The development of squint (strabismus)

Squint is the condition in which there is a failure of the visual axis (the line which passes from the fovea to the fixation object) of one eye (the *squinting eye*) to be directed at the same time to the object which is being observed by the other eye (the *fixing* or *non-squinting eye*), although this failure may occur only under certain circumstances. In general a squint is the result of a failure in the development of normal binocular vision, and the 'obstacle' which induces this failure may arise in any of the complex mechanisms which have been discussed above:

1.   One eye may have a defective form of central vision as the result of some structural anomaly of the cornea, lens, retina, etc.

2.   There may be difficulty in promoting fusion. Fusion is obviously defective if the vision of one eye is poor, but fusion is prevented, even when the corrected vision of each eye is good, if there is a significant difference (usually more than 5%) between the sizes of the retinal images transmitted to the brain (a condition termed *aniseikonia*, p.14), usually the result of a marked difference in the refractive errors of the two eyes (anisometropia), but sometimes because of a difference in the retinal mosaic in the central parts of the two eyes. Weakness of the fusion mechanism may be the result of some severe general illness or of certain psychological states affecting the stability of the cerebral mechanisms. A loss of fusion mechanism may occur after a head injury which induces a state of concussion, even in the absence of any disorder of the extrinsic ocular muscles, and the reason for this is obscure. In general, however, weakness of the fusion mechanism is most often the *result* of the squint; the failure of the eyes to be directed at the same time to the same object inhibits the promotion of the fusion mechanism.

3.   A defect may prevent the eyes from maintaining the correct positions relative to one another at rest or during movement; such defects may be of a structural nature (e.g. a defect in the shape of the orbit), of a neurogenic nature (this accounts for the paretic or paralytic type of squint), or of a myogenic nature (this accounts for many of the squints of congenital origin, but also may be of acquired origin as in exophthalmic ophthalmoplegia).

4.   A defect may prevent the establishment of a harmony between the accommodation and convergence reflexes so that there is an abnormal AC/A ratio. The frequent occurrence of fairly high degrees of hypermetropia in a young child leads to an excessive use of accommodation, with a tendency to overconvergence, thus favouring the development of a convergent squint, the so-called *accommodative squint*, but a convergent squint may occur also in the absence of excessive hypermetropia when there is a high AC/A ratio (*convergence excess esotropia*). Conversely, in myopia there is a diminished use of accommodation which may lead to a decreased convergence of the eyes and thus favour the development of divergent squint.

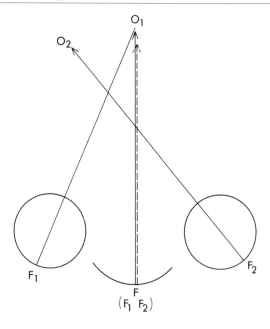

Fig. 58. The occurrence of confusion in a right convergent squint: the stimulation of corresponding retinal points in each eye (F_1 and F_2) by two different objects (O_1 and O_2) causes a superimposition of the two images which are projected straight ahead from the fovea of the binoculus (F)—the binoculus is a perceptual concept which represents the two eyes considered as one (the median eye).

It is apparent that many factors may adversely affect any part of the complex mechanisms responsible for the development of binocular vision and produce a squint, but it must be appreciated that these adverse effects vary greatly; in the very young child with poorly developed binocular vision, a relatively trivial defect may cause a squint, particularly when the child is unwell, but in the older child with good binocular vision development of such a squint may be avoided.

Adaptations to the development of squint

It might be assumed that the development of squint is the final event in a chain of events which leads to a failure in the proper establishment of binocular vision, but in fact the squint only represents the beginning of a new series of events which take place because of the occurrence of double vision. Double vision is the direct result of the squint as it causes the visual axes of the two eyes to be directed to two different objects, thereby causing (a) a superimposition of two different images (this form of double vision is called *confusion* and is the result of a

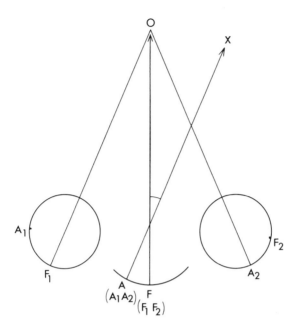

Fig. 59.   The occurrence of diplopia in a right convergent squint: the stimulation of non-corresponding retinal points in each eye (F_1 and A_2) by one object (O) causes a separation of the two images, one of which (the left one) is projected straight ahead from the fovea of the binoculus (F) and the other (the right one) is projected to the right of the straight ahead position from a peripheral point of the binoculus (A). It should be noted that the angle between the projection from F on the binoculus (which represents F_1 in the left eye) and the projection from A on the binoculus (which represents A_2 in the right eye) is equal to the angle of the squint.

stimulation of corresponding retinal points by two different objects, Fig. 58); and (b) the stimulation by one object of retinal areas in the two eyes which do not correspond with one another, thereby causing a separation of the two images (the true image and the false image) of the object (this form of double vision is called *diplopia*, Fig. 59). The nature of confusion and diplopia is illustrated with relation to the *binoculus*; this is a perceptual concept which represents two eyes considered as one (the median eye). Certainly in the normal binocular act there is no mental impression of a synthesis of two separate images and it seems that the binocular image is projected from somewhere behind the eyes.

The changes which follow the development of double vision represent attempts by the brain to overcome its troublesome effects and may be called *adaptations*; they are produced subconsciously, particularly in the young child. The following adaptations may occur:

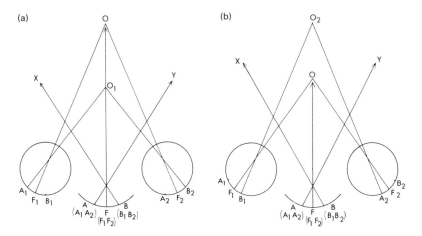

Fig. 60. The phenomenon of physiological diplopia: when an object (O) is viewed by the fovea of each eye (F_1 and F_2) it is projected from the fovea of the binoculus (F) so that the image of the object is a single one. (a) An object which is nearer to the eyes (O_1) than the fixation object (O) is perceived by disparate retinal points (A_1 and B_2) so that the two images are projected from the binoculus (from A to Y and from B to X) with the awareness of a crossed form of physiological diplopia (unless one of the images is suppressed). (b) An object which is farther from the eyes (O_2) than the fixation object (O) is perceived by disparate retinal points (B_1 and A_2) so that two images are projected from the binoculus (from B to X and from A to Y) with the awareness of an uncrossed form of physiological diplopia (unless one of the images is suppressed).

Suppression

The vision of the squinting eye may be ignored by a process of active neglect of the eye by the visual cortex (suppression), but this is a temporary phenomenon which occurs only when both eyes are given the opportunity of acting visually; it is a feature of the early stages of a uniocular squint and persists in an alternating or intermittent squint, but on transferring fixation from one eye to the other spontaneously or by covering the fixing eye there is an immediate cessation of the suppression. Suppression is a feature also of normal binocular vision whereby the diplopia of objects nearer to or farther from the object of fixation (*physiological diplopia*)is ignored (Fig. 60).

Amblyopia

The vision of the squinting eye may be ignored by a process of active neglect of the eye by the visual cortex, but unlike suppression this cortical inhibition is a progressive and permanent phenomenon (in the absence of treatment) so that it persists during an enforced fixation of the squinting eye (*strabismic amblyopia*). It follows that in an amblyopic eye there is a loss of central vision which cannot be explained wholly on the basis of a structural defect of the eye or of the afferent visual pathways. In this context it is appropriate to consider other related forms of amblyopia:

1. *Stimulus deprivation amblyopia (amblyopia ex anopsia)* occurs when an eye is deprived of visual stimuli at an early stage of life (as in congenital cataract, p.171 or in complete ptosis), and the amblyopia is intense and accompanied by a loss of fixation. Experimental work on kittens and monkeys indicates that this form of amblyopia is related to a lack of integration of the complex visual pathways in the cortex, which seems dependent on adequate stimuli in early life.

2. *Anisometropic amblyopia* is the result of an inhibition of the vision of one eye because of a significant difference in the refractive errors of the two eyes, so that one eye is favoured at the expense of the other.

3. *Ametropic amblyopia* occurs in the presence of an uncorrected refractive error of sufficient magnitude that correction of the refractive error at some later stage only produces a partial improvement in the vision. It may occur in both eyes.

4. *Nystagmic amblyopia*, a defective form of vision, occurs in nystagmus (p.270), which is frequently unrelated to any structural defect of the eye.

Eccentric retinal fixation

The fixation of the squinting eye may become abnormal by the development of an eccentric type of retinal fixation. In many cases of squint the retinal elements may retain their normal projections despite a marked amblyopia of the squinting eye, but sometimes, particularly when the squint occurs at an early age and when there is a prolonged interval between the development of the squint and the start of effective treatment, this ability is lost and some other retinal area assumes the principal visual direction and becomes a point of *eccentric retinal fixation*. The nature of the eccentric fixation may be designated according to the position on the retina of the eccentric point: parafoveal (within 3° of the fovea), paramacular (within 4 to 5° of the fovea), and peripheral (beyond 5° of the fovea), and in each case the eccentric fixation may be steady or unsteady. *Wandering fixation* may also occur in which there is no fixed point of retinal fixation (central or eccentric).

The nature of the retinal fixation is detected by the *visuoscope*, a special type of ophthalmoscope which incorporates a target in the form of a star; this target is projected onto the fundus and the patient attempts to fix the star.

Anomalous (abnormal) retinal correspondence

The eyes may develop an anomalous association with one another in order to obtain a form of binocular vision (albeit of an anomalous type)

232   *Ophthalmology*

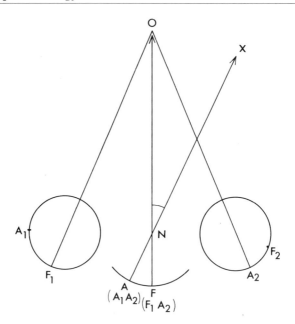

Fig. 61. The phenomenon of harmonious anomalous retinal correspondence in a right convergent squint: the stimulation of non-corresponding retinal points (F_1 and A_2) by the fixation object (O) would create two projections from the binoculus (from F to O and A to X) in the presence of normal retinal correspondence, but in harmonious anomalous retinal correspondence, A_2 in the right eye assumes an anomalous relationship with F_1 so that both projections are from F on the binoculus in a straight ahead direction to O. The angle between the normal and abnormal projections of A_2 (ONX) represents the angle of anomaly; it is identical with the angle of the squint (ONX). The angle of anomaly may also be regarded as the difference between the subjective angle of the squint (which is zero) and the objective angle of the squint (ONX).

despite the presence of a squint; this implies that the retinal area of the squinting eye which is stimulated by the object of fixation assumes an anomalous relationship with the fovea of the non-squinting eye, so that it is projected anomalously from the fovea of the binoculus. It should be noted that the retinal area of the squinting eye which assumes the anomalous relationship with the fovea of the non-squinting eye is not necessarily a point of eccentric fixation because in anomalous correspondence (a sensory anomaly of a binocular nature) there may be no eccentric fixation (a sensory anomaly of a uniocular nature) or there may be eccentric fixation, which is not compatible with the anomalous correspondence, during the use of the squinting eye alone. Sometimes, however, in small-angle esotropia (*microtropia*), the two conditions are compatible so that the angle of anomaly is equal to the angle of eccentricity.

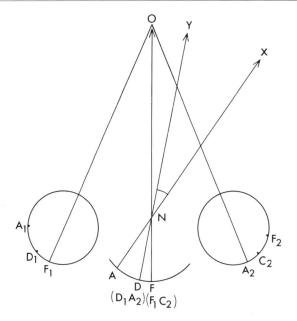

Fig. 62. The phenomenon of inharmonious anomalous retinal correspondence in a right convergent squint: the stimulation of non-corresponding retinal points (F_1 and A_2) would create two projections from the binoculus (from F to O and from A to X) in the presence of normal retinal correspondence, but in inharmonious anomalous retinal correspondence, C_2 in the right eye assumes an anomalous relationship with F_1 so that the projection from A_2 is from D on the binoculus to Y in contrast with the projection from F_1 which is from F on the binoculus in a straight-ahead direction to O. The angle between the normal and abnormal projections of A_2 (YNX) represents the angle of anomaly; it is less than the angle of squint (ONX). The angle of anomaly may be regarded also as the difference between the subjective angle of the squint (ONY) and the objective angle of the squint (ONX).

Anomalous correspondence is termed *harmonious* when there is a precise relationship between the retinal point stimulated by the fixation object and the fovea of the non-squinting eye; the angle between the abnormal projection of the stimulated point of the squinting eye (in the presence of a harmonious anomalous retinal correspondence) and its normal projection (in the presence of a normal retinal correspondence) is regarded as the angle of anomaly (Fig. 61). The angle of anomaly is equal to the angle of the squint, and it also represents the difference between the subjective angle of the squint (which is zero in a harmonious anomalous retinal correspondence) and the objective angle of the squint. Anomalous retinal correspondence is termed *inharmonious* when there is a less precise relationship between the two eyes, so that a retinal area of the squinting eye (other than that stimulated by the object of fixation) assumes an anomalous relationship with the fovea of the non-squinting eye; in this way the angle of anomaly is less than the angle of squint, and the subjective angle of the squint is no longer zero, although it is less than the objective angle (Fig. 62); the subjective and objective angles of a squint are equal only in normal retinal correspondence. It is most unlikely that the inharmonious type of anomalous retinal correspondence exists in everyday seeing, and it is found more or less only in certain diagnostic tests which introduce an element of dissociation of the eyes (such as test using the synoptophore, p. 238).

Bagolini striated glass test Inevitably any test of binocular function causes some degree of dissociation of the eyes, but the Bagolini striated glass test—which uses, in front of each eye, plane glass with fine striations adjusted in such a way that the striations produce linear streaks of light which are at 90° to each other—creates a minimal degree of dissociation. When the two striated glasses are arranged to produce a cross with one streak of light at 45° and the other streak of light at 135°, this cross bisects the fixation light under normal conditions—that is, in an absence of any squint and in the presence of bifoveal fixation. This is found also in a small angle squint, which is an indication of the presence of harmonious retinal correspondence so that there is a new anomalous sensorial relationship of the two eyes which is in keeping with the squint; the absence of any findings which would indicate an inharmonious retinal correspondence is simply because of the minimal dissociation of the eyes during the test. The absence of one streak of light in whole or in part indicates a state of suppression of one eye in a binocular situation.

Compensatory (abnormal) head posture

This may be adopted in certain forms of incomitant squint, usually when it involves one of the vertically acting muscles, in order to avoid diplopia, particularly in the primary position and on looking down. There are two main components in this abnormal posture: (a) *face turning* (up, down, right or left) in order turn the eye as far away as possible from the field of action of the affected muscle—this involves turning the face into the direction of this field of action because the eye then turns automatically into the opposite direction; and (b) *head tilting* (right or left) to diminish the vertical separation of the true and false images and to compensate also for any abnormalities of torsion which are usually the result of a weakness or overaction of one of the oblique muscles. Sometimes, a compensatory head posture is adopted in a concomitant squint if there is an associated A or V phenomenon (p.249).

A compensatory head posture also occurs in cases of severe bilateral ptosis (p.193), when it is necessary to turn the face up in order to retain a reasonable level of vision; in congenital nystagmus (p.270) to secure the eyes in the so-called 'neutral zone'; and in homonymous hemianopia (p.341), when an attempt is made to centralize the remaining field—in a right homonymous hemianopia this consists of a turning of the eyes to the right.

The term *ocular torticollis* may be used to denote the various forms of compensatory head posture discussed above, but the term *torticollis* is reserved for the head posture induced by a contracture of the sternocleidomastoid muscle which is usually of congenital origin. The head is tilted to the affected side, the torticollis persists during sleep, and is difficult or impossible to relieve manually.

Increase in the angle of squint

Sometimes the development of a small degree of squint may be followed by a much greater degree of squint (the *purposive squint*) because diplopia is less troublesome when the two images of the one object are widely separated from one another as it is easier for the patient to distinguish between the true and false images. This occurs also in some paretic squints when the patient may fix with the paretic eye to make use of the secondary deviation of the unaffected eye (p.253).

Types of squint

There are four main types of squint: *concomitant (heterotropia)*, *intermittent*, *latent (heterophoria)*, and *incomitant (paresis or paralysis)*.

Concomitant squint (heterotropia)

This is a manifest squint in which the angle of the squint remains more or less the same in all positions of gaze and irrespective of which eye is used for fixation. The nature of a concomitant squint is designated by the direction of the squint: *convergent* when the squinting eye turns in (*esotropia*), *divergent* when it turns out (*exotropia*), *sursumvergent* when it turns up (*hypertropia*), and *deorsumvergent* when it turns down (*hypotropia*). Sometimes a squint may show both horizontal and vertical features, although the presence of a vertical element frequently implies some incomitant element in the squint originally. It should be appreciated, however, that this distinction is in no way rigid, so that the horizontal and vertical aspects in the squint frequently co-exist, and the one may arise from the other. This is evident in *alternating hypertropia* which may accompany esotropia or exotropia—in addition to the convergent or divergent deviation, each eye rotates upwards when the other eye is fixing; this vertical element is evident also in the upshoot (or updrift) of each eye in adduction (when the action of the inferior oblique is especially effective). Less commonly there is an *alternating hypotropia* which may accompany esotropia or exotropia—in addition to the convergent or divergent deviation, each eye rotates downwards when the other eye is fixing; this vertical element is evident also in the downshoot (or downdrift) of each eye in adduction (when the action of the superior oblique is especially effective). It is evident that these forms of alternating hypertropia or hypotropia differ from the usual forms of hypertropia and hypotropia (in which one eye deviates in an opposite direction to the other eye – one eye upwards and the other eye downwards – to more or less equal extents) because each eye deviates in the same direction (upwards or downwards) and quite frequently to unequal extents (see p.249).

A concomitant squint is also designated by the terms *right* or *left* according to the eye which is the squinting one (as distinct from the fixing one) or by the term *alternating* when either eye may squint in turn or indiscriminately.

The development of a concomitant squint is essentially the result of some obstacle in the development of normal binocular function as discussed above. The only presenting symptom is an awareness of confusion and diplopia, but these are seldom appreciated except by the older and more introspective child and are rapidly eliminated by the mechanism of suppression. The complications of concomitant squint— amblyopia, eccentric retinal fixation and anomalous retinal correspondence—are discussed above.

False squint (pseudostrabismus). Quite frequently there is a false appearance of a convergent squint in early childhood; the presence of well-marked folds on either side of the nose (epicanthic folds) and the characteristically flat base of the nose in early childhood combine to give an impression of a convergent squint. Much more rarely a narrowing of the lateral canthi causes a false appearance of a divergent squint. Sometimes there may be an undue increased distance between the medial canthi (*telecanthus*) so that there is a spreading out of the tissues of the medial canthi, and this contributes to the false impression of a convergent squint. The cover test (see below) is of great value in determining the absence of any squint, and this is confirmed by a positive response to the *prism vergence test*; when a prism (usually 12Δ) is placed base out in front of either eye there is a movement of convergence to eliminate the diplopia which is induced by the prism in the presence of binocular vision.

The management of concomitant squint

The methods of investigation and treatment should proceed as soon as possible after the onset because the aim is to restore binocular function whenever possible. Obviously in very young children some methods are inapplicable, but this is no valid reason for deferring certain forms of examination in all cases.

History of the squint. This is important because an accurate determination of the age of the child at the time of onset of the squint, of the length of time during which the squint remained only occasional before becoming constant, and of any previous forms of treatment is of great value in assessing the chances of obtaining a binocular result after treatment.

Diagnosis of the type of squint. This is achieved by the following methods of examination:

1. An *observation of the corneal reflexes.* The presence of a squint may be established by careful judgement of the positions of the reflexes which are visible on the cornea of each eye when a light shines on the eyes. In the absence of a squint these reflexes lie on symmetrical parts of the cornea of each eye, but in a convergent squint the reflex on the cornea of the squinting eye is displaced towards its outer side and in a divergent squint the reflex is displaced to its inner side. A vertical type of squint is associated similarly with an alteration in these reflexes.

2. *The cover test.* This test is composed of two parts: the *cover and uncover test* and the *alternate cover test.* The cover and uncover test consists of covering each eye in turn with the hand or some form of occluder during the fixation of the other eye on the target. In the absence of any squint there is no movement of either eye during this test. If a convergent squint is present, on removing the cover from one eye and transferring it to the other eye, the uncovered eye moves outwards to take up its correct central position because it was turned inwards during the time it was covered. Conversely, if a divergent squint is present, on transferring the cover the previously covered eye will move inwards from an outwards position to become straight. A vertical type of squint is also determined by this method.

The alternate cover test consists of rapidly and repeatedly transferring the occluder from one eye to the other so that there is dissociation of the eyes; this reveals a latent squint which is controlled only by the corrective fusion reflex (p.225); the rapidity of recovery on removing the dissociating influence is a measure of the strength of this reflex.

The extent of the deviation (manifest or latent) may be measured by the *prism and cover test* in which prisms of increasing strength are placed before one eye (with the base of the prism in a direction which is opposite to the direction of the squint; i.e. base out in a convergent squint, etc.) until there is an absence of any deviation.

The cover test is of supreme value in early childhood when reliance must be placed solely on an objective assessment, but it is of equal value in a rapid evaluation of any form of squint at any age, particularly as it is a reliable test which requires no form of instrumentation.

3. *Prism vergence tests.* The ability of an eye to overcome the effect of a base-out prism has been discussed above in relation to the

238   *Ophthalmology*

determination of a false squint (p.236), but special mention is made here
of the 4Δ test. This is of particular value in the presence of a small-
angle squint (*microtropia* or *esoflick*), when there is a negative response
when the 4Δ prism is placed base-out in front of the affected eye
because the prism moves the image of the target into the central part of
the fundus where there is a suppression scotoma. The test is also of
value when there is some form of amblyopia in the absence of a squint,
such as in certain forms of anisometropia, when there is a similar
negative response. This is of special value in the young child in whom
some amblyopia of one eye is suspected at an age before it is possible to
determine this by a subjective test.

4. *Ocular movements.* This should be carried out in all directions
of gaze for each eye separately and for both eyes together. In a
concomitant squint the range of movement of each eye is usually
normal. Sometimes, however, there is weakness of movement of the
squinting eye in a direction away from the squint; for example, in a
right convergent squint there may be an apparent weakness of the right
lateral rectus muscle because of habitual disuse of the eye in a position
of full abduction, and the absence of any true paresis is demonstrated
by the recovery of movement which follows a short period of occlusion
of the left fixing eye unless contractural changes have developed in the
right medial rectus muscle (the ipsilateral antagonist). Weakness of
movement of the squinting eye also occurs in a squint which becomes
concomitant after starting originally as an incomitant one (p.252).
Sometimes a previous limitation of movement as the result of a paresis
is shown by an exaggeration of the so-called *end-point nystagmus* even
when there has been a restoration of a normal degree of movement in
the field of action of the previously affected muscle.

5. *The nature of the potential binocular function.* This is assessed
most readily by the *synoptophore (major amblyoscope)* which involves
the principles of the stereoscope. In this instrument there is an eyepiece
for each eye and the position of the eyepieces may be adjusted to
compensate for the angle of the squint—this adjustment is correct when
the examiner observes that the corneal reflections on the eyes are in
central and symmetrical positions—and it provides an objective
measurement of the angle of the squint. Pictures on slides are then
presented to each eye and the patient adjusts the eyepieces to obtain a
superimposition of these pictures; this provides a subjective
measurement of the angle of the squint. Various types of pictures are
used to provide information on the grades of binocular vision:

Grade I. Simultaneous macular perception is the simplest form of
binocular vision and implies the ability of each eye to superimpose two
dissimilar objects—the classical example is to put the bird (seen with
one eye) into the cage (seen with the other eye) (Fig. 63). A failure to
see one of the objects indicates suppression or amblyopia. The concept
of simultaneous macular perception is essentially an instrumental one;
it is not possible to have simultaneous macular perception without a

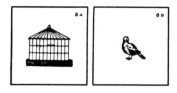

Fig. 63. Slides for testing simultaneous macular perception on the synoptophore.

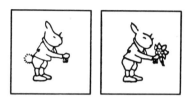

Fig. 64. Slides for testing fusion on the synoptophore.

form of fusion, although the fusion is a very limited type with an absence of any signficant range of fusion.

Grade II. This was regarded as the possession of *fusion,* but as indicated above in the context of simultaneous macular perception, fusion is not unique to Grade II. However, in Grade II, fusion is a more elaborate form of binocular vision and implies the ability of the eyes to produce a composite picture from two similar objects, each of which is incomplete in one detail—the classical example is the rabbit with a tail but without a bunch of flowers and the rabbit without a tail but with a bunch of flowers (Fig. 64). The range of fusion is then tested by moving the arms of the synoptophore so that the eyes have to converge and diverge to maintain fusion; under normal conditions this should be possible over at least 25° of convergence and 3° of divergence. It is obvious that simple fusion without any range of fusion is of little or no practical value.

Grade III. Stereopsis is the highest form of binocular vision and implies the ability to obtain an impression of depth by the superimposition of two pictures of the same object which have been recorded from very slightly different angles so that there is a small degree of dissimilarity—the classical example is the bucket which is appreciated in its true dimensions (Fig. 65). However, stereopsis is determined to only a limited extent by the synoptophore; *stereoacuity,* which is the smallest amount of horizontal retinal image disparity which provides a sensation of depth, is a more reliable measurement of stereopsis. This is expressed as the visual angle (in seconds of arc) of this disparity, with a normal figure of 100″ or less; a figure greater than this is regarded as evidence of a defective form of stereopsis such as

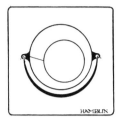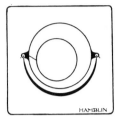

Fig. 65.   Slides for testing stereopsis on the synoptophore.

occurs when there is some degree of amblyopia of one eye. In the Frisby stereotest the presence of stereopsis is shown by the ability to see a circle of pattern elements which is lying in depth to the surrounding pattern elements; the variations of plate thickness and viewing distances at which this may be achieved provide a measurement of the stereoacuity. The TNO test for stereoscopic vision is of similar value. The Titmus fly test is less reliable.

The synoptophore also provides accurate information on the state of retinal correspondence; when there is normal retinal correspondence the subjective and objective angles are equal, but when there is an abnormal retinal correspondence the subjective angle is less than the objective angle and this difference is termed the *angle of anomaly*.

Determination of the health of each eye. It is important to establish the fact that each eye is free from any disease which would affect its visual function, for example, a scar of the cornea, a cataract or some retinal disorder like a retinoblastoma. This is a further reason why all infants with a suspected squint must have an early examination.

Determination of the refraction of each eye. It is an essential part of the treatment of squint to carry out an accurate assessment of refraction in order to prescribe glasses if these will be in any way helpful in ensuring that the vision of each eye is brought up to as normal a level as possible and in ensuring that a satisfactory relationship is achieved between the mechanisms of accommodation and convergence. This necessitates the estimation of refraction by retinoscopy (p.14) after the use of a cycloplegic drug, and when possible, the recording of the uncorrected and corrected vision of each eye for distance and for near vision.

Treatment of defective vision of the squinting eye by occlusion. If the vision of the squinting eye remains defective despite the provision of a corrective spectacle lens, whether in the older child, when it is possible to measure the visual acuity by the Snellen's test chart or by the Sheridan Gardiner test (see p.6), or in the younger child, when a visual defect is suspected simply because of a reluctance to fix with the squinting eye when the non-squinting eye is covered, it is necessary to carry out occlusion of the non-squinting (fixing) eye.

At one time it was deemed necessary to carry out this occlusion for prolonged periods of time—weeks or even months—but it is now recognized that this is unnecessary, quite apart from the fact that in certain cases prolonged occlusion of the fixing eye may create a reversal of the amblyopia so that the previously fixing eye becomes amblyopic. As a general rule a short period of occlusion (10 to 15 minutes) a few times each day is equally effective, provided a supreme effort is made during the times of occlusion in encouraging the child to make full use of the non-occluded eye by indulging in various games which are appropriate for the particular age of the child.

There has been uncertainty about the value of occlusion of the fixing eye when the amblyopia of the squinting eye is associated with an eccentric retinal fixation. An anomaly of retinal fixation in no way precludes the carrying out of occlusion of the fixing eye (*conventional occlusion*); as a general rule there is shifting of the retinal fixation towards a more normal type, although some degree of eccentricity in the parafoveal region may remain as a permanent feature, particularly when the amblyopia of the squinting eye became determined at an early age.

Sometimes when there is no change in the eccentric fixation of the squinting eye, and, therefore, no improvement in the vision of the amblyopic (squinting) eye, it has been suggested that this should be followed by a prolonged period of occlusion of the squinting eye (*inverse occlusion*) but this is of doubtful value. In such cases it has also been suggested that visual tasks should be carried out by the squinting eye (during occlusion of the non-squinting eye) with a red filter placed in front of the squinting eye because this enforces the use of the more central part of the fundus—a red filter permits the use of the retinal cones only—but any improvement in the vision is of a limited nature.

Management by orthoptic methods. Treatment is carried out by *orthoptists* who are medical auxiliaries with a function which is akin to radiographers, physiotherapists, etc., and their professional status is in the context of a 'profession supplementary to the practice of medicine'. In the early days of orthoptic practice great emphasis was placed on 'orthoptic exercises' with various instruments which were designed specifically for binocular training, such as the synoptophore which is based on the principle of the stereoscope; the aim of such treatment is essentially to achieve fusion. Naturally this is an attempt to achieve a restoration of a normal form of fusion (bifoveal fixation), but it is now realized that in most cases of manifest squint developing in early childhood there is little or no prospect of restoring normal fusion, and an anomalous form of fusion in the presence of a minimal angle of residual squint (microtropia) represents a successful result in such cases.

It follows that there has been a swing in the 'orthoptic exercise pendulum' over the years, and it is important to re-define the vital role of the orthoptist in the overall management of the patient with a squint. They are responsible for: (a) a careful measurement of the deviation by the prism and cover test method; (b) an assessment of the visual acuity of each eye by a method appropriate to the age of the patient—the Sheridan-Gardiner test (p.6) is the most reliable test which may be carried out on the young child, but sometimes the E test (p.6) is more appropriate, although it must be appreciated that this tends to provide a level of vision which is better than would be achieved by other methods; (c) an assessment of the potential binocular function by the Bagolini striated glass test and by such instruments as the synoptophore; (d) the detection of suppression in the absence of any obvious squint by the 4Δ test; and (e) the supervision of occlusion.

Mention should be made of a special form of orthoptic treatment which is described as *pleoptic treatment*. This is designed to attempt to deal as far as possible with eccentric fixation. Pleoptic treatment is concerned mainly with the creation of various forms of after-images in the squinting eye which are projected incorrectly because of the eccentric fixation; by various means an attempt is made to secure a more normal form of projection of the after-images. It is obvious, however, that any treatment of this kind demands a considerable degree of co-operation and concentration so that it is only appropriate for the older child (certainly after the age of five or six years), and by this time the eccentric fixation is of such an established nature that there is likely to be only a limited response to treatment which is seldom maintained when the treatment is discontinued.

It is obvious therefore that pleoptic treatment has only a limited application in cases of squint which occur in early childhood, and the whole emphasis on treatment must be on the prevention of complications such as established eccentric fixation, by the early treatment of the squint, and particularly of the amblyopia which follows a uniocular squint in childhood.

Pleoptic treatment, however, is of distinct value in obtaining improved vision in an amblyopic eye in later life when the vision of the good eye is lost as the result of some injury or disease. It is interesting that in cases of this kind there may be only a very limited improvement in the visual acuity in the distance as judged using the Snellen's test chart (p.6), but there may be a distinct improvement in the close reading vision as judged by the N reading types (p.7) which is of obvious importance. A distinct improvement in the visual status on distant fixation following pleoptic treatment may be related simply to a change towards a more normal type of fixation, so that, although there is only a limited improvement in the distant visual acuity, there is distinct enhancement of visual confidence so that there is a greater degree of visual independence.

Surgical correction of the squint. In some cases the use of glasses may be sufficient to correct the squint, but in many cases it is necessary to correct the deviation by carefully planned surgical treatment on one or more of the eye muscles of one or both eyes, sometimes in more than one stage. It is important to take regard of any difference in the extent of the ocular deviation on near as compared with distant fixation; this is discussed in relation to latent squint (see below).

As a general rule children stand up to this operation very well; the child leaves his bed in hospital for the operating theatre in a relaxed state because of the use of modern sedatives, the operation is carried out under general anaesthetic and the operated eye as a rule only requires to be covered for a few hours or often not at all, particularly when an operation is carried out on both eyes. Ideally this surgical treatment enables the restoration of binocular function, but the operation is justifed purely on cosmetic grounds because a person with an obvious squint or, in the case of a child, the parents, may have problems of a psychological nature, quite apart from the fact he may be prejudiced in obtaining many forms of employment in later life.

There follows a simple outline of surgical treatment of squint in general; surgical treatment is discussed later in the context of intermittent and latent squints (p.248), dissociated vertical divergence (DVD) (p.265), the A and V phenomena (p.251), myogenic disorders (p.261) and neurogenic incomitant squint (p.258).

As a general rule the operation involves recession and resection procedures: a medial rectus recession and a lateral rectus resection in esotropia, and a lateral rectus recession and a medial rectus resection in exotropia. A medial rectus recession is limited to 5 mm in a child and 6 mm in an adult, otherwise there is limitation of adduction (and, therefore, also of convergence) of the operated eye because the medial rectus is then inserted behind the functional equator which is represented by the main arc of contact of the medial rectus with the globe; this is in front of the anatomical equator because of the outwards as well as forwards direction of the orbital axis (Fig. 52, p.218). More than one operation may be necessary in certain cases; sometimes a further operation may be required because the previous operation creates an overcorrection—consecutive exotropia in esotropia or consecutive esotropia in exotropia.

It is sometimes difficult to obtain a satisfactory surgical result, particulary when there is no form of potential binocular function (normal or anomalous), despite careful planning of the surgical procedure. Recently an adjustable rectus recession technique (*adjustable suture*) has been introduced so that the suture is externalized over the conjunctiva which permits an adjustment (advancement or further recession) on the day following the operation; obviously in the case of a child this is only applicable when the child is sufficiently old enough to be co-operative.

Use of botulinus toxin. This toxin when injected into an extrinsic ocular muscle creates a temporary paralysis. It is a relatively new and highly specialized technique in the management of certain forms of squint, and it is difficult at this stage to evaluate its potential value. However, it is possible that it may prove to be a method of treatment of fundamental importance because, at a certain stage of the temporary paralysis, it may enable a restoration of some form of binocular association and the eyes are then maintained in a 'straight ahead' position. The toxin may also be used in the management of essential blepharospasm (p.198).

Use of miotic drugs. Drugs which have a cyclospastic effect create some degree of contraction of the ciliary muscle with enhancement of the peripheral mechanism of accommodation, so that there is a reduction in the activity of the central mechanism which induces accommodation. This is followed inevitably by a reduction in the mechanism which produces a convergence of the eyes. This is a measure of a change in the accommodative convergence and accommodation relationship (AC/A ratio) (see p.226); a reduction in the accommodative component causes a reduction in the accommodative convergence response with a lowering of the AC/A ratio. It follows that such drugs are of value in the management of certain forms of accommodative or convergence excess esotropias.

However, as a method of treatment in isolation (in contrast to the wearing of spectacle lenses to correct any underlying refractive error) they are of value only in a limited number of cases because their use must fulfil two criteria: first, the esotropia on distant fixation must be controlled by the ordinary spectacle correction; and, secondly, the esotropia on near fixation must be controlled by enhancement of the influence of the spectacle correction by the use of the cyclospastic drug. Even when such criteria are attained, the use of the drugs may be limited because their discontinuance may be followed by a re-establishment of the esotropia on near fixation since any alteration in the AC/A ratio is only effective during the persistent use of the drugs, and they can only be used for a limited period, as discussed below. However, sometimes the use of a cyclospastic drug may be sufficient to create an improvement in the binocular status, so that after a period of time it is possible to maintain binocular function, even after discontinuance of the cyclospastic drug and despite persistence of an abnormally high AC/A ratio.

A more important use of cyclospastic drugs is in the postoperative management of esotropias in young children; over a period of a few weeks in the presence of a small residual deviation such drugs help to consolidate the surgical result by reducing the residual esotropia and thus foster the development of a useful form of binocular function (normal or anomalous).

Pilocarpine 1% drops may be used, but these have only a temporary effect so that they have to be instilled at least four times each day; phospholine iodide 0.06 or 0.125% drops used once each day (preferably in the morning, so that their greatest influence occurs during the day) are more effective. However, phospholine iodide drops should only be used for limited periods because their prolonged use may lead to a proliferation of iris pigmentation which is shown by the occurrence of pigmentary nodules around the pupillary margins. It is difficult to establish the safe period, but certainly the drops may be continued for six to eight weeks without any risk. Also general anaesthesia should be carried out with care during the use of these drops because they have an adverse effect if any form of muscular relaxant is used by the anaesthetist.

Use of bifocals. Bifocals are of value in the accommodative type of squint when the deviation is controlled by ordinary glasses for distant fixation but not for near fixation because of the extra accommodative effort which is then required, provided the reading segment (which may be as much as +3 D stronger than the distant segment) permits a control of the deviation for near. It is essential to make the reading segment sufficiently large so that the child is forced to use it for all close work and is not tempted to rely simply on the distant segment.

In general the aim of treatment of a manifest squint is to achieve a functional result, that is, establishment of binocular function, rather than simply amelioration of a cosmetic blemish. When the squint is of relatively late onset, when it shows a prolonged intermittent phase, or when treatment is applied at an early stage, it may be possible to restore normal binocular function (bifoveal fixation), but quite frequently even when various lines of treatment result in a scarcely perceptible residual deviation (microtropia) there is evidence on critical methods of examination of an anomalous retinal correspondence; in certain circumstances, however, this is a perfectly satisfactory result because it provides an adequate form of binocular association with an anomalous form of fusion which is usually sufficient to stand up to the rigours of the visual demands on the eyes in adult life.

Intermittent squint

This is a squint which is present only at certain times. By convention this term is reserved for the squint which is manifest at one distance of fixation but latent at another distance of fixation. The term is applied largely to esodeviations (convergent squints) and exodeviations (divergent squints), and these may be classified according to the position of fixation at which the deviation is manifest.

Intermittent convergent squint (intermittent esotropia)

    1.   *Convergence excess esotropia*—the esotropia is manifest on near fixation, but latent on distant fixation.
    2.   *Divergence weakness esotropia*—the esotropia is manifest on distant fixation, but latent on near fixation.

Intermittent divergent squint (intermittent exotropia)

    1.   *Divergence excess exotropia*—the exotropia is manifest on distant fixation, but latent on near fixation.
    2.   *Convergence weakness exotropia*—the exotropia is manifest on near fixation, but latent on distant fixation.

The various forms of vertical squint (hypertropia and hypotropia) may also show intermittent phases.

The methods of diagnosis and treatment of intermittent squint are essentially based on those for manifest squint (discussed above) and latent squint (discussed below).

Latent squint (heterophoria)

This is a condition in which there is an imbalance of the extrinsic ocular muscles so that under conditions of stress there is failure of the fusion mechanism to function adequately, with the development of a squint. The nature of the latent squint is designated by the direction of the occasional squint: a tendency for the eye to turn in (*esophoria*), which is of three main types—*convergence excess* when the deviation is greater for near than for distant fixation, *divergence weakness* when the deviation is greater for distant than for near fixation, and *basic* when the deviation is more or less equal on near and distant fixation; to turn out (*exophoria*), which is also of three main types—*divergence excess* when the deviation is greater for distant than for near fixation, *convergence weakness* when the deviation is greater for near than for distant fixation, and *basic* when the deviation is more or less equal on near and distant fixation; to turn up (*hyperphoria*); to turn down (*hypophoria*); to wheel-rotate in (*incyclophoria*); or to wheel-rotate out (*excyclophoria*). An alternating hyperphoria and alternating hypophoria may also occur as in the alternating hypertropia and alternating hypotropia (p.235). These imbalances are produced by the same obstacles which cause a manifest squint, but in the latent squint they are sufficiently minor to be controlled (*compensated*), often in the absence of any feeling of strain, except under conditions of stress, illness, advancing age, etc., when they tend to become uncontrolled (*decompensated*) so that the latent squint is converted to a manifest one. It follows that some forms of heterophoria are associated with symptoms (unlike heterotropia), when an effort is required to maintain control of the latent deviation, which are essentially those of eyestrain: headache, ocular discomfort, redness of the eyes, blurring of vision at certain times, or even intermittent diplopia, particularly after intensive use of the eyes.

Diagnosis

The diagnosis of heterophoria is dependent on inducing the latent deviation by a dissociation of the eyes and this is achieved in various ways:

The alternate cover test. The test (p.237) is of great value because it dissociates the eyes so that a latent deviation becomes converted into a manifest one during the rapid transference of the cover from one eye to the other; the rapidity of the recovery of the eyes to a binocular position after the removal of the cover is a useful method of assessing the strength of the fusional vergence. The degree of the control of the latent deviation may be measured accurately by placing prisms of increasing strength (with the base of the prism in a direction opposite to that of the deviation) in front of one eye until there is no further breakdown— the so-called *prism and cover test.* The test is carried out for near fixation (33 cm) and for distant fixation (6 m) because of the marked difference which may occur in these positions.

The Maddox rod test. The Maddox rod is an optical appliance which consists of a series of red-coloured glass rods which converts the appearance of a white spot of light into a red line. This rod is placed in front of one eye—the red line cannot be fused with the unaltered image of the white spot of light which is viewed by the other eye, so that the eyes become dissociated and the extent of the dissociation is measured by obtaining a superimposition of the two images by the use of prisms (with the base of the prism in a direction opposite the direction of the deviation). The Maddox rod may be rotated to make the red line run vertically or horizontally in order to measure latent horizontal and vertical forms of squint respectively, and an abnormal tilting of the line when the Maddox rod is placed correctly in the trial frame indicates a cyclophoria. The Maddox rod test is usually carried out for distant fixation (6 m), but it may be used at other distances of fixation.

The Maddox wing test. This is an instrument which dissociates the eyes on near fixation (33 cm); the amount of the horizontal dissociation is indicated by the apparent position of a vertical arrow (seen by one eye) on a horizontal tangent scale (seen by the other eye), and the amount of vertical dissociation is indicated by the apparent position of a horizontal arrow (seen by one eye) on a vertical tangent scale (seen by the other eye). There is also a movable wire which is adjusted by the patient until it appears horizontal; any cyclophoria is detected by incorrect placement of the wire.

The synoptophore. This instrument (p.238) is used to measure the fusional vergence in cases of heterophoria; when the heterophoria is not well compensated the fusional vergence is poor.

Occlusion. The occlusion of one eye for a few days is a useful diagnostic test in cases when it is uncertain if the symptoms of eyestrain are the result of heterophoria; a disappearance of the symptoms on occlusion is an indication of their association with muscle imbalance.

Treatment

The treatment of heterophoria is often limited to correction of the refractive error and orthoptic treatment, as discussed for heterotropia. If these measures prove to be inadequate, it is necessary to carry out carefully planned surgical treatment on the extrinsic ocular muscles in order to provide a satisfactory degree of control. This must take account of any difference in the extent of the deviation on near as compared with distant fixation: in convergence excess esophoria, a bilateral medial rectus recession is performed; in divergence weakness esophoria, a unilateral (or rarely a bilateral) lateral rectus resection; in basic esophoria, a limited unilateral medial rectus recession and lateral rectus resection; in divergence excess exophoria, a bilateral lateral rectus recession; in convergence weakness exophoria, a unilateral (or rarely a bilateral) medial rectus resection; and in basic exophoria, a limited unilateral lateral rectus recession and medial rectus resection. Sometimes, however, if surgical treatment is contraindicated (as in the very elderly), prisms may be incorporated in the spectacle lenses because these permit the eye to be deviated in the direction of the phoria, without producing an awareness of diplopia, by causing an appropriate deviation of the light rays before they enter the eye. It should be noted, however, that this method of treatment has two great disadvantages; first, it tends to perpetuate the imbalance by forcing the eye into the deviated position, thereby preventing any attempt by the patient to control the imbalance so that there is a further weakening of the fusional vergence; and, second, many forms of heterophoria vary in degree in different positions of gaze so that, although a prism may be able to control symptoms of the deviation in one position of the eyes, it is ineffective in other positions. Prismotherapy is discussed further in relation to incomitant squint (p.259).

In this discussion on manifest and latent squints a distinction has been made between a horizontal type of deviation (esotropia, esophoria, exotropia and exophoria) and a vertical type (hypertropia, hyperphoria, hypotropia and hypophoria). It should be appreciated, however, that this distinction is in no way rigid; the two frequently coexist and the one may arise from the other. The first association is seen particularly in the alternating hypertropia or alternating hyperphoria which may accompany an esotropia or esophoria so that, in addition to the convergent deviation, either eye rotates upwards when the other eye is fixing This vertical element is evident also in the upshoot of each eye which occurs in adduction (where the action of elevation of the inferior oblique is especially effective), and less commonly in the alternating hypotropia or alternating hypophoria in which either eye rotates downwards when the other eye is fixing with a downshoot of each eye in adduction (where the action of the superior oblique is especially effective).

It is evident that these forms of alternating vertical squint differ from the usual forms of hyperphoria, hypertropia, hypophoria or hypotropia (in which each eye deviates in opposite directions—one eye upwards and the other eye downwards—to more or less equal extents) because each eye deviates in the same direction (upwards or downwards) and quite frequently to unequal extents.

The A and V phenomena

Normal eyes on looking up and looking down retain the same degree of 'parallelism' when binocular vision is retained on a series of targets equidistant from the eyes. However there is usually a change in the parallelism because when the eyes turn up they tend to regard a distant object, whereas when the eyes turn down they tend to regard a near object, and thus there is a relative divergence of the eyes on looking up and a relative convergence of the eyes on looking down; this may be regarded as a physiological form of the *V phenomenon*. However, when there is esodeviation (latent or manifest) of the eyes in the primary position with a significant increase in the esodeviation on looking down and a decrease in looking up, or where there is exodeviation (latent or manifest) in the primary position with a significant increase in the deviation on looking up and a decrease on looking down the V phenomenon is pathological. The presence of the *A phenomenon*, that is when there is esodeviation (latent or manifest) in the primary position with an increase in the esodeviation on looking up and a decrease on looking down or when there is exodeviation (latent or manifest) with an increase in the exodeviation on looking down and a decrease on looking up, is invariably pathological.

The extent of the A and V phenomena is assessed by the measurement of the deviation on looking directly up and directly down by the prism and cover test method. From a practical point of view these measurements are made readily on near fixation by shifting the fixation target directly up and down, but on distant fixation it is more expedient to move the face down and up so that the distant fixation target remains stationary.

It is also essential to note any vertical movement of each eye in turning into a position of adduction, because of the characteristic downdrift (or rarely downshoot) of each eye in adduction in association with the A phenomenon and updrift (or quite frequently upshoot) of each eye in adduction in association with the V phenomenon. These movements may be readily visible on a straight forward examination of the movement of the eyes, but sometimes they are only apparent when each eye is moved into a fairly extreme position of adduction. Sometimes it is also necessary for the eye to be very slightly below the horizontal plane to show the downdrift in the A phenomenon, or very slightly above the horizontal plane to show the updrift in the V phenomenon.

The horizontal recti muscles play a role in the development of the A and V phenomena. In general terms the A phenomenon is the result of underaction of the horizontal recti, so that the A esodeviation is the result of weakness of the lateral recti, and the A exodeviation is the result of weakness of the medial recti, whereas the V phenomenon is the result of overaction of the horizontal recti, so that the V esodeviation is the result of overaction of the medial recti, and the V exodeviation is the result of overaction of the lateral recti. The oblique muscles also play a significant role: in the A phenomenon (esodeviation or exodeviation) there is an overaction of the superior obliques, and in the V phenomenon (esodeviation or exodeviation) there is an overaction of the inferior obliques; these overactions are of a primary nature. When the angle between the line of action of the superior oblique and the vertical meridian is significantly less than that of the inferior oblique, there is an enhanced vertical effect of the superior oblique over the inferior oblique, with the development of the A phenomenon. Similarly when the angle between the line of action of the inferior oblique and the vertical meridian is significantly less than that of the superior oblique, there is an enhanced vertical effect of the inferior oblique over the superior oblique, with the development of the V phenomenon.

As a general rule an overaction of an extrinsic ocular muscle is secondary to underaction of another muscle, such as the ipsilateral antagonist. However, there is anatomical evidence that in the A and V phenomena the overactions are of a primary nature due to an anomaly of development of the lines of pull of the superior oblique and of the inferior oblique. These are normally fairly similar (p.220), but sometimes significantly different; the superior oblique has an advantage over the inferior oblique in its vertical action in the A phenomenon, and the inferior oblique has an advantage over the superior oblique in its vertical action in the V phenomenon. This anomaly of the oblique muscles determines the necessity to include them in the surgical correction of the phenomena (see below).

The presence of an A or V element in an esodeviation or exodeviation necessitates a modification of the usual surgical treatment of the horizontal squint. There are many different procedures, but in general a strengthening operation (resection) of the underacting horizontal muscles (lateral recti in an A-esotropia and medial recti in an A-exotropia) and a weakening operation (recession) on the overacting horizontal muscles (medial recti in a V-esotropia and lateral recti in a V-exotropia) are effective measures, but it is frequently necessary also to carry out a weakening operation (recession) of the overacting oblique muscles (superior obliques in an A-esotropia or A-exotropia and inferior obliques in a V-esotropia or V-exotropia), that is, the obliques which are the ipsilateral antagonists of the underacting obliques.

In the A phenomenon a simple recession of each superior oblique may be sufficient, but a partial posterior tenotomy of the tendon at its insertion, leaving only the most anterior part of it, is more effective. In the V phenomenon a simple recession of each inferior oblique may be sufficient, but a moving forwards of the new insertion, so that it is in front of the equator (an anteroposition) in contrast to its normal insertion behind the equator, in addition to the recession is more effective.

Convergence insufficiency

This implies a failure of both eyes to be directed to a near object in the absence of any true paresis of the medial recti. Normally the mechanism of convergence is carried out without any effort of will because it is essentially a reflex phenomenon (p.225), although there is also a voluntary form of convergence, but symptoms of eyestrain are likely to occur if a conscious effort is required for this movement, as in exophoria of the convergence weakness type.

Convergence is tested objectively by bringing an object (like the examiner's finger) from a distance of about 33 cm towards the patient's nose and asking the patient to direct both eyes towards the approaching object; under normal conditions an equal degree of convergence of each eye should be maintained without undue effort until the object is about 7 cm from the eyes, but when there is convergence insufficiency this position may only be achieved with considerable difficulty—so that there is a subjective awareness of ocular discomfort—or there may be a failure of one eye (or even both eyes) to carry out the movement adequately. Convergence is tested subjectively by an instrument such as the Livingston binocular gauge. It is important, however, to distinguish between reflex convergence and voluntary convergence because a difficulty in inducing the latter does not necessarily indicate any defect of the reflex components.

Incomitant squint

This is a condition in which there is a *paresis* (partial loss of function) or *paralysis* (complete loss of function) of one or more of the extrinsic ocular muscles; the squint is an *incomitant* one, that is, the angle of the squint is variable (and often even absent) in certain positions of gaze according to the particular muscle (or muscles) involved in the dysfunction, so that there are varying degrees of external ophthalmoplegia. The nature of the defect is determined by methods (discussed below) which take account of the facts that (a) two muscles—one from each eye—are concerned primarily in the movements of the eyes in the six main positions of conjugate gaze; and (b) that a paresis of one extrinsic ocular muscle is followed by changes in some of the other muscles: overaction (and often later contractural changes) of the ipsilateral antagonist (the muscle of the same eye which opposes the action of the paretic muscle), overaction of the contralateral synergic muscle (the muscle of the opposite eye which is normally concerned with the paretic muscle in a conjugate movement), and secondary underaction of the antagonist of the contralateral synergist (the muscle of the opposite eye which normally opposes the action of the contralateral synergic muscle). It should be noted that an incomitant squint seldom remains incomitant indefinitely; many cases recover spontaneously or are relieved by treatment, and those which persist tend ultimately to become concomitant.

Assessment of the range of uniocular and binocular movements. This shows any area of restricted movement or of excessive movement which indicates underaction or overaction of a particular muscle. In cases of minor disturbance the anomaly may not be detected when the unaffected eye is covered because of the greater effort which is possible in uniocular movement.

Assessment of the nature of the diplopia. Diplopia is a feature of incomitant squint, and it is termed *pathological diplopia* in contrast to physiological diplopia (p.230). The separation of the images (the true image from the fixing eye and the false image from the paretic eye) is in a horizontal direction when one of the horizontally acting muscles is affected and in a vertical direction when one of the vertically acting muscles is affected; often in a vertical displacement there is also some horizontal displacement, so that there is an oblique separation of the images. Horizontal separation is detected by moving an object like a pencil held vertically into the two main positions of horizontal gaze (to the right and to the left,) and vertical separation is detected by moving the object held horizontally into the four main positions of vertical gaze (up and to the right, down and to the right, up and to the left, and down and to the left). The false image is the one which is farther from the eye, so that covering the affected eye causes a disappearance of the farther away image; when the paresis is only slight the recognition of the two images is facilitated by the use of red (for one eye) and green (for the other eye) goggles. In a case of multiple pareses or in a case of a single paresis with secondary overaction and underaction of other muscles, when diplopia is present in more than one of the six main positions of conjugate gaze, an assessment of the diplopia is made in each position with particular emphasis on the position in which there is a maximum separation of the images. A determination of the affected extrinsic ocular muscle from an assessment of the diplopia is dependent on a knowledge of the main field of action of each muscle.

The cover test. It is useful to carry out this test (p.237) in all six positions of conjugate gaze in addition to the primary position to determine the positions in which the deviation is evident. The extent of the deviation differs according to the eye which is used for fixation, with the smaller deviation occurring in the affected eye during the fixation of the unaffected eye (the so-called *primary deviation of the affected eye*) and with the greater deviation occurring in the unaffected eye during the enforced fixation of the affected eye (the so-called *secondary deviation of the unaffected eye*) which is the result of the increased innervational effort of the affected eye during fixation being passed also to the unaffected eye by the phenomenon of reciprocal innervation.

The field of binocular fixation. Measurement of the field of binocular fixation (p.221) indicates the area of the field in which the two eyes are unable to function binocularly because of the paresis.

The Hess screen. This is a projection test in which records are made of the direction of the paretic eye when the unaffected eye is fixing in each of the cardinal positions of gaze (the primary deviation of the affected eye), and of the direction of the unaffected eye in these positions when the paretic eye is fixing (the secondary deviation of the unaffected eye). During the tests the eyes are disssociated by the use of red and green goggles; the cardinal positions (p.221) are 15° (or 30°) from the primary position.

Assessment of abnormal head posture. The nature of the head posture is sometimes diagnostic of a particular paresis (p.234).

False projection. In an incomitant squint there is an upset of the normal appreciation of an object in space so that it is incorrectly located by the paretic eye; this is the so-called *past-pointing* which occurs when the finger points beyond the object of fixation in the direction of the field of action of the paretic muscle during its attempted localization. This occurs because the effort which is made to try to turn the eye into the affected field is interpreted by the brain as evidence that the eye has moved into the desired position so that the subsequent stimulation by the object of a peripheral point on the retina, instead of the fovea, gives the impression that the object is displaced still farther from the eye. The failure of the brain to appreciate the absence of any movement of the eye is explained by the fact that in any active (as distinct from passive) movement of the normal eye from point A to point B there is no impression of a sensation of movement of the objects between A and B, despite the fact that these objects flit over the retina, as the result of a perceptual adjusting mechanism.

There are two main forms of incomitant squint—*neurogenic,* due to some lesion of the complex nervous network which is concerned in the control of ocular movement, and *myogenic,* due to some lesion of the muscle or its fascial tissues.

Neurogenic disorders

There is a wide variety of conditions which may produce neurogenic lesions; only a limited number in each main category is mentioned:

1. *Congenital abnormalities* (these are very rare)
    (a) Nuclear aplasia
2. *Inflammatory conditions*
    (a) Encephalitis (septicaemia, poliomyelitis)
    (b) Neuritis (meningitis, herpes zoster)
    (c) Neurosyphilis (meningo-vascular, tabes dorsalis or general paralysis of the insane)
    (d) Osteoperiostitis (syphilis)
3. *Toxic disorders*
    (a) Bacterial toxins such as tetanus and botulism
    (b) Intoxications such as lead, carbon dioxide, alcohol (particularly methyl alcohol), snake venom, spinal anaesthesia
4. *Demyelinating diseases*
    (a) Disseminated sclerosis
5. *Metabolic disorders*
    (a) Vitamin B deficiency (beri-beri and pellagra)
    (b) Diabetes mellitus—the ophthalmoplegia in this condition is almost invariably the result of involvement of a nutrient artery to one of the cranial motor nerves. It is frequently short-lived, but in the absence of effective control of the diabetes it may be recurrent

6. *Vascular lesions*
   (a) Intracerebral haemorrhage
   (b) Subarachnoid haemorrhage (p. 329)
   (c) Congenital and acquired intracranial aneurysms (p. 328)
   (d) Vertebro-basilar insufficiency (p. 127)
   (e) Thrombosis
   (f) Embolism
7. *Neoplastic diseases*
   Many different forms of primary and metastatic tumour formations, particularly those involving the midbrain, the middle cranial fossa and the region of the superior orbital fissure
8. *Degenerative lesions*
   (a) Amyotrophic lateral sclerosis
   (b) Hereditary ataxia
9. *Traumatic lesions*
   May be direct involvement of a nerve in the lesion (as in a fractured base of skull).
   Involvement is usually of an indirect nature, as the result of a pressure on the nerve by associated haemorrhage or oedema

The diagnostic features of different forms of neurogenic incomitant squint depend on the motor nerves which are involved:

Third cranial nerve involvement. This causes the affected eye to be maintained in a position of abduction due to the unopposed action of the intact lateral rectus (innervated by the sixth cranial nerve) with a failure of the eye to move into positions of adduction, elevation or depression. It might be expected that the intact superior oblique (innervated by the fourth cranial nerve) would cause the eye to be somewhat depressed, but this is not so because it acts as a depressor mainly when the eye is in an adducted position, although its integrity is demonstrated by the obvious intorsion of the eye which occurs on attempting to look down. There are also other features: a drooping of the upper lid (ptosis) caused by paralysis of the levator muscle, a dilatation of the pupil (mydriasis) with a failure to respond to light directly or consensually or to respond to a near stimulus because of a paralysis of the sphincter muscle of the pupil, and a failure of accommodation (cycloplegia) due to paralysis of the ciliary muscle. Sometimes, however, there is only *external ophthalmoplegia* (involvement of the extrinsic ocular muscles and the levator) without *internal ophthalmoplegia* (involvement of the sphincter of the pupil and the ciliary muscle), and at other times there is only a partial involvement of the nerve (paresis) so that there is a sparing of the action of some of its muscles.

The *misdirection-regeneration syndrome (aberrant regeneration)* may follow a third nerve ophthalmoplegia after some degree of recovery; typically there is retraction of the upper eyelid on down-gaze, and sometimes there are abnormal pupillary movements on a gaze movement in a particular direction. The syndrome is generally regarded as a misdirection of axons from the distal to the proximal parts of the nerve across the area of damage.

Fourth cranial nerve involvement. This causes a loss of depression in an adducted position, with frequently a latent or manifest upward displacement of the affected eye in the primary position (*hyperphoria* or *hypertropia*), and also a defective intorsion of the eye, so that it becomes extorted because of the unopposed action of the inferior oblique (the ipsilateral antagonist). The overactions of this muscle and also of the inferior rectus of the unaffected eye (the contralateral synergist) increase the hyperphoria or hypertropia of the affected eye, which is increased further by a weakness of the superior rectus of the unaffected eye (the antagonist of the contralateral synergist).

A bilateral fourth nerve paresis occurs mainly in severe concussional head injury as the result of a disruption of the nutrient vessels to both fourth nerve fibres as they decussate on the dorsal surface of the midbrain in the medullary velum. Sometimes this bilateral paresis affects almost exclusively the action of intorsion so that there is a torsional type of diplopia which increases on looking down.

Sixth cranial nerve involvement. This leads to an absence of abduction and the affected eye is usually convergent because of the overaction of the medial rectus (the ipsilateral antagonist), which is increased by an overaction of the medial rectus of the unaffected eye (the contralateral synergist) and by a weakness of the lateral rectus of the unaffected eye (the antagonist of the contralateral synergist).

Involvement of all the motor nerves to the extrinsic ocular muscles. This is associated with a complete external ophthalmoplegia; the paralysed eye usually assumes the *'position of rest'* which is one of divergence because of the forwards and outwards direction of the orbital axis. There may also be an internal ophthalmoplegia (p.103) *(total ophthalmoplegia)*.

The promixity of the third, fourth and sixth cranial nerves to other nervous structures during their passage from the nuclei to the extrinsic ocular muscles (Fig. 66) determines the occurrence of certain syndromes.

Brainstem lesions. Brainstem lesions include the following four syndromes:

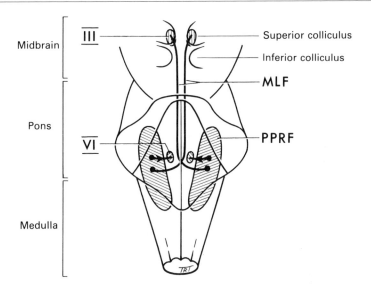

Midbrain

III — Superior colliculus

Inferior colliculus

MLF

Pons

VI — PPRF

Medulla

Fig. 66. Horizontal gaze centres—brain stem nuclei. MLF = medial longitudinal fasciculus. PPRF = parapontine reticular formation.

1. *Benedikt's syndrome (tegmental syndrome)* follows a lesion in the dorsal part of the cerebral peduncle in the tegmental part of the midbrain. It causes involvement of the ipsilateral third cranial nerve (see above), of the red nucleus (causing contralateral hemitremor of the face and limbs and sometimes also an impairment or hesitancy of conjugate lateral gaze), and occasionally of the medial lemniscus, which represents the ascending sensory fibres to the thalamus after their decussation (causing contralateral hemianaesthesia).

2. *Weber's syndrome (syndrome of the cerebral peduncle* or *alternating oculomotor hemiplegia)* follows a lesion in the posterior end of the cerebral peduncle. It causes involvement of the ipsilateral third cranial nerve (see above) within the brainstem or as it emerges from the brainstem, and of the pyramidal tract in the cerebral peduncle (causing contralateral hemiplegia of face and limbs).

3. *Foville's syndrome* follows a lesion in the pons. It causes involvement of the ipsilateral sixth nerve (see above), of the corticofugal fibres from the frontal motor cortex after their decussation in the region of the posterior commissure (causing loss of conjugate deviation to the side of the lesion), of the seventh (facial) cranial nerve (causing ipsilateral facial palsy), and of the pyramidal tract (causing contralateral hemiplegia).

4. *Millard-Gubler syndrome* follows a lesion in the lower part of the pons. It causes involvement of the sixth and seventh cranial nerves, as in Foville's syndrome, but with sparing of the corticofugal fibres so that

there is no loss of movement of the contralateral medial rectus on attempted conjugate movement to the side of the lesion.

Trunk lesions. This category includes the following five syndromes:

1.   *Basal palsy* follows a lesion of the base of the brain. It causes involvement of the third, fourth and sixth cranial nerves and often also involvement of the fifth, seventh and eighth cranial nerves.
2.   *Gradenigo's syndrome* follows a lesion of the apex of the petrous temporal bone. It causes involvement of the sixth cranial nerve.
3.   *Cavernous sinus syndrome* follows a lesion of the cavernous sinus. It causes involvement of the third, fourth and sixth cranial nerves, involvement of the fifth nerve (the ophthalmic division of the nerves when the lesion is placed anteriorly and the maxillary and mandibular divisons when the lesion is placed posteriorly), and sometimes a pulsating type of exophthalmos.
4.   *Sphenoidal fissure syndrome* follows a lesion in the region of the superior orbital fissure. There is progressive involvement of the third cranial nerve (sometimes only the superior or inferior division is involved—the superior division supplies the levator and superior rectus and the inferior division supplies the medial rectus, inferior rectus, inferior oblique, the ciliary muscle and the sphincter of the pupil), of the fourth and sixth cranial nerves, and of the fifth cranial nerve (sometimes only the ophthalmic division but often also the maxillary division), causing a combination of anaesthesia and severe neuralgic pain and with an associated proptosis.
5.   *Orbital apex syndrome* follows a lesion in the posterior part of the orbit near its apex, with involvement of the second cranial nerve (causing optic disc swelling or optic atrophy) in addition to the features of the sphenoidal fissure syndrome.

Treatment of neurogenic ophthalmoplegia. This is directed at the cause of the ophthalmoplegia, although in many conditions (e.g. fracture of the skull, disseminated sclerosis) there is often spontaneous recovery in the absence of any specific treatment; during the waiting period diplopia may be avoided by occlusion of one eye. Persistence of a significant degree of ophthalmoplegia after an interval of six months demands surgical intervention, provided repeated examinations confirm that the condition is not in a progressive or regressive phase; the main object is to restore comfortable binocular single vision in the primary position and also in as much of the field of binocular fixation as possible, particularly on depression (because this is the conventional reading position). In complicated forms of paralysis the operative treatment may need to be carried out in several carefully planned stages. There are various methods involved: an increase in the effectiveness of a paretic muscle by its resection, a decrease in the

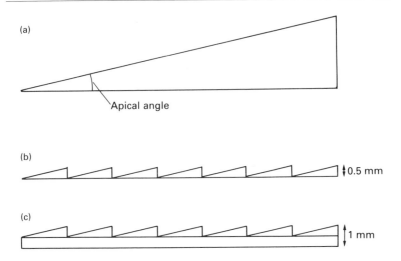

Fig. 67. (a) The power of a prism depends on the size of the apical angle. (b) Multiple small prisms with the same apical angle produce the same optical effect as in (a). (c) The Fresnel prism—multiple small prisms of the same apical angle with a 0.5 mm base width, attached to a 0.5 mm membrane.

effectiveness of an overacting muscle (ipsilateral antagonist or contralateral synergist) by its recession or by its division—myectomy or tenotomy (usually only of the superior or inferior oblique)—an increase in the range of movement of the eye by a recession of a muscle in a state of contracture (usually the ipsilateral antagonist), and sometimes the restoration of some degree of movement in the paralysed muscle by a transplantation type of operation with slips from unaffected muscles.

In a sixth nerve palsy with a persistent loss of abduction, a union between slips of the superior and inferior recti to the lateral rectus may provide some degree of abduction, but this should be carried out separately from a recession of the medial rectus (the more effective procedure because of the contractural state of the ipsilateral antagonist muscle) because of the risk of causing anterior segment ischaemia (p.99). In a third nerve palsy, with persistence of an abducted position of the eye despite a recession of the lateral rectus (the ipsilateral antagonist) and a resection of the affected medial rectus, a shift of the superior oblique to the region of the insertion of the medial rectus may be of limited value.

Prisms are of value in the management of certain cases in order to eliminate diplopia on looking straight ahead, particularly in any case when diplopia is troublesome at a stage before surgical treatment can be carried out (i.e. during the six months after the onset of the ophthalmoplegia), and in the elderly as a permanent procedure when surgical treatment is not advisable or not acceptable by the patient. Conventional prisms are of limited value because of the cumbersome nature of sufficiently strong prisms which are cosmetically unsightly and optically inefficient unless maintained consistently in the correct position. Fortunately these difficulties are overcome by the use of Fresnel prisms which were developed and adapted from the original hand-ground lenses designed for lighthouses by Augustin J. Fresnel early in the nineteenth century. The Fresnel prism makes use of the fact that the power of a prism is related only to the apical angle of the prism, and not to the size of its base which is determined by the length of the prism. Thus a series of small prisms has the same prismatic effect as a single large prism because of constancy of the apical angle (Fig. 67). It is now possible to obtain a Fresnel type of prism which is composed of a series of small membranous plastic prisms (each with a base of only 0.5 mm) lying adjacent to one another on a thin membranous plastic platform (with a thickness of only 0.5 mm) so that the total thickness is 1 mm. This membranous prismatic lens can be adhered to a spectacle lens, and replaced readily if a different prismatic power is required, However, it is cosmetically noticeable, and it causes some reduction in the clarity of vision.

Myogenic disorders

Myogenic disorders causing ophthalmoplegia are much less common than neurogenic disorders. They may be of a congenital or acquired nature.

Congenital abnormalities. These are termed *musculo-fascial anomalies* in which there may be restriction of movement of the eye in the direction of action of the affected muscle (or muscles) because of fibrosis of the muscle or its sheath, and also some defect of movement of the eye in the opposite direction because of failure of the affected muscle to relax adequately as the result of its fibrotic state or as the result of rigidity of the muscle sheath.

There are two main congenital conditions of this kind—*Duane's retraction syndrome* and the *superior oblique tendon sheath syndrome*, but it must be conceded that they may not be the same thing because of the uncertainty of the origin of Duane's retraction syndrome, as discussed below.

1. *Duane's retraction syndrome.* In the typical form the lateral rectus is involved primarily in the fibrotic process, with only a minor involvement of the medial rectus (Type A) or sometimes no involvement of the medial rectus (Type B), so that there is failure of abduction and a defect of adduction with retraction of the eye on attempted full adduction because of failure of the lateral rectus to relax; this failure may be confirmed accurately at operation by the resistance

which is experienced on attempting to move the globe manually into a position of adduction—the *forced duction test.* The retraction is not simply the result of the mechanical effect of the fibrotic lateral rectus but is produced also by the combined actions of the medial, superior and inferior recti which, in trying to achieve a position of full adduction, produce the effect of retraction (sometimes regarded less accurately as an enophthalmos) with a slight narrowing of the palpebral fissure. There is also ptosis of the upper lid during the retraction of the eye, but this is simply the result of a failure of the retracted eyeball to support the upper lid. A slight protraction of the eyeball occurs on attempted abduction because the superior and inferior obliques which, in trying to exert their abducting influences following the loss of abduction by the lateral rectus, produce protraction with a slight widening of the palpebral aperture. In the primary position there is usually only a slight degree of manifest (or latent) convergent squint, which is in contrast to the gross loss of abduction; this is characteristic of a myogenic lesion as compared with a neurogenic one (in which there would be obvious overaction of the ipsilateral antagonist and contralateral synergist, particularly on dissociation of the eyes as in the cover test) and is a feature of great diagnostic significance.

In the atypical form of the syndrome (Type C), the medial rectus is more affected than the lateral rectus by the fibrosis so that adduction is more limited than abduction and a manifest (or latent) divergent squint is present in the primary position; the retraction of the eye on attempted adduction and the protraction of the eye on attempted abduction occur as in the typical form of the syndrome.

However, there is increasing evidence that the features of Duane's retraction syndrome as described above are the result of a peculiar congenital anomaly of innervation (perhaps of the brainstem centres concerned in the control of ocular movement) so that there is co-contraction of the lateral and medial recti. This has been demonstrated quite conclusively by electromyographic (EMG) studies so that, although the description of Duane's retraction syndrome is correct, it is almost certainly no longer appropriate to regard it as a musculo-fascial anomaly, except in a few isolated cases, and this explains the relative infrequency of finding a positive forced duction test in such cases.

Treatment. Attempts have been made to restore some degree of abduction in Type A of the syndrome, but these are usually unsuccessful, which is explained by an understanding of the basic nature of the condition. As a general rule surgical treatment is limited to a restoration of binocular single vision in the primary position when there is an esotropia which is not controlled or when there is an esophoria which becomes an esotropia in the absence of a compensatory head posture. This demands a recession of the medial rectus of the affected eye and sometimes also a recession of the medial rectus of the other eye; a lateral rectus resection of the affected eye is indicated only when the esotropia is marked, an unusual event.

2. *Superior oblique tendon sheath syndrome.* In this syndrome there is an abrupt cessation of movement of the affected eye in the field of action of the inferior oblique (elevation in a position of adduction) because of a failure of relaxation of the superior oblique (the antagonist of the inferior oblique) as a result of its abnormal sheath; this is sometimes associated with a sensation of pain in the region of the trochlea (around which the superior oblique hooks) because the sheath may be attached to the pulley. This fascial anomaly is distinguished from a congenital neurogenic palsy of the inferior oblique by the forced duction test (which demonstrates the resistance on attempted manual movement of the eye into the field of action of the inferior oblique), and also to some extent by the absence of any marked deviation of the eyes in the primary position (often there is no deviation or only a very slight hypotropia) because of an absence of the secondary overactions which occur in a neurogenic palsy with the development of a marked deviation of the affected eye when the unaffected eye is fixing in the primary position; in the superior oblique tendon sheath syndrome any hypotropia is usually controlled by a compensatory head posture.

Treatment. Myectomy of the superior oblique or preferably removal of the abnormal sheath of the superior oblique is followed by restoration of some movement of the inferior oblique, but such treatment is usually reserved for cases in which there is a significant deviation in the primary position (a rare event), and particularly for bilateral cases.

Acquired conditions. There are five acquired myogenic disorders to be considered:

1. *Myasthenia gravis.* Paresis of one or more of the extrinsic ocular muscles, which is less common than paresis of the levator muscle of the lid (p.199), is characterized initially by fleeting episodes of diplopia which ultimately become more persistent, particularly towards the end of the day or after periods of fatigue, although they remain variable in extent. The functions of elevation and convergence are most frequently affected and both eyes are seldom involved to equal degrees. The intrinsic ocular muscles are not affected in this condition.

2. *Progressive external ophthalmoplegia (ocular myopathy).* In this condition there is a gradual and progressive loss of ocular mobility which usually causes a disturbance of elevation before involving the other forms of movement, although a ptosis is often the first feature. The disturbance is bilateral and, although it starts to some extent in adolescence, it is seldom obvious before early adult life or even middle age, except for a few cases which are advanced in childhood. Rarely there may be similar changes in the peripheral skeletal musculature. Its myopathic nature accounts for the absence of any involvement of the intrinsic ocular muscles. An ocular myopathy in childhood may be associated with tapetoretinal degeneration (retinitis pigmentosa, p.144).

3. *Ocular myositis.* An acute form occurs in an orbital cellulitis (p.284), but there is a rare chronic form with exophthalmos, lid oedema, multiple extrinsic ocular muscle pareses, photophobia, and sometimes a disturbance of vision because of a defect of the vascular supply of the optic nerve due to the raised intraorbital pressure with the production of some degree of optic atrophy. It probably represents one of the collagen diseases and this explains the good response obtained sometimes to the use of steroids. An acute myositis follows an infestation of the muscle by the nematode *Trichinella spiralis*.

4. *Dermatomyositis.* A myositis of the extrinsic ocular muscles may occur in association with the other features of the condition (see p.134).

5. *Ophthalmoplegia in thyrotrophic exophthalmos.* This is discussed on p.292.

It should be noted that in addition to the neurogenic and myogenic forms of incomitant squint, an abnormality of ocular movement with the features of incomitancy may occur simply as the result of displacement of the eye or as the result of a limitation of movement for purely mechanical reasons; this type of paresis or palsy is liable to occur in any lesion of the orbit, for example, a fracture of the floor of the orbit or a tumour of the orbit.

Ocular deviations

The term ocular deviation is applied to a supranuclear lesion which causes a disturbance of ocular movement that, unlike a lower motor neuron lesion which causes an incomitant squint, is not capable of being resolved in terms of a disorder of individual muscles because it represents a disorder of one of the combined movements of the eyes—conjugate movements (versions) or disjunctive movements (vergences)—causing conjugate gaze palsies or disjunctive gaze palsies.

A gaze palsy may follow a lesion of the frontal motor centres (or their corticofugal nerve fibres) or of the occipital motor centres (or their corticofugal nerve fibres).

Frontal lesion causing a lateral gaze palsy

This shows a diminution or abolition of conjugate movement to the side away from the lesion (a right-sided lesion causes a failure of laevoversion) when the attempt to carry out the movement is of a voluntary nature or in response to a command. A slight conjugate movement of the eyes to the side of the lesion occurs because of the unopposed action of the centres in the unaffected side of the brain in the unconscious patient and a slight turning of the head to the side away from the lesion in the conscious patient. There is retention of the conjugate movements which follow the reflex fixation of an object; this may be intensified so that the gaze becomes anchored to the moving object, provided it is moved sufficiently slowly. There is retention and intensification of the conjugate movements which follow proprioceptive reflexes from the labyrinthine mechanisms and neck muscles, provided the lesion is above the level of the midbrain; in a right-sided frontal lesion a sudden turning of the patient's head to the right causes the eyes to move conjugately to the left (the doll's head, or doll's eye, phenomenon), or the conjugate movement may be induced by caloric or galvanic stimulation of the labyrinthine mechanism. There is also retention of reflex convergence (provided the lesion is above the level of the pons). The condition is not accompanied by any awareness of diplopia because the defective motility is equally represented in each eye.

Paralysis of vertical movements (Parinaud's syndrome)

A supranuclear lesion affecting vertical movement is rare and is usually the result of a lesion in the subthalamic region. The persistence of Bell's phenomenon—the ability of the eyes to turn up on attempted closure of the lids—is retained. The syndrome is not associated with any awareness of diplopia.

Paralysis of convergence

Paralysis of convergence in the absence of any defective movement of either eye during ductions or lateral versions is a rare occurrence, and this is in marked contrast to a functional disturbance of the convergence mechanism (p.251) which is common. The site of the lesion is uncertain. It is characterized by persistent diplopia for near objects, but an absence of any diplopia when looking in the distance. There is no satisfactory treatment of the defect, but the diplopia may be avoided on close work by the provision of glasses incorporating prisms (base in). Fresnel prisms (p.259) are of particular value.

Spasm of convergence

Spasm of convergence, usually in association with spasm of accommodation, is a rare occurrence in children and young adults as the result of some disturbance of a psychological or hysterical nature. More frequently it is a feature of the convergence excess type of esophoria or intermittent esotropia (p.246).

Occipital lesion causing a lateral gaze palsy

This shows a disorientation of the psycho-optical reflex, so that there is an inability to turn the eyes conjugately towards an object on the side away from the side of the lesion; the eyes may remain staring ahead or carry out awkward rolling movements. There is retention of the conjugate movements induced by the frontal centres and by proprioceptive stimuli from the labyrinthine mechanism and from the neck muscles.

Dissociated gaze palsies

These palsies represent a form of supranuclear disturbance which is of an irregular nature, so that diplopia is a feature at times. They follow lesions of the medial (posterior) longitudinal bundle which is concerned in providing a link between the various motor nuclei which supply the extrinsic ocular muscles (internuclear palsy) (see Fig. 66).

In a *bilateral anterior internuclear palsy* there is defective movement of the adducted eye and nystagmus of the abducted eye on attempted movements of lateral gaze to either side, but there is usually retention of normal convergence, except when there is also involvement of the descending nerve fibres which subserve the convergence reflex. In a *unilateral anterior internuclear palsy*, the defective movement of the adducted eye and the nystagmus of the abducted eye occur on lateral gaze to the side away from the lesion; there may also be a skew deviation on attempted lateral gaze with the ipsilateral eye becoming higher than the contralateral eye. A bilateral internuclear palsy is usually the result of a demyelinating lesion as in disseminated sclerosis (multiple sclerosis); a unilateral palsy may follow a vascular lesion or a brainstem tumour. (A *posterior internuclear palsy* has been described in which there is a loss of abduction with a retention of adduction, but it is doubtful is this is an established entity.)

Dissociated vertical divergence (DVD)

In this condition, when the vision of an eye is embarrassed by occlusion or by a reduction in light (as with a tinted glass in front of the eye) the eye turns slowly upwards with some extorsion, and reverts slowly to its previous position when the dissociating factor is removed; this may also occur even in a period of inattention without any dissociating factor. Usually there is symmetrical involvement of each eye, but sometimes it is asymmetrical, even rarely to such an extent that it is virtually unilateral. It frequently occurs in association with congenital esotropia and with congenital nystagmus so that it is almost certainly a congenital anomaly, but oddly it is seldom detected until the age of two to three years.

Dissociated vertical divergence is also termed *alternating sursumduction*, but this is a less appropriate term because it is liable to be confused with alternating hypertropia (p.249) which is an entirely different condition. In both conditions there is an upshoot of each eye in adduction; in alternating hypertropia this is the result of overaction of the inferior oblique, whereas in DVD it is simply the result of a normal action of the inferior oblique when the adducted eye is in a position of dissociation.

Surgical intervention in DVD gives a limited result. A recession of the inferior oblique of each eye is no value, and a recession of the superior rectus of each eye is of little value, but an improved effect is obtained by combining the recession with the placement of posterior fixation sutures (Faden operation) because this procedure, by anchoring the superior rectus to the globe behind the equator, increases the weakening effect of the muscle without reducing significantly its ability to move the eye into a position of elevation.

Skew deviation

This may follow a destructive lesion of the cerebellum. The eyes at times become deviated in opposite directions; one eye turns up and out whilst the other eye turns down and in.

Oculogyric crisis

This is liable to occur in paralysis agitans (Parkinson's disease) which is a degenerative condition of the corpus striatum. Initially there is a weakness of conjugate and disjunctive movements of the eyes in association with a diminution of movement of the skeletal musculature, but this is followed by a muscular rigidity which is associated with jerky movements of the eyes (cog-wheel rigidity) and with a stiffness and tremor of the other muscles. Sometimes marked conjugate spasms of the eyes occur so that they move violently into a certain position (usually upwards) and are maintained there for a variable length of time, the so-called *oculogyric crisis*. This alarming state may occur with the use of the phenothiazine group of drugs, and resolves with withdrawal of the drug.

Nystagmus

Nystagmus is a disordered state of ocular posture in which the eyes exhibit involuntary oscillatory movements. It has been suggested that there are two main types of nystagmus as far as rhythm is concerned: *pendular*, in which the undulatory movements are equal in speed and amplitude in both directions of gaze, and *jerky*, in which the undulatory movements are unequal in speed and amplitude so that there is a slow movement in one direction (the fundamental movement of the nystagmus) and a rapid movement in the opposite direction (the compensatory movement of the nystagmus to regain fixation). However, more recent sophisticated studies of the ocular movements in nystagmus such as the use of electromyography (EMG) or electrooculography (EOG) have shown that this is not a rigid distinction; for example, a pendular type of nystagmus when the eyes are in the primary position may become a markedly jerky type of nystagmus on movement of the eyes away from the primary position. The importance of this recognition about the rhythm of nystagmus is that it is no longer valid to regard a pendular rhythm as an indication of an ocular type of nystagmus.

The nystagmus may occur in different planes: horizontal, vertical, oblique or rotatory; in jerky nystagmus the direction of the nystagmus is designated by the direction of its rapid phase— right, left, up, down, oblique (with right or left and up or down components), clockwise rotatory, or anticlockwise rotatory. Fine degrees of nystagmus which are not detected readily on direct viewing are demonstrated on ophthalmoscopic examination because of the magnification of the movement; however they are, of course, more readily determined by electrodiagnostic methods (EOG and EMG).

Other features may be associated with nystagmus:

1. A sensation of apparent movement of stationary objects is not a feature of nystagmus which develops in early life (congenital nystagmus), but it is feature sometimes of the acquired forms of nystagmus. This is the result of the development of a perceptual adjusting mechanism, as discussed under false projection (p.254).

2. An awareness of diplopia is only a feature of nystagmus when it is induced by some lesion of the central nervous system. This is because the nystagmus is associated with some incomitancy of the ocular movements.

3. Head nodding may occur in the ocular type of nystagmus in children, the so-called *spasmus nutans*; it seldom occurs before the age of four months and usually disappears spontaneously before the age of three years, although it may recur to some extent when the child is in dim illumination. This head nodding is not compensatory to the nystagmus because it has a slow and inconstant rhythm in contrast to the nystagmus which is fast and steady.

Nystagmus is rarely confined to one eye. The most common form of nystagmus occurs in both eyes in a conjugate manner (i.e. in a position of version), but it may occur also in both eyes in a disjunctive manner (i.e. in positions of vergence—convergence or divergence—or when one eye turns up and the other eye turns down—the *see-saw nystagmus*), or it may even occur in a dissociated manner (i.e. the nystagmus of the two eyes is unrelated to one another because each is dissimilar in direction, extent and speed).

Nystagmus is liable to occur in many circumstances, but in general there are three main aetiological types: *ocular, vestibular,* and *central* (or *neurological*). There is also an idiopathic congenital nystagmus which is not related precisely to any of these three groups.

Ocular nystagmus

This type of nystagmus is the result of a defective form of central vision which mitigates against a normal type of steady central fixation, perhaps because inadequate visual sensations lead to a failure of the normal tonic control of the extrinsic ocular muscles. Ocular nystagmus is usually of the pendular variety, but it may become jerky on lateral gaze. It should be noted, however, that the occurrence of nystagmus after the loss of central vision depends largely on the age of the patient at the time of the visual failure; in the newborn or young infant nystagmus develops invariably within a few weeks; between the ages of two months and two years nystagmus usually but not invariably develops; between two and six years nystagmus seldom develops, except for a few irregular unsustained fixation movements; and after the age of six years, nystagmus is absent.

There are certain distinct forms of ocular nystagmus:

Deviational nystagmus. This occurs as a normal phenomenon when the eyes are turned conjugately to the limits of the binocular field of fixation; it has been described as nystagmoid jerks rather than nystagmus, but an exaggeration of the normal end-point nystagmus is a more accurate description. It occurs pathologically in the field of action of the affected muscle in an incomitant squint and in certain positions of gaze in a supranuclear lesion.

Latent nystagmus. This becomes obvious only on dissociation of the eyes, so that the binocular visual acuity is significantly better than the uniocular visual acuity. It is sometimes of congenital origin.

Optokinetic nystagmus. This is a physiological type of nystagmus which is induced by viewing a drum with alternate black and white lines which may be rotated vertically or horizontally; this is sometimes called *railway nystagmus* (*railroad nystagmus* in USA) because it also occurs in such activities as looking out of the window of a moving train. An optokinetic response may be elicited at an early age of life (certainly after the age of three months) and it forms a reliable method of determining the presence of visual function in an infant with suspected blindness. The integrity of the reflex is disturbed in lesions of the visual cortex or affecting the association pathways from the region of the visual centres to the motor centres in the brain stem, as well as in ocular blindness.

Miner's nystagmus. This is an acquired type of nystagmus which is due largely to working for prolonged periods in conditions of dim illumination (as in a coal mine), but there are other contributory factors including the crouched attitude of the miner with the persistent adoption of an upward gaze, the repeated exposure to noxious gases, and the mental stress of such work. There may be associated tremor of the head and spasm of the eyelids.

Vestibular nystagmus

This type of nystagmus is the result of a disturbance of the elaborate labyrinthine mechanism which exerts a proprioceptive influence on the extrinsic ocular muscles. It may be induced in the normal person on causing movements of the fluid within the labyrinth by rotating the subject or by caloric stimulation, or by galvanic stimulation. It occurs pathologically in any lesion (congenital or acquired) of the labyrinth or its subcortical pathways and centres. The nystagmus is of the jerky type with fine rapid horizontal and rotatory movements.

Neurological nystagmus

This type of nystagmus is the result of a disturbance (congenital or acquired) of any part of the complex nervous mechanisms—visual, proprioceptive and motor—which control the posture of the eyes. It is jerky in type. There are obviously many different causes of this nystagmus but mention is made of only two distinctive conditions: *see-saw nystagmus* and *ataxic nystagmus*.

See-saw nystagmus. In this form of nystagmus there is a turning up of one eye with some degree also of intorsion, and a turning down of the other eye with some degree of extorsion; this unusual form of nystagmus is associated characteristically with lesions of the optic chiasm.

Ataxic nystagmus. This form of uniocular nystagmus with impairment of conjugate lateral gaze has been described as pathognomonic of disseminated sclerosis (multiple sclerosis). In this condition there is some limitation of adduction of one eye with nystagmus of the other eye in abduction. However, it is essentially a form of the dissociated palsy which occurs in an internuclear palsy which is the result of a lesion of the medial (posterior) longitudinal bundle as discussed earlier (p.265).

Idiopathic congenital nystagmus

This is a form of nystagmus which is almost certainly present shortly after birth, but seldom becomes noticeable until the age of about three months when it increases in amount because of increased visual interest. It may be differentiated into two types according to the rhythm of the nystagmus—*pendular* or *jerky*.

Pendular congenital nystagmus. This is almost invariably the result of some ocular abnormality such as congenital tapetoretinal degeneration (p.143), cone monochromatism (p.21) and ocular albinism (p.79) when it is of an inherited nature, so that the prefix 'idiopathic' is not appropriate, although the nature of the underlying ocular defect may be difficult to detect. The visual prognosis depends on whether the cause of the pendular nystagmus is susceptible to treatment, but almost inevitably the distant vision is restricted because the pendular nystagmus tends to persist even after the elimination of the cause. It should be noted, however, that, as discussed above, the prefix 'pendular' must not be regarded too rigidly because away from the primary position a pendular type of nystagmus almost invariably assumes jerky features.

Jerky congenital nystagmus. This is almost invariably of unknown origin (except when it is of an inherited nature) so that the prefix 'idiopathic' is appropriate. It is reasonable, however, to regard it as some form of exaggeration of the fine movements of the normal eyes (high frequency eye tremors, rapid eye flicks—*saccades*—and slow motion drifts) and the fixation movements which occur persistently during steady fixation and which are essential to the maintenance of a clear image of the fixation target; these movements are co-ordinated by the complex centres in the brain stem (p.223), and presumably a slight derangement of the centres as the result of an inherited factor or some adverse neonatal influence may produce nystagmus in the absence of any other obvious neurological disorder. It is characteristic of this nystagmus that it varies greatly in different positions of gaze, and the position of least nystagmus (the neutral zone) provides the best form of vision, so that a compensatory head posture is frequently adopted (unless the neutral zone happens to be in the straight ahead position). The nystagmus tends to be greatest in the early years of life and then becomes progressively less, but even in adult life it is prone to sudden increases during times of stress and strain; this is of practical significance, for example, during an interview for a job or during an attempt to pass the visual part of a driving test. The close reading vision is usually remarkably good, although it may be necessary for the book to be held fairly near the eyes; this utilizes the reduction in the nystagmus which occurs in a position of marked convergence, and the position also provides magnification.

The jerky form of congenital nystagmus may be ameliorated by surgical treatment. This is of two main types.

First, when the congenital nystagmus is associated with congenital esotropia (the so-called *convergence blockage of the nystagmus*) any relief of the esotropia by a bilateral medial rectus recession is followed inevitably by an unmasking of the nystagmus so that it becomes increased to a considerable extent; this unmasking may be reduced significantly by combining each recession of the medial rectus with the Faden operation (posterior fixational sutures) because this procedure, by suturing the medial rectus muscle to the globe behind the equator, increases the weakening effect on the muscle without reducing significantly its ability to move the eye into a position of adduction.

Second, when the congenital nystagmus is associated with a significant degree of compensatory head posture, an operation may be carried out on both eyes in order to 'shift' the so-called *neutral zone* into a more straight ahead position. This involves a recession and resection procedure on the horizontal recti of both eyes, and the aim is to move the eyes so that they become 'straight' in relation to the compensatory head posture. Thus, if the neutral zone is to the left so that there is a compensatory head posture to the right, the operation consists of a right medial rectus recession, a right lateral rectus resection, a left medial rectus resection, and a left lateral rectus recession; the amount of each recession and resection is determined by the degree of compensatory head posture.

14

The Orbit

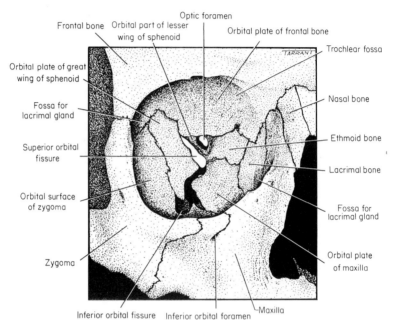

Fig. 68. The right bony orbit viewed from in front.

Structure and function

The bony orbit (Fig. 68) is formed by four walls—roof, floor, lateral wall and medial wall; there is no posterior wall because the roof slopes down to meet the floor and because the lateral wall slopes backwards and medially to meet the medial wall at an angle of about 45°. The medial walls of the two orbits are more or less parallel with one another; the angulation of the lateral and medial walls determines the forwards and outwards direction of the orbital axis (Fig. 52, p.218). There are three spaces in the orbital walls which transmit various structures: the *optic canal*, the *superior orbital fissure*, and the *inferior orbital fissure*.

The optic canal. This is the space which is formed by the union of the two roots of the lesser wing of the sphenoid which arise independently from the body of the sphenoid. It transmits the optic nerve with its meningeal coverings (dura mater, arachnoid mater and pia mater), the ophthalmic artery, and some sympathetic fibres from the carotid plexus.

The superior orbital fissure. This is a gap between the posterior part of the roof (lesser wing of the sphenoid) and the lateral wall (greater wing of the sphenoid); part of this is closed by dura mater but its wide part is open and provides a communication between the orbit and the middle cranial fossa for the transmission of several structures: the third, fourth and sixth cranial nerves, the lacrimal, frontal and nasociliary branches of the ophthalmic division of the fifth cranial nerve, the superior and inferior ophthalmic veins, and sympathetic nerve fibres.

The inferior orbital fissure. This is a gap between the posterior part of the lateral wall (greater wing of the sphenoid) and the floor (maxilla and orbital process of the palatine bone) which provides a communication between the orbit and the infratemporal (zygomatic) fossa in front and the pterygopalatine (sphenomaxillary) fossa behind for the transmission of several structures: the maxillary division of the fifth cranial nerve, the secretomotor nerve to the lacrimal gland from the sphenopalatine ganglion, the infraorbital artery, and communications from the inferior ophthalmic vein to the pterygoid venous plexus.

The orbital fascia

This consists of six different components:

1. *The bulbar fascia (Tenon's capsule)* covers the sclera from the limbus to the exit of the optic nerve from the eye. It provides two potential spaces: a subconjunctival space between the fascia and the overlying conjunctiva, and an episcleral space between the fascia and the underlying sclera.

2. *The check ligaments of the extrinsic muscles* are developed to any great extent only in relation to the lateral and medial recti, with attachments to the lateral and medial orbital margins, respectively. Each check ligament acts by preventing undue freedom of movement of the eye away from the field of action of its associated muscle.

3. *The fascial sheaths of the extrinsic ocular muscles* closely invest each muscle. Superiorly in the orbit there is a close association between the sheaths of the superior rectus and superior oblique muscles and the sheath of the levator muscle which extends medially and laterally to become anchored at the orbital margins (thus forming the *superior transverse fascial expansion of Whitnall*); inferiorly there is a close association between the sheaths of the inferior rectus and inferior oblique muscles which also extend medially and laterally to the orbital

margin (thus forming the *inferior transverse fascial expansion* or *suspensory ligament of the eyeball of Lockwood*). These expansions act as checking mechanisms which prevent undue upwards and downwards movements of the eyes because they become taut by bowing forwards or backwards during such movements.

4. *The periorbital membrane* lines the inner surface of the orbit and is continuous with the outer layer of the dura mater, which lines the inner surface of the cranial cavity, and with the periosteum, which covers the outer surface of the bones of the skull.

5. *The orbital septum* represents a fascial membrane which passes from the upper (and lower) orbital margins to the tarsal plate of the upper (and lower) eyelids so that the orbital space is separated from the lid substance.

6. *The connective tissue of the orbital fat* forms a supporting network within the orbital fat which fills the free space of the orbit.

The other constituents of the orbit—the eye, the optic nerve, the extrinsic ocular muscles and the lacrimal gland—are discussed in other chapters.

Assessment of the orbit

Examination of the orbit demands attention to detail, for many indirect clues, together with the history, radiology and ultrasonography, will give information about the site and size and, to some extent, the nature of the disorder, and dictate the choice of operation if necessary. For convenience the diagnostic values of ultrasonography and computerized tomographic scanning are discussed here on a broad basis and not just as applied to the orbit.

Ultrasonography

This non-invasive investigative technique has great application in ocular and orbital disease. Sound behaves in a similar fashion to light waves, with reflection, refraction and scattering occurring at sites of tissue discontinuity; the equivalent of refractive index for light is *acoustic impedance* for sound. In ultrasonography it is the reflected ray that is principally recorded.

Delivery of high frequency pulses of sound of short duration from a transducer produces echoes from tissue interfaces which are recorded by the transducer, displayed on an oscilloscope, and photographed.

The transducer is coupled to the patient by direct contact on the lid well-lubricated with hypromellose, or by the immersion technique when the zone between the cornea and transducer is filled with saline. Of the several modalities possible, two which are commonly used are known as the 'A' and 'B' scans.

(a)

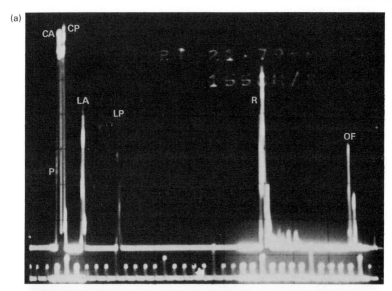

(b)

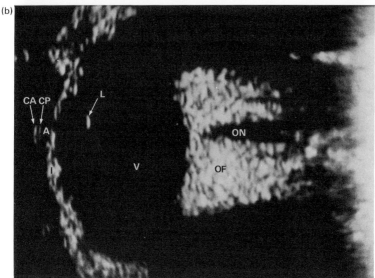

Fig.69. Ultransonography. (a) Normal A-scan—one-dimensional scan. P= probe; CA= corneal epithelium; CP = corneal endothelium; LA = anterior lens capsule; LP = posterior lens capsule; R = retina; OF = orbital fat. (b) Normal B-scan—two-dimensional scan. CA = corneal epithelium; CP = corneal endothelium; A = aqueous; I = iris; L = lens; V = vitreous; OF = orbital fat; ON = optic nerve. Note the acoustically empty aqueous and vitreous. (c) Collar-stud malignant melanoma of choroid. CA = corneal epithelium; CP = corneal endothelium; L = lens; MM = malignant melanoma. (d) Total retinal detachment with fibrosis. C = cornea; LA = anterior lens surface; LP = posterior lens surface; arrowheads = two folds of total fibrotic retinal detachment. (Figure continued overleaf.)

Fig. 69 continued

(c)

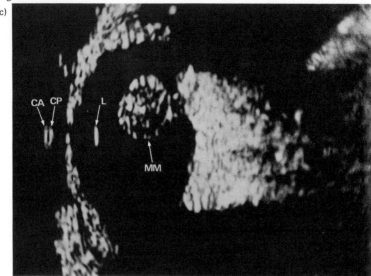

(d)

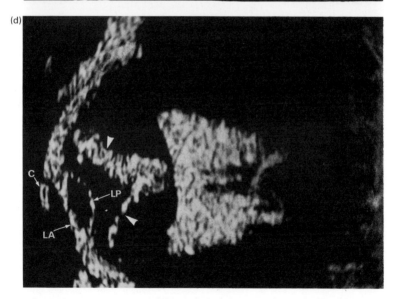

The 'A' scan gives a one-dimensional representation (Fig. 69a) where the time for echoes to return to the transducer is a measure of distance and therefore localizes a tissue interface, and the height of the deflection represents the echo intensity and may vary according to the consistency of the tissue. 'A' scanning has distinct advantages in orbital disease for, to some extent, it can differentiate histology by the patterns of reflected echoes within a mass lesion.

'B' scanning, by contrast, is two-dimensional (Fig. 69b) so that a composite representation of the globe and orbit is built up by multiple positions of the transducer. It is particularly useful for assessing vitreous dynamics and thereby areas of vitreoretinal traction. Ultrasound has several clinical applications. Its biometric value— measuring axial length, anterior chamber depth, scleral thickness, etc.—has become popular for estimation of the appropriate strength intraocular lens by computing the axial length and keratometer readings. When opacities in the ocular media preclude an examination of the posterior segment, 'B' scanning gives valuable information about the vitreous, retina and choroid, the site of blood, the presence of tumours (Fig. 69c) and of detachments (Fig. 69d) or traction membranes.

Computerized tomographic (CT) scanning

The advent of this non-invasive radiological technique has not only provided remarkable soft-tissue detail of intracranial and orbital contents, but has reduced the need for procedures such as arteriography, venography or pneumoencephalography, which carry a definite morbidity.

Transverse and coronal cross-sections of the brain and orbits are produced by computerized analysis of the density patterns of multiple layers of collimated X-rays (Fig. 70). In combination with the history, physical signs and prevalence patterns, the CT scan has permitted accurate identification of mass lesions and their extent, thus facilitating management, not least the choice of surgical approach. Present resolution of the scans gives details not only of the extrinsic ocular muscles (Fig. 70a,b), optic nerve or vascular anomalies but also of intraocular structures such as the lens, the presence of intraocular foreign bodies or tumours (Fig. 70c,d) and, by the demonstration of scleral thickening, has facilitated the often difficult diagnosis of posterior scleritis.

Radiology

Routine skull X-rays, including views of the optic foramina, provide details of the bony orbit, and show an increase or decrease in size, or evidence of destruction or reactive sclerosis, while tomography (axial hypocycloidal) will give details of the optic canal and paranasal sinuses.

Nuclear magnetic resonance

A further imaging system which, like computerized tomography, is non-invasive, but has the added advantage of no exposure to ionizing radiations, is the technique of computerized nuclear magnetic

(a)

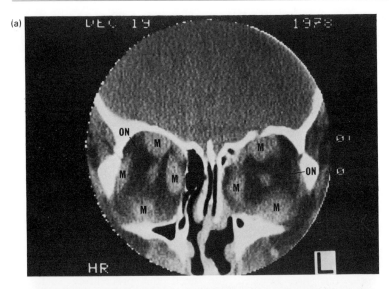

(b)

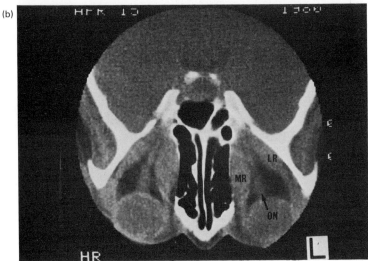

Fig. 70. Computerized tomography. (a) Dysthyroid eye disease—coronal section. Note the markedly enlarged rectus muscles (M); ON = optic nerve. (b) Same patient as in (a)—horizontal section. Note muscle enlargement maximal in posterior orbit and adjacent to optic nerve exit. MR = medial rectus; LR = lateral rectus; ON = optic nerve. (c) Haemangioma (H)—coronal section. (d) Haemangioma (H)—horizontal section. Note (i) intraconal position, and (ii) muscle size in comparison to (a) and (b).

(c)

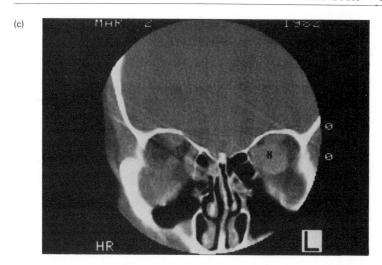

(d)

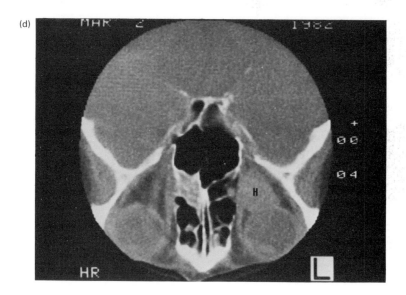

resonance. It is based on the principle that tissue hydrogen ions can be displaced from their alignment when placed in a magnetic field, and exposed to a radio frequency pulse. The energy released on removing the pulse is emitted as a radio frequency signal whose pattern and duration are analysed by computer to create an image. A particular advantage of this technique is the potential for identifying different histological types within imaged tissue.

Congenital anomalies

Craniofacial dysostosis

A dysostosis of the skull is the result of a failure in the development of the primitive mesoderm which is concerned in the formation of the bones of the skull (including the orbit), whereby there is premature synostosis of one or more of the sutures of the skull at a time when the brain is still expanding (most of this expansion occurs in the first decade of life). It is likely that the condition is determined early in intrauterine life (sometimes as an inherited disorder), so that the defects are evident in the newborn but the full effects occur in the early years of life. Males are more commonly affected than females. There may be other associated bony defects such as syndactyly and synarthroses.

Oxycephaly (tower skull). A premature synostosis of the craniofacial sutures results in a vertical elongation of the head, with a shortening of its anteroposterior diameter and, to a lesser degree, of its transverse diameter. The synostosis of the base of the skull determines the upwards expansion of the brain towards the patent anterior fontanelle with the formation of a dome-shaped head which tapers to its summit (and sometimes with the production of a meningocele or even a cerebral hernia). The associated upwards displacement of the optic nerves is liable to cause optic atrophy. Optic atrophy may also follow papilloedema due to an increased intracranial pressure; this increased pressure also causes headaches. The vertical direction of the forehead is accentuated by the absence of obvious supraciliary arches, and the face shows characteristic features: prominence of the nose, hypoplasia of the maxillae (flatness of the cheeks), and prognathism (prominence of the lower jaw). The orbits are shallow with a marked loss of the roof, so that proptosis (or even a true forwards dislocation of the eye) and a divergent squint are common features; rarely there is an associated narrowing of the optic canals with consequent damage to the optic nerves. Mental retardation is a common feature because of brain damage. In severe cases the removal of large parts of the bones of the vault of the skull may relieve pressure on the optic nerves, provided it is carried out sufficiently early.

Dolichocephaly. This represents a variant between oxycephaly and scaphocephaly (a long narrow head with elongation of the anteroposterior diameter and a narrowing of the transverse diameter) and is represented characteristically by *Crouzon's craniofacial dysostosis* (parrot head) in which there is marked frontal bossing, a prominent hooked nose, very marked recession of the maxillae, very marked prognathism of the lower jaw with irregularly spaced dentition and persistent salivation, marked proptosis, and sloping of the palpebral apertures in an outwards and downwards direction.

Hypertelorism. This is characterized by an excessively wide separation of the two eyes, with the production of a bovine appearance; the interpupillary distance often exceeds 80 mm (as compared with a normal distance of about 60 mm). It follows a premature ossification of the greater wings of the sphenoid which remain extremely small, so that the lateral directions of the orbits which are features of fetal life persist after birth; a divergent squint is a common feature. The optic nerves are not affected. The forehead is extremely shallow and the nose is characteristically upturned (retroussé).

Underdevelopment

A small orbit occurs characteristically when the eye is microphthalmic or absent (*anophthalmos*). It seems likely that the normal growth of the orbit in the child is dependent on an eye of normal size; this is evident also when an eye is enucleated in early childhood because the orbit tends to remain relatively small. A shallow orbit occurs sometimes in hydrocephalus.

Overdevelopment

An enlargement of the orbit is liable to occur in association with the expanding eye in buphthalmos (p.303) and in any form of expanding mass in the orbit.

Facial asymmetry

This may follow undue pressure on the face during a difficult labour. It is also a feature of the torticollis which occurs as the result of tautness of the sternocleidomastoid muscle on one side of the neck, so that the affected side of the face develops to a lesser extent than the other side; as a rule there are no associated ocular complications. Extrinsic ocular muscle palsies and lid displacement may occur in the rare condition of unilateral facial atrophy, a maldevelopment of both the bones and the soft tissues of the face.

Dermoid cyst

This occurs in the orbit as an inclusion cyst, usually in association with the suture lines, particularly in the upper and outer part of the orbit, with an attachment to the underlying bone. The cyst contains many different tissues, such as sebaceous material, hair and fat. It commonly causes ptosis of the upper lid, but it may also cause some degree of proptosis when it extends into the orbit. Leakage from a dermoid cyst may lead to the formation of a pseudotumour (see p.285). The cyst may be removed by simple excision, but sometimes the operation proves to be quite extensive; a failure to secure complete removal may cause a

granulomatous reaction of the surrounding tissues. Rarely, there may
be a direct communication through the bone with the dura.

Meningoencephalocele

This represents a herniation of a meningeal sac containing
cerebrospinal fluid (a meningocele) and usually also some brain tissue (a
meningoencephalocele) through a defect in the orbital wall, usually
between the frontal and ethmoid bones. It is readily determined on
radiological examination. Both orbits may be involved in the anomaly.
The cystic herniation is usually pulsatile because it contains circulating
cerebrospinal fluid; it increases in size when there is an increase in
venous pressure, it may transmit a detectable bruit, and it is readily
reducible by external pressure, although this may cause serious side-
effects (such as convulsions or a decrease in the pulse rate). The
pressure of the cyst on the overlying skin is liable to lead to ulceration
with an obvious risk of a spreading infection in the meninges
(meningitis).

Orbital varices

Congenital venous malformations may occur in the orbit with the
production of a proptosis in childhood which is aggravated by pressure
on the neck or by performing the Valsalva manouevre, and may be
intermittent; there may also be some venous dilatations in the
conjunctiva and skin of the affected eye. Sometimes there is a marked
increase in the proptosis as the result of a haemorrhage which
eventually forms a blood cyst of the orbit. A radiograph may show
enlargement of the orbit and sometimes concentric rings of calcification
(phleboliths); orbital venography provides more detailed information
and ultrasonic examination and CT scanning are also of value in
localizing the lesion.

Haemangioma

Haemangioma is discussed below on p.293.

Injuries

Orbital haemorrhage

Severe contusion of the eye or orbit (sometimes in association with a
fracture) may produce an intraorbital haemorrhage, so that the eye
becomes proptosed and there is an associated haemorrhage within the
lids (ecchymosis) and the conjunctiva; it may also occur in the sudden
venous congestion which follows strangulation. The proptosis of the

eye causes a restriction of ocular movement, although this is usually only temporary unless the haemorrhage becomes organized by a process of fibrosis before its absorption is complete. Visual loss from sudden and persistent elevation of intraorbital pressure can be relieved by a full-thickness lid incision.

Perforation

Perforating injuries of the orbit by pointed objects, such as a pair of scissors or a knife, are liable to cause orbital haemorrhage, but they may also produce more serious effects as the result of damage to other structures in the orbit (nerves, arteries, veins, extrinsic ocular muscles or optic nerve) or as the result of the introduction of infection (orbital cellulitis), particularly when there is retained foreign material within the orbit. A deep injury may even involve the membranous coverings of the brain, with a subsequent leakage of cerebrospinal fluid through the wound.

Treatment. Any infective element is treated by systemic antibiotics; a retained foreign body may be removed by an exploration of the orbit (orbitotomy, p.296), but sometimes it is expedient (particularly when the foreign material is of a relatively inert metallic nature) to leave it alone unless it produces obvious adverse effects. Tetanus immunoglobulin is advisable in perforating injuries of the orbit, particularly when wood or vegetable material is introduced into the tissues.

Orbital fractures

Blow-out fracture. A fracture of a wall of the orbit is liable to follow a direct blow on the eye which causes a marked increase in the intraorbital pressure during the sudden backward displacement of the eye, with rupture of the floor in the region of its weakest part (the region of the infraorbital groove), or rupture through the thin medial wall into the ethmoidal sinuses. Some of the orbital connective tissue, fat or one of the extrinsic ocular muscles may become trapped in the fractured area. Patients usually present with a vertical diplopia, swollen lids and, although there is usually a slight hypotropia of the eye when the other eye is looking straight ahead (or even no deviation), there is a dramatic disturbance of elevation associated with globe retraction and an abrupt cessation of movement of the eye. Palpable tissue emphysema may occur with ethmoidal fractures, and, if the infraorbital nerve is damaged, the sensation of the lower lid and adjacent cheek will be impaired. It is very important to look for evidence of intraocular contusion injury. Suitable X-rays including tomography delineate any fracture of the orbital walls. Prophylactic systemic antibiotics are prescribed and the patient instructed neither to blow the nose or rub the eye. Serial measurements of the ocular movements using the Hess chart, and of the field of binocular single vision using the perimeter, provide essential data in planning surgical intervention. Unless there is extensive herniation of orbital contents into the maxillary antrum, surgery is delayed for 14 days. If at this stage the diplopia has not begun to lessen, or there is retraction of the globe with upgaze associated with an elevation of intraocular pressure, suggesting significant tethering, or if there is 3 mm or more of enophthalmos, then surgical exploration of the orbital floor is required. This is performed through an incision in the skin of the lower eyelid in the region of the inferior orbital margin and then through subperiosteum to relieve the incarceration, with the insertion of a silicone sheet over the site of the fracture. When the medial wall of the orbit is involved, the incision and freeing of the incarcerated tissues is in that region.

Facial fractures involving the orbital margins (Le Fort types II and III). These may be widespread in their effects because they may extend into the skull base, leading to intracranial and neurological complications, or into the nose or into the paranasal sinuses, often producing CSF rhinorrhoea or otorrhoea. Disorders of ocular movements and contusion to the globe may result if bony fragments become impacted into the orbital tissues. Treatment is by disimpaction and external fixation of the bones. A depressed fracture of the zygoma requires early elevation and wire fixation. Orbital roof fractures may extend into the optic canal and damage the optic nerve, either directly or indirectly because of a disruption of its nutrient vessels. Fractures of the skull base may extend forwards to involve the optic nerve and sphenoid bones and are often associated with retro-orbital haemorrhage. Detailed radiography and tomography is the best way to delineate the fractures and the trapping of soft tissue masses.

Inflammatory conditions

Orbital cellulitis

This is an acute inflammatory condition of the orbital tissues which may be in front of the orbital septum (*preseptal cellulitis*) or, more seriously, behind (*postseptal cellulitis*). The infection may spread directly into the orbit from a periostitis (of the periorbital membrane) or from a paranasal sinusitis. It may also reach the orbit indirectly by the bloodstream from some neighbouring or remote source of infection, or it may be introduced into the orbit in association with a perforating wound (particularly when there is a retained foreign body) or during an intraorbital operation. There is marked swelling and redness of the eyelids, and in the postseptal variety, chemosis of the conjunctiva, a tense form of proptosis, severe pain and restricted ocular movement. The increased intraorbital pressure causes oedema of the optic disc, congestion of the retinal veins, and sometimes obstruction of part of the vascular supply to the optic nerve resulting in a variable visual field defect. Infection of the exposed cornea is liable to occur and may lead to a panophthalmitis. There may be an associated pyrexia. Sometimes the infection may spread backwards with the production of the *orbital apex syndrome* or the *sphenoidal fissure syndrome* (p.258), a meningitis or a cavernous sinus thrombosis (see p.286).

A more localized form of orbital cellulitis occurs when the inflammatory process is limited largely to Tenon's capsule (*tenonitis*), although this condition is more commonly secondary to a severe inflammatory change of the eye (panuveitis or panophthalmitis).

Treatment. The condition may be relieved by intensive systemic antibiotics, but the formation of an abscess demands its incision and drainage.

Orbital granulomas

There is a group of different clinical conditions which present in a manner similar to an orbital neoplasm, but in the absence of any neoplastic change. These conditions represent orbital granulomas in association with a specific disease such as tuberculosis, sarcoidosis, syphilis, Wegner's granulomatosis, leakage from a dermoid cyst, fungal or parasitic disorders, or after trauma. There is evidence also that a granuloma may follow the release of lipids in the orbital tissues following a focus of fat necrosis, and it may also occur as a tissue reaction to an underlying adenocarcinoma of the lacrimal gland or to an underlying lymphoma.

The term *inflammatory pseudotumour of the orbit* is applied to another group of conditions with similar presentation for which no cause can be found, although the histological pattern invokes a disorder of the lymphocytes, displaying a continuum from reactive hyperplasia to neoplasia. The usual features are proptosis with pain, swelling of the lids, chemosis of the conjunctiva, and limitations of ocular movement with diplopia. The proptosis may be sufficiently severe to cause optic disc swelling or exposure keratitis. Radiological examination of the orbit, in particular the CT scan, shows an absence of any bony abnormality but a discrete soft tissue orbital shadow which may be intraconal, extraconal, or simply involving a muscle (myositis) or the orbital apex (orbital apex syndrome). A- and B-scan ultrasonography are also useful aids in diagnosis.

Management. Surgical removal usually necessitates exploration of the orbit by a lateral approach, but this is liable to be followed by postoperative scar tissue and extensive surgical interference is seldom worthwhile. Therefore, the administration of systemic steroids for a trial period is of value; where there is no improvement, orbital biopsy is then justified. Should the tissue reveal a non-neoplastic lymphocytic response, then further treatment with steroids with irradiation may be used, while those biopsies that demonstrate lymphoproliferative disorder require irradiation and in some cases chemotherapy.

It is important to bear in mind that a non-neoplastic lymphocytic response may in due course proceed to a neoplastic response and, therefore, these patients must be investigated for systemic lymphoma, preferably under the care of an oncology department.

Cavernous sinus thrombosis

This usually results from an infection which spreads directly to the sinus by the bloodstream from various sources—the face, orbit, middle ear, mouth or paranasal sinuses—or which occurs in association with a generalized infection (pyaemia or septicaemia). There is usually some proptosis of the globe with loss of all movements as the result of involvement of the motor cranial nerves (the third, fourth and sixth) to the extrinsic ocular muscles; the involvement of the third cranial nerve also leads to a fixed dilated pupil and the absence of accommodation. The cornea is anaesthetic because of involvement of the ophthalmic division of the fifth cranial nerve. There is usually, but not invariably, engorgement of the retinal veins and oedema of the optic disc. The patient is generally acutely ill. The condition is liable to become bilateral because of the vascular communication which exists between the two cavernous sinuses.

Treatment. Intensive treatment with antibiotics and anticoagulants usually prevent a fatal termination to the disease, which is therefore becoming rare.

Mucocele of the paranasal sinuses

This follows blockage of the accessory nasal sinuses by a polyp or by catarrhal inflammatory changes. It may enlarge sufficiently to extend into the orbit with a gradual displacement of the eye in a particular direction, depending on the situation of the affected sinus; a sphenoid sinusitis is liable to involve the optic nerve.

Lipodystrophies

Hand–Schüller–Christian syndrome

In this disorder of histiocytes, which is one of the reticuloendothelial granulomatoses, xanthomatous deposits may occur in the orbits (sometimes within the sheaths of the optic nerve). Similar deposits may occur in the membranous bones of the skull (showing radiologically as large deficient areas) and less commonly in the long bones. Pituitary disorders (diabetes insipidus, dwarfism, etc.), pressure effects on the optic nerves or optic chiasm, and ophthalmoplegia may also occur in some cases.

The deposits respond to irradiation, with frequently a restoration of bony contours.

Eosinophilic granuloma

The rare eosinophilic granuloma represents a related condition.

Vascular disorders

Orbital haemorrhage

This may occur after trauma (p.282) and in severe blood dyscrasias such as leukaemia and chloroma.

Caroticocavernous fistula

A severe head injury may cause rupture of the internal carotid artery as it lies within the cavernous sinus (a venous chamber) with the formation of an arteriovenous communication (caroticocavernous fistula). The rupture may be delayed for several weeks because it is usually preceded by the formation of an aneurysm; such an aneurysm may also occur spontaneously. There is a pulsating form of proptosis which is synchronous with the pulse beat and accompanied by a rhythmical throbbing within the head because of the disruption of the orbital venous drainage which passes predominantly to the cavernous sinus; the conjunctival (and even the retinal) veins are darkened and dilated, and the optic disc may be oedematous. A secondary optic atrophy, or ocular ischaemia or glaucoma may develop later. The condition is often self-limiting because the free arteriovenous communication becomes obliterated by the development of a thrombosis, but a more speedy resolution may be obtained by a ligation of the ipsilateral internal (or common) carotid artery in the neck.

Orbital varices

This is discussed on p.282.

Bony disorders

Osteopetrosis (Albers-Schönberg disease)

In this condition, which usually becomes evident in early life, there is an excessive formation of osseous tissue (osteosclerosis) so that radiographically the bones appear unduly thickened. This is liable to produce various pareses (or palsies) of the extrinsic ocular muscles as the result of compression of the motor cranial nerves, and optic atrophy as the result of compression. Other general abnormalities may occur such as hydrocephalus.

Osteitis deformans (Paget's disease)

In this condition, which usually becomes evident in later life, there is a progressive enlargement of the bones. The vault of the skull is particularly affected (the presenting feature may be an elderly person's need for a larger hat size); similar changes are liable to occur in the vertebral column and in the long bones. The progressive narrowing of the foramina of the skull leads to compression of the cranial nerves— the optic nerve is particularly liable to be affected—and headaches are common. Brainstem compression may occur due to platybasia.

Exophthalmos and proptosis

These terms are applied to an eye which is more prominent than normal; there is no precise distinction between them but there is a tendency to reserve the term exophthalmos for the prominence which is the result of an endocrine disorder and to apply proptosis to all other forms of prominence.

Diagnostic methods. It is difficult to diagnose the presence of proptosis (or exophthalmos) on straightforward examination, particularly as a marked difference in the width of the palpebral fissures of the two eyes gives a false impression, but viewing the apices of the corneae from above by looking over the patient's head gives an accurate assessment of the relative prominence of one eye (or of the relative recession of the other eye). There are various forms of instruments (*exophthalmometers*) which measure the degree of prominence of each corneal apex from the lateral margin of the orbit.

Endocrine exophthalmos

Dysthyroid eye disease may occur clinically as a purely ocular disorder (*ophthalmic Graves' disease*) or with hyperthyroidism (*Graves' disease*), or rarely with hypothyroidism; all are due to an autoimmune process with the production of organ-specific antibodies.

In a discussion of the occurrence of exophthalmos (and its related phenomena—lid retraction and ophthalmoplegia) in thyroid dysfunction, it is expedient to consider the manifestations which are associated directly with thyrotoxicosis (*thyrotoxic manifestations*) and those which are only indirectly associated with thyrotoxicosis (*thyrotrophic manifestations*).

Thyrotoxic manifestations

In thyrotoxicosis an excessive amount of thyroid hormones (thyroxine and triiodothyronine) is responsible for two main effects:

1. An increased excitability of the sympathetico-adrenal system (*sympathicotonia*), probably as a result of a sensitization of the tissues by thyroxine to the circulating catecholamines. This accounts for many of the general features of the disease, such as tremor, increased excitability, increased sweating and tachycardia, and also frequently for the lid retraction, which follows overaction of the well-developed smooth muscle in the upper eyelid and of the less well-developed smooth muscle in the lower lid; this concept is endorsed by the temporary decrease which occurs in the degree of lid retraction following the administration of a sympatholytic drug such as hexamethonium or guanethidine which, even when administered in the form of drops, has a dramatic effect on lid retraction, but this tends to be short-lived and can be toxic to the corneal epithelium. The occurrence of lid retraction has led to the description of several clinical signs: a staring and frightened appearance of the eyes, which is particularly marked on attentive fixation, and a lagging of the upper eyelid on downward movement of the globe (*von Graefe's sign*).

2. A generalized weakness of the striated muscles, which accounts for some degree of ophthalmoplegia and even possibly for some degree of exophthalmos, on the assumption that the weakness of the recti muscles which normally exert a retracting influence on the eye may allow the increased activity of the smooth muscle fibres of the periorbital and peribulbar tissues to exert a slight protracting influence on the eye. It should be noted, however, that ophthalmoplegia is mainly, and exophthalmos is almost invariably, of a thyrotrophic nature, as discussed below.

Lid retraction, apart from that due to hypersensitivity to catecholamines, occurs as a result of overaction of the levator palpebrae superioris muscle. This is due to the tethering of the inferior ocular muscles, which induces a hypotropia so that a compensatory overaction of the superior rectus muscle occurs, and because the superior rectus and levator palpebrae have a common innervation, this overaction is translated into a lid retraction which disappears on downgaze.

The diagnosis of thyrotoxicosis may be obvious clinically, but ocular signs may occur in the euthyroid state, although minor biochemical and endocrinological changes are usually demonstrable. Currently it is possible to estimate serum thyroxine and triiodothyronine, as well as the thyroid stimulating hormone (TSH) response to thyrotrophin releasing hormone (TRH) and the T3 suppression test, while demonstration of a variety of thyroidal antibodies supports the immune basis of the disorder.

Thyrotrophic manifestations

These may occur at any stage of a thyrotoxicosis; sometimes they arise or become intensified after various forms of antithyroid treatment (surgical, medical or irradiational), and in other cases they may develop without any preceeding general manifestations of the disease. There is some evidence that the changes are related to the activity of a fragment of thyrotrophic hormone (TSH), a product of the basophil cells of the anterior pituitary body. Under normal conditions there is a close relationship between the hypothalmus, the pituitary and thyroid glands, the so-called *hypothalamic–pituitary–thyroid axis*, and, therefore, between the thyrotrophic and thyroid hormones. TSH stimulates the production of thyroid hormone (thyroxine) which is utilized by the tissues so that there is a gradual fall in the thyroxine level of the blood until a critical point is reached when there is a resumption of TSH secretion. TSH is under the control of thyrotrophin releasing hormone (TRH) which is derived from the hypothalamus.

Recent research has shown that a variety of organ-specific antibodies and antigen–antibody complexes cause, not only the inflammatory disorder within the thyroid gland, but also the increased output of thyroid hormones and are responsible for the exophthalmos and the ophthalmoplegia.

Complement fixing antibodies are found to thyroid gland constituents, while a group of non-complement fixing IgG antibodies, by binding to TSH receptor sites on the thyroid where they stimulate cyclic AMP, are believed to induce the excessive and inappropriate release of thyroid hormones. These thyroid stimulating antibodies (TSAb), known originally as long-acting thyroid stimulator (LATS) and LATS-protector (LATS-P), which compete for the TSH receptor site are present in the majority of patients with thyrotoxicosis. LATS is associated with pretibial myxoedema and thyroid acropachy, a subperiosteal inflammation of the phalanges.

Thyrotrophic exophthalmos is produced by an increase in orbital contents due to changes in the extrinsic ocular muscles, orbital fat, and mucopolysaccharides, with a concomitant increase in the vascular supply. It is suggested that LATS may stimulate orbital fat production. A substance known as exophthalmos producing substance (EPS) is now believed to be a fragment of TSH, which has a marked increased affinity for orbital connective tissue in the presence of LATS-P. This induces an increase in mucopolysaccharides, the hydrophilic nature of which induces oedema so that there is an increase in bulk.

A third immune mechanism, that of immune complex deposition with complement activation, accounts for the chronic inflammation of the extrinsic ocular muscles, principally the fibroelastic element that increases in size due to the resultant oedema (see Fig. 70a, b; p.279). This process mainly affects the inferior extrinsic ocular muscles. It is suggested that because the thyroid and the orbit share a lymphatic drainage, together with an extrinsic ocular muscle affinity for thyroglobulin, the immune complexes from the thyroid are filtered in the orbit. The fact that the degree of exophthalmos and ophthalmoplegia are often asymmetric is explained by the typically irregular anatomical arrangement of the lymphatic channels. With time an extensive fibrosis occurs within the muscles and connective tissues.

Dysthyroid eye signs

Exophthalmos. It is worth recalling that the commonest cause of unilateral or bilateral proptosis is dysthyroid eye disease. Twenty-five per cent of patients with Graves' disease and 90% with ophthalmic Graves' disease have exophthalmos; it is often unilateral, or markedly asymmetrical in the latter condition. It is measured as discussed above. The extent of orbital congestion may be determined by the degree of retro-ocular resistance, measured by gently applying pressure through the lids on to the eye in an attempt to retroplace the globe; often this may provide more important information than an assessment only of the degree of exophthalmos. The severity of the exophthalmos does not relate necessarily to the potential severity of the disease because miminal exophthalmos may be associated with a sudden decrease in visual acuity because of an increase in the intraorbital pressure which, because of an intact orbital septum preventing forwards movement of the orbital contents or because of markedly enlarged extrinsic ocular muscles at the orbital apex, may compress the optic nerve or more usually its nutrient vascular supply.

The changes in the orbit are reflected in the surface tissues of the eye with a marked oedema of the lids and chemosis of the conjunctiva, particularly over the extrinsic ocular muscle insertions, often in the presence of dilated vessels over these muscles. A retraction of the swollen eyelids may follow the protrusion of the eye, but this form of lid retraction is purely mechanical and is unrelated to the retraction which occurs in thyrotoxicosis as discussed above.

Superficial keratitis is liable to develop in the exposed cornea, and this may lead to severe hypopyon keratitis; sometimes superficial keratitis affecting the upper limbal region and the adjacent tarsal and bulbar conjunctiva is associated with thyroid disorders but its precise aetiology is unknown.

Ophthalmoplegia. The oedema and infiltration of the muscular and connective tissues leads to symptoms of stiff muscles and diplopia, especially noticeable in the mornings with some improvement during the day. Because the inflammatory disease principally affects the inferior orbital muscles, the resulting fibrosis and tethering restricts upgaze and lateral gaze most commonly, so that the squint has both vertical and horizontal components. The vertical squint is usually a hypotropia so that the patient may adopt an abnormal head posture with chin elevation, and the attempted superior rectus overaction may lead to lid retraction because the levator and superior rectus have a common innervation. The impaired movement of the affected muscle is accompanied by a gross overaction of the ipsilateral antagonist (although this is masked when the agonist muscle is fibrotic) and of the contralateral synergic muscle (unless this is also affected), and subsequent fibrosis with contracture of other affected muscles decreases the ocular mobility still further.

Ophthalmoscopy may show choroidal striae or optic disc swelling due to a congestive ophthalmopathy, but visual loss due to compression may occur with minimal signs. The advent of the CT scan has greatly facilitated examination of the orbit in thyroid disease with accurate delineation of the site and size of the extrinsic ocular muscles.

Treatment

The thyrotoxic state may be mild or fulminating. Treatment is with beta-blockers and thyroid hormone blocking agents, whose success can be monitored by estimation of serum TSH or better still of thyroid stimulating anitbodies as measured by the activation of cyclic AMP.

The effects of stiff ocular muscles and orbital oedema may be relieved to some extent by instructing the patient to sleep with the head elevated and by taking a weak diuretic at night. The gritty sensation due to exposure, incomplete and less frequent blinking, may be improved by artificial tear supplements. The integrity of the cornea must be maintained by the use of local antibiotics and by a tarsorrhaphy when it is necessary to reduce the exposure. Fixed lid retraction may be relieved by levator muscle recession. The diplopia may be correctable in the early stages with suitable prisms, but surgery may be required for large deviations; this is only considered when the deviation has remained static for at least six months.

An acute congestive ophthalmopathy, due to a rise in the intraorbital pressure because of an increase in bulk of the orbital contents with a compression on the optic nerve or its vascular supply, requires emergency treatment—in the first instance by medical decompression with high doses of systemic steroids (prednisolone 80 to 120 mg/day), but should this fail then surgical decompression of the orbit is required, usually through the inferior or medial walls. Irradiation may be used to decompress the orbit, but the effects are usually delayed for days or weeks, so that it is not appropriate when the decompression needs to be urgent.

Proptosis

Proptosis may occur in a wide variety of conditions: congenital disorders (craniofacial dysostosis, meningoencephalocele); traumatic disorders (orbital haemorrhage, orbital fracture); inflammatory disorders (orbital cellulitis, pseudotumour of the orbit, cavernous sinus thrombosis, mucocele of the paranasal sinuses); and vascular disorders (orbital haemorrhage, caroticocavernous fistula, orbital varices), as discussed above. It also occurs in a wide variety of tumour formations. A form of false proptosis occurs when the eyeball is unduly large (e.g. due to high axial myopia, buphthalmos or staphyloma) and this is particularly obvious when it is unilateral.

Tumours

There are various forms of orbital tumour; they may be primary, secondary (by direct spread from an adjacent structure) or metastatic (by indirect spread from a distant source).

Primary tumours

Dermoid cyst. This condition is discussed on p.281.

Haemangioma. This represents a collection of abnormally formed vessels and is essentially of congenital origin, although its full effect may not be apparent in the early weeks of life. A capillary haemangioma seldom causes any interference with the other structures in the orbit and is often best left alone, particularly as it may become slowly less marked. Complications in childhood relate to involvement of the lid, with secondary ptosis, or an induced astigmatism resulting in anisometropia, both of which may induce amblyopia. Thus, careful refraction is essential, with the provision of a spectacle or contact lens together with occlusion of the unaffected eye. If the bulk of the tumour is such as to occlude the central part of the vision, a debulking procedure using cutting diathermy is used. Systemic steroids have been used, while irradiation is of limited value, and attempted surgical excision may prove unwise because of the difficulty of removing the whole mass without endangering the integrity of the many structures in the orbit and because of the liability to postoperative fibrosis. Sometimes a ligature of feeding vessels may be indicated following their delineation by angiography.

In adults a cavernous haemangioma is the commonest primary tumour presenting as a painless proptosis due to a discrete intraconal mass. It is well seen on CT scan (see Fig. 70c,d; p.279) and ultrasonography. Treatment is by surgical excision.

Lacrimal gland tumours. Benign mixed and adenoid cystic tumours are described on p.216.

Optic nerve tumours. Glioma, meningioma and fibroma are described on p.162.

Neurofibroma. This may develop in one of the peripheral nerves in the orbit, sometimes in association with other manifestations of von Recklinghausen's disease (see p.149).

Reticuloses. This term comprises several related tumours of the haemopoietic system—lymphoma (lymphosarcoma), lymphadenoma (Hodgkin's disease), and reticulum cell sarcoma. Occasionally the tumour may occur as an isolated mass, but usually similar deposits occur elsewhere because of their multicentric nature or because of an associated blood dyscrasia (leukaemia). Lymphomas may present with bilateral orbital signs. These tumours almost invariably respond to irradiation, but if the condition is widespread it is necessary to attempt systemic treatment with chemotherapeutic drugs. Burkitt's lymphoma is a malignant lymphoblastic lymphoma affecting children between the ages of 2 and 15 years and is related to three main factors: (a) the geographical location, which is mainly in tropical Africa; (b) the association with endemic malaria; and (c) the implication of the Epstein–Barr virus. It is believed that endemic malaria alters the immune response to exposure to the Epstein–Barr virus, which then induces neoplasia. The condition is multifocal, rapidly progressive and may respond dramatically to cyclophosphamide. The orbit is commonly involved from direct maxillary spread.

Chloroma. This is a malignant tumour of the haemopoietic system which is liable to involve the bones of the orbit (and skull) and is usually associated with myelogenous leukaemia. It is more common in young children, particularly males. It spreads rapidly and almost invariably ends fatally, despite a temporary response to irradiation and chemotherapy.

Multiple myelomatosis. This is a multifocal tumour of plasma cells associated with a monoclonal gammopathy and Bence-Jones proteinuria. Orbital lesions may occur as an isolated phenomenon, but are usually part of a general myelomatous process. Chemotherapeutic agents are the mainstay of treatment.

Sarcoma. This primary malignant tumour occurs particularly in young people, especially males; the round-celled sarcoma has a higher degree of malignancy than the fibrosarcoma. It may rarely occur as a long-term complication of extensive irradiation for retinoblastoma.

Embryonal sarcoma (rhabdomyosarcoma). This tumour, arising from soft tissue, usually occurs in the orbit in early childhood (rarely after the age of ten years). It may start in the eyelid or in the region of one of the conjunctival fornices before spreading to the orbit, with rapid development of proptosis, chemosis of the conjunctiva and oedema of the eyelids so that it may be difficult to observe the eye. Differential diagnosis from acute orbital cellulitis may be difficult, but pain is an uncommon feature of embryonal sarcoma. It is essential to have a tissue diagnosis by transconjunctival or lid biopsy prior to treatment. Irradiation of the orbit usually causes rapid resolution and is combined with chemotherapy, irrespective of the size of the primary tumour, to debulk the neoplasm, to eradicate micrometastases early and to secondarily decrease the vascular supply; this effects a 75% complete remission. There are, of course, complications of the chemotherapy such as alopecia, bone marrow depression and increased susceptibility to infection, while the radiation induces bone growth retardation which may be disfiguring, keratoconjunctivitis, impaired tear secretion and cataract. Surgery (*exenteration*) is now reserved for a recurrence after conservative treatment.

Endothelioma. This primary malignant tumour arises from the endothelium of the blood vessels or lymph vessels; they are sometimes extremely vascular so that the term *haemangioendothelioma* may be used. A variant of this tumour is the *perithelioma.*

Melanoma. This is a rare primary tumour of the orbit. It necessitates exenteration but the prognosis is poor.

Secondary tumours

From the nasal sinuses. This is usually a carcinoma.

From the nasopharynx (postnasal space). This, too, is usually a carcinoma, but sometimes a sarcoma, a plasma-cell tumour or rarely a chordoma. The orbit may be invaded directly, with the development of proptosis and involvement of the structures in the posterior part of the orbit with the features of the sphenoidal fissure syndrome or the orbital apex syndrome (p.258), or it may be invaded indirectly after an intracranial extension, so that the proptosis is preceded by a disturbance of one or more of the cranial nerves (the *hypophyseosphenoidal syndrome* or the *petrosphenoidal syndrome*).

From the cranial cavity. This may be due to spread of, for example, a meningioma, glioma or chordoma.

From the ocular tissues. Spread of, for example, a uveal melanoma or a retinoblastoma may occur.

Metastatic tumours

These are rare and include a neuroblastoma from the adrenal gland or from the abdominal ganglia in early childhood, or a carcinoma from the breast, bronchus, etc. in the adult.

Surgery to the orbit

Orbitotomy

The orbit may be explored from four different directions:

Anterior orbitotomy. An incision through the eyelid and orbital septum along the upper (or lower) orbital margin is appropriate for lesions which are readily palpable through the eyelids and which are unlikely to extend deeply into the orbit.

Lateral orbitotomy (Krönlein's operation). An incision through the skin along the lateral orbital margin, with an extension from the centre of this incision laterally to permit the removal of a quadrilateral part of the bone of the lateral orbital wall after reflection of its periosteal covering, allows good exposure of the lateral and posterior parts of the orbit; sometimes a skin incision alone may be sufficient.

Transfrontal orbitotomy (Naffziger's operation). Removal of a portion of the orbital roof after exposure of the frontal lobe of the brain (which is then elevated) through a quadrilateral opening in the frontal bone is sometimes necessary in extensive lesions of the upper and posterior parts of the orbit.

Subconjunctival approach. Sometimes when a lesion responsible for proptosis lies within the core of the extrinsic ocular muscles, an approach to this region by a *subconjunctival approach* is sufficient for diagnostic (biopsy) purposes.

Exenteration

This involves the removal of the entire orbital contents (including the eye, the eyelids and the orbital part of the optic nerve) within their periorbital coverings, by an incision with cutting diathermy through the skin, muscle and periosteum around the entire orbital margin. The exposed bony orbit may be covered by a split-skin graft from the medial surface of the thigh, but this is not essential and spontaneous epithelialization of the orbital surface occurs from the skin edges within a few months; it is usually expedient to omit the skin graft when there has been previous (or liable to be subsequent) irradiation of the area.

Enophthalmos

This term is applied to an eye which is less prominent than normal. It occurs when the eye is unduly small (microphthalmos, phthisis bulbi, or atrophia bulbi) or when a fracture of the floor of the orbit leads to a displacement of some of the orbital contents into the underlying antrum. A form of enophthalmos occurs when the eyeball is retracted in Duane's retraction syndrome (p.260), but the enophthalmos which is described in Horner's syndrome is a misnomer; it is a false impression due to the narrowing of the palpebral fissure.

15

Glaucoma

The principal determinant of the integrity of the optic disc and therefore the retinal ganglion cell nerve fibres, is its perfusion, which is dependent on two main factors: first, the end-artery system of vascular supply to the optic nerve head which is from the choroidal circulation, apart from the innermost or nerve fibre layer which is supplied by the peripapillary plexus derived from the retinal circulation; and second, the haemodynamic state of equilibrium between the ophthalmic artery blood pressure, the intraocular pressure and the episcleral venous pressure.

Glaucoma is a condition in which ischaemia of the optic nerve head results in discrete areas of infarction, producing a notching or cupping of the optic disc resulting in typical nerve fibre bundle field defects, and usually associated with an elevation of intraocular pressure. Some patients, however, have typical glaucomatous field defects and cupped discs, but a normal intraocular pressure (low-tension glaucoma), while others have elevated pressures without disc or field changes (ocular hypertension). There is thus a spectrum of disease determined by the susceptibility of the optic nerve to ischaemia.

The aqueous humour

This is a clear fluid which is formed within the processes of the ciliary body by filtration (and therefore dependent on ciliary artery blood pressure), modified by the pigmentary layer of the ciliary body, and finally secreted into the posterior chamber by a process of active transport across the epithelium requiring ATPase and carbonic anhydrase, at a rate of 2 μl/min. Secretion is independent of the ciliary artery pressure and to some extent of the intraocular pressure. The aqueous passes forwards from the posterior chamber into the anterior chamber through the pupillary opening and also percolates backwards through the vitreous. It is concerned with the metabolic requirements of the cornea and the lens which are avascular structures and contributes to the maintenance of the intraocular pressure. The aqueous leaves the eye through the trabecular meshwork in the angle of the anterior chamber (*trabecular outflow*), and also, but to a small extent, through the anterior surface of the iris and ciliary body to gain access to the suprachoroidal space (*uveoscleral outflow*). Trabecular outflow is pressure dependent and facilitated by pilocarpine and

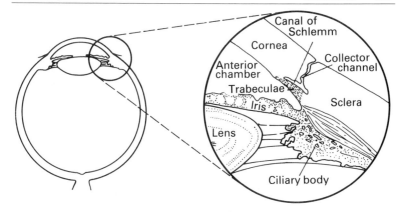

Fig. 71. Section of the anterior segment of the eye to show the anterior chamber, the trabeculae of the filtration angle, the canal of Schlemm and a collector channel.

inhibited by atropine, while the reverse is true for the uveoscleral outflow.

The posterior chamber

This is the narrow space which lies between the anterior surface of the lens and the posterior surface of the iris; it contains aqueous (0.06 ml).

The anterior chamber (Fig. 71)

This is the space in the anterior segment of the eye which lies between the inner surface of the cornea and the anterior surface of the iris and lens and which is bounded laterally by the filtration angle; it contains aqueous (0.25 ml).

The filtration angle. The angle of the anterior chamber is bounded by a sieve-like structure (the *trabecular meshwork*) through which the aqueous passes to an endothelium-lined canal (the *canal of Schlemm*) within the sclera immediately behind the corneoscleral junction (the *limbus*); from this canal the aqueous passes to the episcleral veins on the surface of the eye by way of small veins, some of which contain only aqueous (aqueous veins) and others a mixture of blood and aqueous. The angle of the anterior chamber is not visible on straightforward examination because it lies under the sclera beyond the limits of the cornea, but the use of a special corneal contact lens (a *gonioscope*) which incorporates an angled mirror provides an indirect view of the angle (Fig. 72). The detailed inspection of this region is facilitated by the use of the slit-lamp microscope, and the following structures are visible in sequence: the inner surface of the cornea ending at the

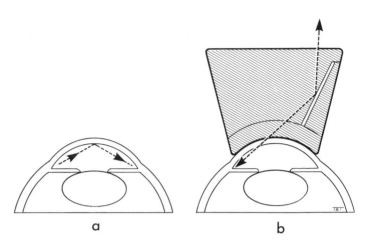

Fig. 72.   The optical principles of gonioscopy. (a) Arrows depict total internal reflection from anterior chamber angle. (b) Gonioscope in position—anterior chamber angle visible.

terminal edge of Descemet's membrane (*Schwalbe's ring*), a greyish area representing the inner surface of the trabecular meshwork of the filtration area which may be pigmented—its posterior limit represents the canal of Schlemm which may be visible particularly if filled with blood, a discrete thin white line representing the scleral spur, the ciliary· body, and finally the root of the iris.

The intraocular pressure (IOP) (ocular tension)

This is dependent on the influences of both the *vitreous,* which fills the posterior part of the eye, and the *aqueous,* which fills its anterior part, but the aqueous is concerned primarily with the variations which may occur in this pressure because the volume of the vitreous tends to remain fairly constant except in gross intraocular disease or after a perforating injury involving the posterior segment of the eye. The influence of the aqueous is determined by three main factors: (a) the rate of entry of aqueous into the eye from the ciliary body; (b) the outflow resistance within the trabecular meshwork and episcleral plexus; and (c) the episcleral venous pressure, which may be increased with superior vena caval obstruction or chronic right-sided heart failure.

The intraocular pressure is measured indirectly by assessing the resistance of the sclera or the cornea to compression; a manometric method involving the insertion of a needle into the anterior chamber would provide a direct and more accurate measurement, but it is obviously unsuitable for routine clinical use. The following methods are in use:

Digital measurement. The pressure is assessed by placing the tips of both forefingers on the surface of the upper lid, with the patient looking down, and then pressing the sclera through the lid with each forefinger in turn so that the resistance of the sclera to indentation is assessed in much the same way as the determination of fluctuation within an abscess. This is obviously only a comparative method whereby the tension of the eye is compared with the tension which is found in the average eye and it requires considerable experience before becoming even remotely reliable. However, it provides a more accurate assessment of the differences in the tension between the two eyes.

Tonometric measurement. This involves the use of an instrument termed a *tonometer* (for example, the *Schiotz tonometer*), the lower end of which is curved so that it may be applied to the outer surface of the cornea after surface anaesthesia with amethocaine 1% drops. A metal plunger passes down the central part of the tonometer and impinges on the anterior pole of the cornea, thereby causing a certain amount of indentation which is recorded by a lever on a scale; the weight of the plunger may be altered in some types of tonometer so that different readings on the scale are obtained in the same eye. The results of these readings are then translated into terms of intraocular pressure using graphs obtained experimentally. This method is fairly accurate in most cases but it assumes, incorrectly sometimes, that the rigidity of the outer coat of the eye (cornea and sclera) has a more or less uniform value in all persons. It is largely superseded by the *applanation tonometer* which measures the amount of pressure which is required to cause a flattening of a small area of the normally curved cornea, and has a much greater degree of accuracy. Ideally the recording of the intraocular pressure of each eye by the applanation method should be a routine procedure in an examination of the eyes, certainly over the age of 40 years. A hand-held applanation tonotmeter is now available which does not require the use of the slit-lamp microscope. More recently a non-contact tonometer which uses the applanation principle by delivering an air pulse to the apex of the cornea until a specific area is flattened has been adopted and it is useful for screening purposes, but it is less accurate than the contact tonometer.

The normal intraocular pressure is between 16 and 22 mmHg, but is not maintained at a constant level in any one individual because of the variations (up to 3–5 mmHg) which occur during each 24 hours, the so-called *diurnal variations*; the highest pressure usually occurs in the early hours of the morning during sleep.

Tonographic measurement. This is a more elaborate form of tonometry whereby the coefficient of the facility of aqueous outflow (C) is estimated by a measurement of the change which occurs in the pressure of the eye from its initial level (Po) during the application of the tonometer, of known weight, to the eye for a given length of time (usually four minutes). It is difficult, of course, to obtain values of C which are strictly comparable between individuals because the method does not take into account the variability of the rigidity of the outer coat of the eye, and a more accurate value is obtained by the applanation tonometer. Furthermore, it is obvious that any pressure on the eye produces modifications in its entire hydrodynamic system so that the significance of this method as a measurement simply of the ease with which aqueous is able to leave the eye must be regarded with some caution. Under normal conditions the value of C, as derived mathematically, should be more than 0.18, although values between 0.12 and 0.18 may sometimes be considered as within normal limits. The value of C may also be considered in relation to the initial intraocular pressure (Po/C) which should be less than 100, although values between 100 and 200 may sometimes be considered as within normal limits. Tonography is presently mainly used in research and in assessing the efficacy of anti-glaucoma medication.

Primary glaucoma

Anterior chamber cleavage syndrome (iridocorneal dysgenesis)

This is a genetic term applied to a number of morphologically distinct abnormalities which are the result of a faulty cleavage between the cornea and iris during embryonic development; in normal development at about the seventh week a split appears in the solid mass of undifferentiated mesenchyme which fills the anterior segment and this split extends laterally so that the cornea becomes separated from the trabecular meshwork and the iris with the formation of the anterior chamber. There are various anomalies which comprise this syndrome: *posterior embryotoxon*, which represents an undue prominence of Schwalbe's ring which lies on the inner surface of the cornea near the filtration angle; *Axenfeld's anomaly*, in which prominent iris processes span the anterior chamber angle and become adherent to Schwalbe's ring; *Rieger's anomaly*, in which there are varying degrees of dysgenesis of the iris stroma; *Rieger's syndrome*, in which Rieger's anomaly is associated with other forms of mesodermal dysgenesis, particularly skeletal defects, hypodontia and partial anodontia; and *congenital anterior synechiae* or *congenital leucoma adherens (Peter's anomaly)*, in which the collarette of the iris is adherent to the pericentral corneal endothelium and stroma—this mimics the leucoma adherens which follows a perforating corneal ulcer (p.52), and in the past many such cases have been regarded incorrectly as following an intrauterine keratouveitis. All these conditions are liable to be associated with the development of infantile glaucoma (see below), or glaucoma which becomes manifest in adult life.

Iridocorneal endothelial syndrome

The three conditions of *progressive essential iris atrophy, Chandler's syndrome,* and the *iris-naevus syndrome* are believed to represent variations of one disorder that is characterized by an abnormal corneal endothelium associated with peripheral anterior synechiae across the trabecular meshwork, distortion of the pupil, iris nodules, iris holes, and impaired visual acuity due to corneal oedema or secondary glaucoma. It is a unilateral condition, occurs predominently in women, and is of unknown aetiology. It presents in young adults and has a progressive course.

Infantile glaucoma (buphthalmos)

This is a form of glaucoma which is determined congenitally as a result of a developmental anomaly of the tissues of the filtration angle, although the obvious effects of the condition are usually not apparent until some months or even a few years after birth. Sometimes only one eye is affected, but usually the condition involves both eyes, although often to varying degrees. It is more common in boys than in girls. There may be a hereditary factor, and rarely it is part of the rubella syndrome (p.171).

A progressive enlargement of the eye is often the presenting feature because the immature outer coat of the infantile eye is unable to withstand the increased intraocular pressure. This causes an increase in the anteroposterior diameter of the eye with an increased curvature of the expanding cornea so that the anterior chamber becomes deep. The eye becomes red and irritable with considerable photophobia, blepharospasm and epiphora. The eye becomes progressively myopic, but this is often unrecognized because of the other changes in the eye. The cornea often remains remarkably clear despite its enlargement, but eventually it becomes hazy as a result of oedematous changes in the epithelium and in the stroma following localized ruptures of Descemet's membrane. The increased intraocular pressure also exerts its effect on the optic nerve head; the optic disc becomes progressively atrophic and cupped with severe and permanent loss of vision, so that eventually blindness may ensue in the absence of effective treatment. Gonioscopy demonstrates a fine transparent membrane across the peripheral iris and trabecular meshwork, often in association with an anterior insertion of the iris, sectors of peripheral iris atrophy, and a prominent Schwalbe's ring.

Other congenitally determined disorders may be associated with buphthalmos or glaucoma presenting later in life: the glaucoma associated with aniridia; the Sturge–Weber syndrome, where the affected eye is on the same side as the vascular anomaly; neurofibromatosis, often in the presence of a plexiform neuroma of the face, numerous iris nodules and ectropion uveae; and Marfan's syndrome.

Treatment. Many forms of drainage operation (e.g. trephine, flap sclerectomy with iris inclusion) have been attempted in this condition, but a goniotomy is the most satisfactory procedure. This consists of stripping away the abnormal tissues from part of the filtration angle using a goniotomy knife. This is inserted at the limbus into the anterior chamber and directed across the anterior chamber to the angle on the opposite side of the point of insertion, under direct view through a gonioscopic lens which lies on the surface of the cornea, aided by the magnification which is provided by the operating microscope and by an intense focal illumination. This operation may be repeated several times if necessary in a different or the same part of the filtration angle. It is desirable for the goniotomy to be carried out at a reasonably early stage before the development of advanced degenerative changes in the eye. When the angle cannot be seen due to corneal oedema, a trabeculotomy may be performed; should these procedures fail then a trabeculectomy is required.

The progressive enlargement of the eye induces an axial myopia, so producing anisometropia with the subsequent risk of amblyopia. This may be prevented by the provision of a spectacle lens or a contact lens in conjunction with occlusion therapy.

Chronic simple glaucoma (open-angle glaucoma)

This condition presents the triad of elevated intraocular pressure, optic disc cupping with visual field defects and an anterior chamber angle that is free of synechiae. The mechanism is inadequately understood, but it seems likely that the defect lies in the region of the filtration angle. This may be the result of: (a) abnormal changes in the tissues of the filtration angle (e.g. of a mucinous nature) which gradually impede the passage of aqueous; (b) a failure of the action of cells in the trabecular meshwork which normally provide transcellular channels for the aqueous to pass into the canal of Schlemm; or (c) an anomaly of the sympathetic (or parasympathetic) nerve complexes in the region. It is essentially a disease of the middle-aged or elderly—only a few cases occur before the age of 40 years—although isolated cases may occur at any age, even in childhood (juvenile glaucoma). It is almost invariably bilateral, but both eyes are seldom affected equally at any one time. There is a definite hereditary component to the condition; other risk factors include myopia, diabetes mellitus, and an elevation in intraocular pressure to a challenge by dexamethasone drops.

Clinical features

In contrast to most other forms of glaucoma this type is practically free from all symptoms, except for an insidious and progressive visual loss which usually only affects the peripheral part of the vision to any marked degree until the later stages, so that it may remain unnoticed by the patient until it encroaches on the fixation area. This lack of awareness is also explained by the fact that the visual fields of the two eyes have a large amount of overlap (the binocular field of vision, see Fig. 76, p.318) so that extensive loss of vision of one eye, even with involvement of the central vision, may be masked by the less affected visual field of the other eye. Very occasionally when there has been a sudden rise of pressure, patients may be aware of an ache and an associated impairment of vision. Early development of presbyopia may occur in chronic simple glaucoma.

There are, however, many objective findings in the disease:

1. *Visual field loss.* Characteristically there is a progressive loss of the peripheral visual field, demonstrated using the perimeter (p.343), particularly in the nasal part of the field—often in the upper nasal quadrant before the lower one—with a gradual spread towards the fixation area so that ultimately there is a permanent loss of central vision. It is important, however, to appreciate that other subtle changes are present in the more central parts of the visual field, as demonstrated on the *tangent screen* (e.g. the *Bjerrum screen*, p.344) at a much earlier stage. For example, there is restriction of the peripheral limit of the field using a very small white target (1 mm in diameter) at a distance of 2 m in the region of the blind spot which becomes isolated (or 'bared') outside the distorted circle (Fig. 73); normally this target would provide a circular field of 25 to 30° so that the blind spot, which lies about 13 to 18° from the fixation point, would lie within the field. There are also sometimes small scotomata (paracentral) within a narrow zone extending in an arcuate form above (Fig. 73) and below the blind spot—when these scotomata become confluent they are termed *arcuate scotomata*. These changes in the central field are of vital importance in the early recognition of the disease but they are detected only by careful quantitative methods of kinetic and static perimetry (p.346).

2. *Increased intraocular pressure.* A characteristic feature is a raised intraocular pressure, but the extent of this is variable in different patients—in some it may be only slightly raised whereas in others it may be high—and it is also variable in any one patient over a period of 24 hours, as there is an exaggeration of the normal diurnal variation; recordings of the pressure every four hours over a period of 24 (or even 48) hours are sometimes necessary to ascertain the true extent of the pressure. An isolated reading may even be normal in some cases.

3. *Abnormal facility of aqueous outflow.* Tonographic measurements show a diminished outflow of aqueous, with C less than

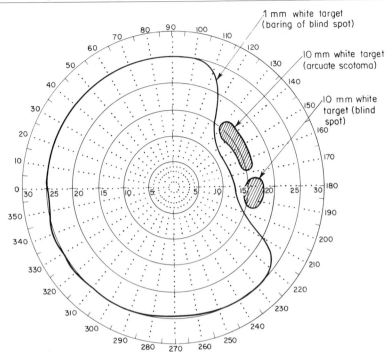

Fig. 73. Visual field chart to show 'baring' of the blind spot and an arcuate scotoma.

0.18 (or in certain cases 0.12) and Po/C more than 100 (or in certain cases 200) in a significant number of cases.

4.   *Optic disc changes.* The effect of the increased intraocular pressure is particularly seen in the optic disc with gradual enlargement of the optic cup due to a progressive degeneration of the optic nerve and glial tissue within the optic disc (Fig. 74); early disc evidence of glaucoma is manifest by the development of a vertically oval cup, in contrast to the normal where the horizontal diameter is the greater. This degeneration is the result of interference with the capillary blood supply of the nerve fibres rather than a direct pressure effect on the fibres. In advanced glaucoma the cup extends to the disc margin so that the retinal vessels dip markedly on crossing it, but it is important to recognize earlier forms of cupping. It is not possible to define the size of the abnormal cup because the size of the normal cup varies in different individuals due to a variation in size of the scleral canal, and in different types of refraction (a large cup in myopia), but there are certain features which should be considered during any ophthalmoscopic examination. It is rare for the size of the normal cup to occupy more than 70% of the area of the disc. This measurement

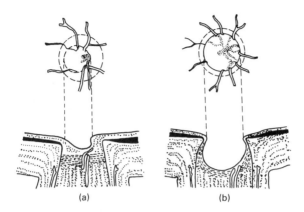

(a)   (b)

Fig. 74. (a) Physiological cupping and (b) pathological cupping of the optic disc, as seen on section of the optic nerve head and as seen ophthalmoscopically.

applies only to the cross-sectional area of the cup; the depth of the cup is of much less significance and the ability to observe the lamina cribrosa which lies beyond the floor of the cup may be a feature even of a relatively small cup.

It is usual for the cups of the two discs in any one individual to be similar in size, except when the two eyes have a marked difference in refractive error when ophthalmoscopic examination inevitably provides a misleading impression. However, with this proviso, asymmetry suggests early cupping.

The occurrence of small haemorrhages on the disc or the disc margin is strongly suggestive of local capillary closure and ischaemia, and in due course is followed by the development of a notch in the optic cup. Haemorrhages tend to occur more in low-tension glaucoma.

The development of pathological cupping is associated with an accentuation of the normal nasal shift of the retinal vessels as they pass through the cup.

5. *Abnormalities of the filtration angle.* Gonioscopic examination usually shows an open angle in chronic simple glaucoma with no demonstrable pathological features, but some cases show areas of angle closure with the formation of peripheral anterior synechiae.

6. *Provocative tests.* The water-drinking test (1 litre of water after 12 hours of fasting) produces a significant rise in the intraocular pressure and a decreased facility of aqueous outflow in the majority of cases.

Low-tension glaucoma. This is a form of open-angle glaucoma when there is pathological cupping of the disc and progressive field loss with intraocular pressures of less than 21 mmHg (monitored over 24 hours) in patients who are on no treatment and who have no evidence of optic nerve compression or of congenital disc anomalies with their associated field defects. These patients typically have large optic cups, an increased frequency of disc haemorrhages and a predominantly upper field defect which is close to fixation and dense. There is often a family history of chronic simple glaucoma. Although this is probably a variant of chronic simple glaucoma, there is usually evidence of generalized microvascular disease, which probably makes the disc more susceptible to the prevailing ocular pressure. A sudden drop in blood pressure, due to massive haemorrhage or an arrhythmia, may result in a permanent arcuate field defect which, however, is non-progressive.

Ocular hypertension. This condition of elevated intraocular pressure with normal discs and fields may never proceed to glaucoma, but certain risk factors increase the likelihood, such as myopia, a family history of chronic simple glaucoma and a pronounced alteration in the intraocular pressure on changing from the sitting to supine position, which demonstrates an instability of ocular haemodynamics. Treatment is not required unless the pressure is more than 30 mmHg or evidence of glaucoma supervenes.

Treatment

Because of the insidious nature of the disease and the familial pattern, it is important to screen family members and patients over 40 years. Established cases require life-long monitoring of visual fields, intraocular pressures and disc signs; the latter is best achieved by sequential colour stereo-photographs.

Medical treatment. Treatment of open-angle glaucoma by the topical application of various drugs has been performed since the later part of the nineteenth century, but in recent years the emergence of new drugs has provided a fresh emphasis of the importance of medical treatment, and the introduction of laser therapy often defers surgical treatment. It is important to emphasize the preventive life-long nature of the treatment to the patient, because the unpleasant side-effects of the medication coupled with perhaps no visual handicap, or no improvement in the vision when there is a visual handicap, induces non-compliance.

The ocular hypotensive drugs may be considered in four groups according to their pharmacological characteristics:

1. *Anticholinesterase drugs.* These drugs, which potentiate the effects of acetylcholine at the myoneural junctions as the result of inhibition of the cholinesterase which normally destroys it, form a large group of pressure-lowering drugs which act primarily by lowering the resistance to aqueous outflow (and also act as miotics and cyclospastics). Eserine (0.25% or 0.5%) drops have a maximum effect

during a period of about six hours, but this is somewhat variable in certain eyes and their prolonged use is liable to cause irritation and even intolerance after a time. DFP (di-isopropyl fluorophosphonate— 0.025%, 0.05%, or 0.1%) and phospholine iodide (0.06%, 0.125% or 0.25%) are powerful drugs which retain their effects for 24 or even 48 hours, but they are also liable sometimes to cause congestion, discomfort and even pain. Because they may induce cataract formation, they are best reserved for aphakic patients. Their long-term use may result in hyperplasia of the pigment layers of the iris, with large nodules of pigment in the pupillary margins. The drug must be discontinued at least six weeks prior to any surgery because of the risk of inducing scoline apnoea.

2.   *Pilocarpine* (1%, 2%, 3% or 4% drops). This drug has a pressure-lowering effect which is limited to about four hours, although its miotic and cyclospastic effects persist for a longer time. It acts directly on the ciliary muscle fibres, thereby pulling on the scleral spur and opening the trabecular meshwork. It decreases uveoscleral outflow. The complications of miosis, darkened vision—especially in poor illumination, impaired acuity in the presence of an axial cataract, and the accommodative spasm are intolerable side-effects for many patients.

3.   *Adrenergic drugs.* Adrenaline is the most potent pressure-lowering drug of this group and is used in the form of drops. It lowers the resistance to aqueous outflow and acts as an inhibitor of aqueous function for at least 24 hours. It has no miotic effect and indeed causes some dilatation of the pupil so that it is useful in glaucoma associated with central lens opacities, although it is contraindicated if there is any element of angle closure. It has no cyclospastic effect. It may be potentiated by combining it with guanethidine which induces a chemical denervation hypersensitivity. Unfortunately it may have certain side-effects including cardiac arrhythmias, increased pigmentation of the conjunctiva, and cystoid macular oedema in aphakic patients.

4.   *Carbonic anhydrase inhibitors.* The administration of acetazolamide (Diamox) (e.g. 125 mg six-hourly) by mouth causes a diminution in the entry of aqueous into the eye from the ciliary body because it inhibits the action of carbonic anhydrase which is concerned with the transference of aqueous across the blood-aqueous barrier. It is of great value in reducing the intraocular pressure for short periods, but is liable to cause complications when used for prolonged periods, including loss of appetite, general malaise, paraesthesia and renal colic; bone marrow depression and exfoliative dermatitis are unusual but severe complications.

5.   *Beta-adrenergic blockers.* The recent introduction of timolol maleate, a topical beta-blocker that is well tolerated, has greatly improved the medical management of glaucoma. It suppresses the formation of aqueous and is given twice daily. Because there is no miosis or spasm of accommodation, it is particularly suitable for those

patients who cannot tolerate pilocarpine. It is contraindicated in patients with asthma or severe cardiovascular disease.

Surgical treatment. In those patients in whom medical treatment has failed to arrest the progression of visual field defects, fistulizing operations to promote drainage of aqueous humour from the anterior chamber to the subconjunctival space have been advised. However, the introduction of *Argon laser trabeculoplasty*—the photocoagulation of the trabecular meshwork as a series of 100 evenly-spaced burns through 360°—has reduced the need for drainage surgery. The facility of outflow is increased, but patients usually have to continue their pre-laser treatment. Occasionally there is an early post-laser increase in intraocular pressure which can be largely avoided by performing two separate 180° treatment sessions.

The drainage operation of choice is *trabeculectomy* where a superficial scleral flap guards a hole into the anterior chamber, created by excising a thin rectangular block of peripheral cornea which includes the scleral spur. It is combined with the removal of the adjacent basal iris (*peripheral iridectomy*) to prevent the iris from sealing the sclerostomy. The aqueous then drains into the subconjunctival space. The advantage of this procedure is the early reformation of the anterior chamber, and a well-covered drainage bleb. In another type of operation the aqueous is drained into the choroidal circulation along a channel which is formed in the suprachoroidal space (*cyclodialysis*); this operation is of particular value in aphakic eyes. More rarely an attempt is made to diminish the production of aqueous by the application of diathermy to parts of the ciliary body (*surface* or *perforating cyclodiathermy*) or the application of intense cold (*cryotherapy*); such an operation is seldom indicated in an uncomplicated case of chronic simple glaucoma, particularly as its effect is frequently rather short-lived.

Closed-angle glaucoma (congestive glaucoma)

This form of glaucoma is caused by a narrowing of the entrance to the angle of the anterior chamber; it is found particularly in the small hypermetropic eye which has a shallow anterior chamber (conversely, it is very rare in the myopic eye with a deep anterior chamber), and this shallowness occurs sometimes as a familial characteristic. The narrow angle by itself, however, is not sufficient to produce glaucoma, so that many such eyes remain normal indefinitely, and various other factors play significant contributory roles (Fig. 75).

First, in normal eyes there is only a small peripupillary zone of iris–lens contact, but this is considerably increased in eyes with shallow anterior chambers. A state of relative pupillary block ensues which

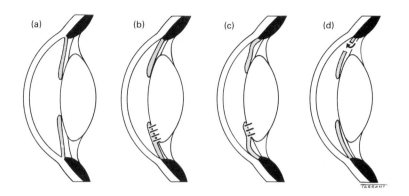

Fig. 75. Mechanism of acute closed-angle glaucoma. (a) Cross-section of the normal eye. (b) Shallow anterior chamber with increased irido-lenticular contact. (c) Pupil block leading to peripheral anterior synechiae. (d) Principle of peripheral iridectomy.

causes a lifting forwards of the peripheral part of the iris against the trabecular meshwork by the pressure of the aqueous which accumulates behind the iris in the posterior chamber. These changes may produce an area of iridocorneal contact at the entrance into the angle so that the passage of aqueous is impeded; the subsequent absorption of the residual aqueous in the angle through the filtration meshwork obliterates the entire angle and, in the absence of effective treatment, leads to the formation of peripheral anterior synechiae in the area of initial iridocorneal contact.

Secondly, with advancing age there is dilator muscle atrophy leading to a laxity of the peripheral iris, which is accompanied by a gradual miosis (*senile miosis*); the former favours a forwards bowing of the peripheral iris, and the latter increases the relative pupillary block.

Third, crowding of the angle of the anterior chamber by dilatation of the pupil may occur after the use of parasympathetic blockers or sometimes merely by exposure to darkness or possibly by emotion, or by an increased thickness and bulging forwards of the lens in an elderly person. It is the position of mid-dilatation that poses the greatest threat to the pressure differential between the posterior and anterior chambers because this is the stage of maximal iris-lens contact; this position tends to occur during recovery from pharmacological dilatation.

Clinical features

The subjective symptoms of closed-angle glaucoma are usually strikingly evident: in a mild subacute attack there is discomfort of the eye (because of a sudden rise in the intraocular pressure) and some degree of generalized mistiness of the vision, often with an awareness of rainbow-like haloes (resulting from the development of corneal oedema). These attacks may be only transient (the prodromal attacks), but usually they tend to become more prolonged and severe so that an acute attack occurs with intense pain in and around the eye, photophobia, lacrimation, marked loss of vision, and sometimes even vomiting; if not relieved, intractable blindness is inevitable (*absolute glaucoma*).

The objective signs of closed-angle glaucoma are also strikingly evident. A redness of the eye, particularly in the circumcorneal region (*ciliary injection*), which varies in intensity according to the severity of the attack, is a characteristic feature; this type of redness may occur also in acute iridocyclitis or even to some extent in intense conjunctivitis. A steamy haze of the cornea caused by varying degrees of corneal epithelial oedema, with eventually an oedema also of the corneal stroma is also a characteristic feature.

There is a shallowness of the anterior chamber; this is a basic feature of the condition which is accentuated by the oedematous state of the iris. The angle of the anterior chamber is obliterated, and it is usually not possible to examine the details of the angle by the method of gonioscopy (p.299) because of the corneal haze.

Usually there is partial dilatation of the pupil which becomes elongated vertically so that it assumes an oval shape, with an obvious whorling of the iris pattern. The direct and consensual reactions of the pupil to light are diminished and even absent in severe cases. Swelling of the eyelids may occur in severe or persistent attacks.

The intraocular pressure is frequently raised to extremely high levels. If the pupil block reverses spontaneously then the intraocular pressure may not be elevated, but some inflammatory signs persist which may lead to an erroneous diagnosis of uveitis; in such a case an examination of the fellow eye, which reveals a narrow angle of the anterior chamber, avoids this error.

Several subacute angle-closure attacks with the formation of peripheral anterior synechiae lead eventually to optic disc cupping. In some cases of closed-angle glaucoma when the intraocular pressure falls and the circulation is re-established to the ischaemic disc and retina, there is development of disc swelling with multiple haemorrhages, mimicking papilloedema or central retinal vein thrombosis. The lens may show discrete anterior subcapsular lens opacities as a result of a focal ischaemic necrosis, a condition known as '*glaukomflecken*'.

Provocative tests. Induction of relative pupillary block by the use of weak mydriatics or more physiologically by confining the patient to a dark room in the prone position for an hour causes a significant rise in the intraocular pressure in the majority of cases of congestive glaucoma, so that it may be used to confirm the diagnosis in doubtful cases; the significance of vague congestive symptoms may be difficult to determine otherwise because the eye remains normal in appearance, except for the narrowness of the angle of the anterior chamber.

Treatment

Medical treatment. A subacute closed-angle attack, which by definition has some preservation of pupillary response, may respond rapidly to the use of a miotic such as eserine 0.25% or pilocarpine 4%, thus drawing the peripheral iris away from the angle, allowing drainage of aqueous and lowering of the pressure. Apart from the danger of recurrent attacks of subacute angle closure, the miotic itself may increase the iris–lens contact, predisposing to further pupillary block and therefore surgical intervention in the form of a peripheral iridectomy is required.

An acute closed-angle attack, by definition, has no pupillary response due to the ischaemic nature of the condition, and demands rapid intensive treatment with aqueous suppressants such as acetazolamide (Diamox) given by the intravenous or intramuscular route, or osmotic agents such as glycerol orally or mannitol intravenously. Once the pressure decreases, the pupil will begin to react and it is at this stage that miotics may be used to decongest the angle, being given at two- to four-hourly intervals. Surgery is ultimately required.

Surgical treatment. In cases which respond to medical treatment, subsequent attacks may be avoided by the performance of a *peripheral iridectomy* which removes the pressure differential between the anterior and posterior chambers and thus pre-empts the development of pupillary block. It is important to ascertain that there is no impairment of the facility of aqueous outflow (at a time when there is no congestive attack) by the absence of cupping or field defects or abnormal tonography, otherwise the peripheral iridectomy should be combined with a drainage procedure as in chronic simple glaucoma.

Congestive glaucoma should always be regarded as a potentially bilateral disease, so that treatment of the affected eye must also include the use of a simple miotic like pilocarpine in the apparently unaffected eye to prevent any risk of angle closure if there is any form of narrow angle, with subsequently a peripheral iridectomy or laser iridotomy, even in the absence of any previous congestive symptoms.

Secondary glaucoma

Secondary glaucoma may occur in a wide variety of conditions (which are discussed elsewhere), usually as a result of a mechanical interference with the circulation of the aqueous humour.

Obstruction of the filtration angle by an accumulation of abnormal materials. This would include:

1.   *Haemorrhage* as the result of trauma (perforating or non-perforating), following some intraocular operation, particularly involving the iris, or as the result of some lesion of the anterior uvea (e.g. an angioma or a leiomyoma) which is liable to bleed. Clotted blood may produce pupillary block, while degenerate red cells–erythroclasts—may block the trabecular meshwork.

2.   *Inflammatory material* (cells or exudate) as the result of an iridocyclitis—sometimes in the acute stage of the disease but more commonly in the later stages after several recurrences. Herpes simplex and herpes zoster uveitis are commonly associated with elevated intraocular pressure, partly as a result of inflammatory material but also as a result of trabeculitis.

3.   *Lens material* as the result of the liberation of lens particles into the anterior chamber following a perforating injury involving the lens, an extracapsular cataract extraction or discission, or phacolytic glaucoma (p.176).

4.   *Abnormal material from the ciliary body.* In this condition the filtration angle becomes embarrassed by the accumulation of white particles, which also collect on the anterior lens capsule, pupillary margin, ciliary body and zonule, where they give the impression of representing exfoliations of the lens capsule, but it is now known that this material, which is of a mucinous nature, arises from the inner surface of the ciliary body and that its occurrence on the pupillary margin is purely coincidental; hence the term *pseudocapsular glaucoma* (or *pseudoexfoliation of the lens capsule*). Gonioscopy demonstrates marked pigmentation of the trabecular meshwork. The condition usually occurs in the elderly.

5.   *Tumour cells.* A malignant melanoma may obstruct the angle of the anterior chamber and rarely may proliferate within Schlemm's canal, the condition of *ring melanoma*.

6.   *Pigment.* A form of glaucoma associated with pigment dispersion occurs in young adult males with moderate myopia who have deep anterior chambers and concave irides. Pigment particles are deposited on all structures bathed by the aqueous. Retro-illumination of the iris shows radial iris atrophy.

Obliteration of the filtration angle by the formation of peripheral anterior synechiae. This is a result of:

1.   The subsequent organization of the abnormal materials discussed above.

2.   The delayed reformation of the anterior chamber after its partial or total loss following a perforating injury or operation.

3.   The occurrence of new vessel formations on the anterior surface of the peripheral part of the iris (*rubeosis iridis*), a complication liable to follow conditions of severe retinal damage, such as central retinal vein thrombosis, diabetic retinopathy, long-standing retinal

detachment, retrolental fibroplasia and ocular ischaemia due to carotid artery disease. It is suggested that the neovascularization is the outcome of an abormal stimulus from the anoxic retina.

Obstruction of the passage of the aqueous from the posterior chamber to the anterior chamber through the pupillary aperture. This is a result of:

1. The occurrence of an *iris bombé* (total adherence of the pupil margin to the lens) after severe uveitis (p.84). This may be termed *seclusion of the pupil* and may also occur as the result of an adhesion between the iris and the prolapsed intact vitreous face following an intracapsular cataract extraction (pupil block).
2. Occlusion of the pupil by the formation of a *cyclitic membrane* following a severe anterior uveitis (p.84).
3. The occurrence of pupil block as a result of a congenital abnormality of the shape of the lens *(spherophakia,* p.166), an anterior subluxation of the lens, or a hernia of vitreous through the pupil in the aphakic eye.

Steroid-induced glaucoma. Some eyes respond to topical steroids with an elevation of the intraocular pressure, a phenomenon which is genetically determined. It occurs in the majority of patients with chronic simple glaucoma and in patients with a family history of glaucoma. Persistent use of steroids may occur in patients with vernal conjunctivitis, recurrent iritis, blepharitis or following corneal graft surgery; intraocular pressures must therefore be carefully monitored for, although the increased pressure usually subsides after the withdrawal of steroids, a few proceed to chronic simple glaucoma requiring medical or even surgical treatment. The recent development of a progestogenic steroid, fluomethalone, with less pressure-elevation effect, has lessened the risks of long-term topical steroids.

Prevention

It is essential to try and prevent secondary glaucoma by the adequate treatment of the conditions which predispose to its occurrence, for example, using full mydriasis in iridocyclitis, the restoration of the anterior chamber after its loss by the use of air or the removal of an extensive hyphaema.

Treatment

In general, treatment should be directed to the cause of the secondary glaucoma, but acetazolamide (Diamox) is of value in obtaining a temporary reduction in the intraocular pressure before the general measures become effective. In intractable cases, operation is necessary—an iridectomy may be of value in certain cases when there is an obstruction in the filtration angle or in the pupillary area, but sometimes a drainage operation or a procedure to reduce the production of aqueous is necessary.

16

The Afferent Visual Pathway

Each component of the afferent visual pathway is discussed with regard to the disposition of the visual fibres, their blood supply, the characteristics of the visual field defects which follow their involvement, and the nature of the lesions which cause such defects, thus providing an opportunity to describe various neuro-ophthalmological conditions together instead of including them in other chapters.

The retina and optic nerve head

The visual fibres arise from the retinal ganglion cells and are divided into four main groups by a vertical line which bisects the macula (the part of the retina concerned with central vision–including both the fovea and the parafovea)—so that there is a *temporal hemiretina* (including a *temporal hemimacula*) and a *nasal hemiretina* (including a *nasal hemimacula*)—and by a horizontal line which bisects the macula—so that there is an *upper hemiretina* (including an *upper hemimacula*) and a *lower hemiretina* (including a *lower hemimacula*). Thus there are four different retinal quadrants—*upper temporal, lower temporal, upper nasal* and *lower nasal*—with fibres subserving central vision (from part of the macula) and peripheral vision (from the rest of the retina) in each quadrant. It should be noted that all the macular fibres and most of the peripheral fibres have corresponding fibres in the other eye which are concerned with the *binocular field of vision*, but the most peripheral fibres of the upper and lower nasal quadrants have no corresponding fibres in the other eye and are concerned with the peripheral *uniocular field of vision* which forms a small extension on each temporal side of the binocular visual field (Fig. 76).

All the retinal fibres converge on the optic nerve head as though it lies at the junction of the nasal and temporal parts of the retina. However, it lies within the nasal part, so that some of the fibres run a complex course (Fig. 77). The nasal peripheral fibres pass more or less directly to the nasal border of the disc, except those arising from the retina above and below the temporal side of the optic disc which curve slightly in passing to the upper and lower aspects of the nasal border of the disc; this curve is accentuated markedly by the nasal fibres from the small portion of the retina between the temporal side of the optic disc

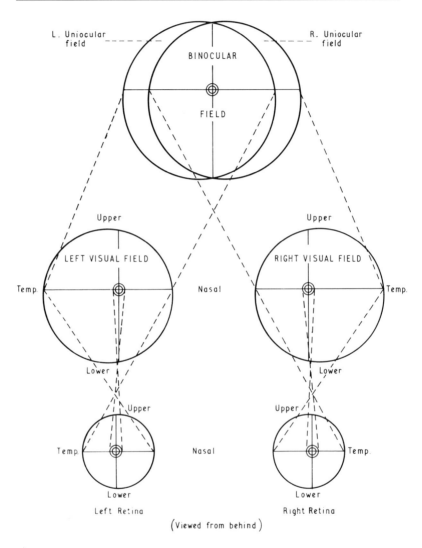

L. Uniocular field

R. Uniocular field

BINOCULAR

FIELD

Upper

LEFT VISUAL FIELD

Temp.   Nasal

Lower

Upper   Right VISUAL FIELD   Temp.

Upper

Temp.   Nasal

Lower

Left Retina

Upper

Nasal   Temp.

Lower

Right Retina

(Viewed from behind)

Fig. 76. The projection of the visual field from each retina, and the relation of the binocular visual field to the right and left uniocular visual fields.

and the macula (the *juxtapapillary fibres*) which pass to the extreme upper and lower aspects of the nasal border of the disc. The temporal peripheral fibres pass by a curved course from their origins above and below the horizontal raphe (which extends from the macula to the temporal periphery of the retina and separates the temporal peripheral fibres into upper and lower groups) to the upper one-fifth and lower one-fifth of the temporal border of the optic disc; this curved course is

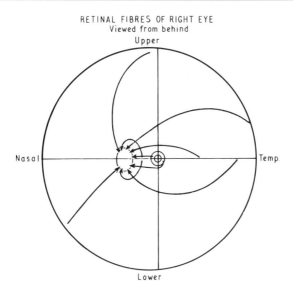

RETINAL FIBRES OF RIGHT EYE
Viewed from behind

Fig. 77. The direction of the visual fibres on passing from the different areas of the retina to the optic disc (right eye viewed from behind, or left eye viewed from in front).

dictated by the presence of the large papillomacular bundle of fibres on the temporal side of the disc. The nasal macular fibres pass directly in closely related upper and lower groups to the temporal aspect of the optic disc. The upper and lower temporal macular fibres curve sharply from their origin to combine with the upper and lower nasal macular fibres to form a large compact oval-shaped bundle which occupies three-fifths of the temporal margin of the disc (the *papillomacular bundle*).

In all quadrants the more peripheral fibres lie deeply in the nerve fibre layer of the retina and peripherally in the optic nerve head, whereas the less peripheral fibres lie superficially in the retina and centrally in the optic nerve head (Fig. 78).

The blood supply of the retina has a dual nature; the inner part, including the nerve fibre layer, is supplied by the central retinal artery, and the outer part, including the visual receptors, is supplied by the underlying capillary layer of the choroid (the *choriocapillaris*), except for the macular area which is nourished only by the choriocapillaris. The terminal branches of the central retinal artery function as endarteries so that each branch supplies a clear-cut bundle of visual fibres. The blood supply of the optic nerve head is derived almost exclusively from the ciliary circulation, with contributions also via the adjacent choroid, while the nerve fibre layer adjacent to the disc is supplied by the peripapillary capillary plexus from the retinal vessels.

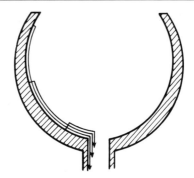

Fig. 78. The relative positions of the peripheral, equatorial and central visual fibres in the retina and in the optic nerve head.

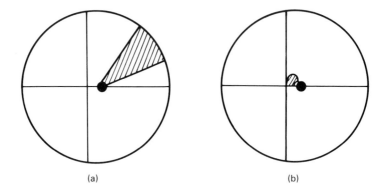

(a)   (b)

Fig. 79. Scotomata (hatched areas) occurring in the temporal part of the visual field following isolated lesions of the nasal visual fibres in the retina (right eye). (a) Scotoma continuous with the blind spot and extending to the peripheral limit of the temporal field. (b) Juxtapapillary scotoma.

Lesions of the retina and optic nerve head

A lesion of the nasal peripheral fibres on the nasal side of the optic disc produces a sector-shaped scotoma which lies in the temporal field of vision and expands as it passes to the periphery; the scotoma is continuous with the blind spot when the lesion borders on the disc, and extends to the peripheral limit of the temporal field when all the nerve fibres in the affected area are involved (Fig. 79a). It is broad when the affected area is large, and narrow when the affected area is small. A lesion of the nasal peripheral fibres which lies between the optic disc and the macula produces a markedly arcuate scotoma which is adjacent to the blind spot (*juxtapapillary scotoma*) (Fig. 79b).

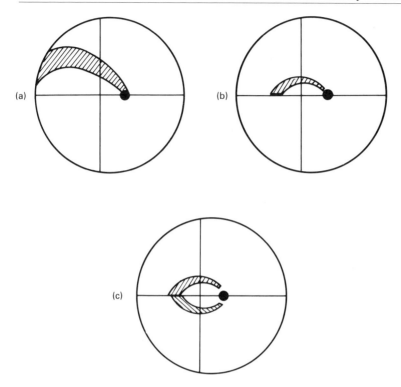

Fig. 80. Scotomata (hatched areas) occurring in the nasal part of the visual field following isolated lesions of the temporal visual fibres in the retina (right eye). (a) and (b) Arcuate scotomata which extend from the region of the blind spot around the fixation area towards the horizontal meridian. (c) Arcuate scotomata in both the upper and lower parts of the field with characteristic nasal step at the horizontal meridian.

A lesion of the temporal peripheral fibres produces an arcuate scotoma which extends from the region of the blind spot around the fixation area towards the horizontal meridian in the nasal part of the field (Fig. 80a, b). Sometimes there may be arcuate scotomata in both the upper and lower parts of the field, although these are often of unequal size so that they produce a characteristic nasal step at the horizontal meridian (Fig. 80c). The arcuate scotoma often fails to reach the blind spot even when the lesion directly involves the upper or lower temporal borders of the disc; this results from the failure of such a lesion to involve the nasal retinal fibres which lie between the temporal border of the disc and the macula because these fibres terminate in the upper and lower parts of the nasal border of the disc. The greater frequency of an arcuate scotoma in the upper rather than the lower part of the visual field in chronic simple glaucoma may be related to the

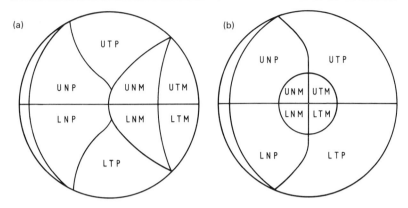

Fig. 81. The distribution of the visual fibres in the right optic nerve (viewed from behind): (a) near the optic nerve head, and (b) midway between the optic nerve head and the optic chiasm. U = upper; L = lower; T = temporal; N = nasal; P = peripheral; M = macular.

increased crowding of the fibres in the lower part of the optic nerve head as a result of its slightly asymmetrical division into upper and lower parts.

A localized lesion of the retina from behind, for example a patch of choroiditis, produces an isolated scotoma in the visual field corresponding to the area which suffers destruction of its visual receptors, but this is followed by an extension of the scotoma towards the periphery due to a subsequent involvement of the nerve fibre layer; at a certain stage there is sometimes a small area of sparing of the visual field between the two defects because of a temporary sparing of the fibres from the retina immediately peripheral to the affected area which lie superficially in the retina. Sectorial damage of the optic nerve produces corresponding defects in the nerve fibre layer of the retina, which are more readily seen in red-free light.

The lesions which affect the retina and optic nerve head are discussed in Chapters 7 and 8.

The optic nerve

In the distal part of the optic nerve, the visual fibres maintain to a large extent the distribution which they assume in the optic nerve head; the upper retinal fibres lie in the upper half of the nerve and the lower retinal fibres in the lower half, the nasal peripheral fibres lie in the upper and lower regions of the medial part with the most peripheral fibres (uniocular fibres) lying superficially, the temporal peripheral fibres lie in the upper and lower regions of the lateral part, and the macular fibres lie in the central region of the lateral part so that they extend to the surface of the nerve (Fig. 81a). In the main part of the

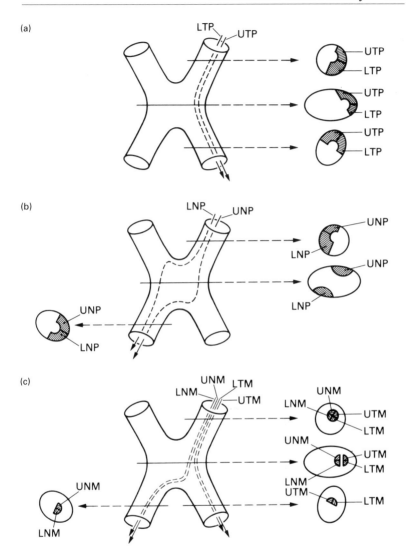

Fig. 82. The distribution of (a) the temporal peripheral, (b) the nasal peripheral, and (c) the macular fibres in the central part of the optic chiasm viewed from above and in cross-section. U = upper; L = lower; T = temporal; N = nasal; P = peripheral; M = macular.

optic nerve the different groups of fibres maintain similar positions, except for the macular fibres which pass to the central region so that the temporal peripheral fibres occupy the whole of the lateral part of the nerve (Fig. 81b). This distribution is continued until the proximal part of the nerve near the optic chiasm where the temporal peripheral fibres move from a lateral position to a ventrolateral one (Fig. 82a), the nasal peripheral fibres move from a medial position to a dorsomedial one (Fig. 82b), and the macular fibres move from a central position to a dorsocentral one (Fig. 82c).

The blood supply of the optic nerve is derived from two systems—a peripheral vascular system of the pial sheath which is formed by various branches from the orbital arteries (ophthalmic, ciliary and lacrimal arteries, and branches from the anterior cerebral and superior hypophyseal arteries contributing to the intracranial part of the nerve), and an axial vascular system formed by the central retinal artery and its branches. There is evidence that the peripheral and axial vascular systems form anastomoses with one another within the nerve.

Lesions of the optic nerve

Lesions of the optic nerve tend to produce field defects which are similar to those which follow retinal lesions, although there is a predilection for the macular fibres to suffer damage, resulting in impaired colour vision, an afferent pupillary defect, central field loss and optic atrophy. This may be the result of involvement of the axial circulation within the nerve. It is important to remember that atrophy of nervous tissue is usually the result of a defect of blood supply rather than a direct pressure effect; this may account for the visual field defects which sometimes occur in severe cases of endocrine exophthalmos when there is a marked increase in intraorbital pressure.

The lesions which affect the optic nerve are discussed in Chapter 8.

The optic chiasm

In the optic chiasm there is a partial decussation of the nerve fibres so that the fibres from the temporal hemiretina (peripheral and macular fibres) pass to the optic tract of the same side, thus constituting the *uncrossed fibres*, and the fibres from the nasal hemiretina (peripheral and macular fibres) pass to the optic tract of the opposite side, thus constituting the *crossed fibres*.

The temporal peripheral fibres (Fig. 82a) from both eyes traverse the lateral parts of the optic chiasm as two widely separated compact masses. In each mass the fibres from the upper temporal retina lie dorsal and slightly medial to those from the lower temporal retina, with the most peripheral fibres lying superficially and the most central fibres lying deeply. It is evident, therefore, that these fibres maintain the same relative positions as in the main part of the optic nerve, although they turn slightly dorsally near the caudal end of the chiasm to enter the dorsolateral part of the ipsilateral optic tract.

The nasal peripheral fibres (Fig. 82b) from both eyes traverse the central part of the optic chiasm; there is considerable intermingling of the fibres from the two eyes, although there is distinct separation of the upper and lower groups of fibres from each eye. The upper nasal peripheral fibres lie in the more dorsal part of the chiasm and travel towards the ipsilateral optic tract before crossing in the posterior part of the optic chiasm to enter the upper dorsomedial part of the contralateral optic tract, whereas the lower nasal peripheral fibres lie in the ventral part of the optic chiasm and, after crossing in the anterior part of the chiasm, travel towards the contralateral optic nerve before looping back to pass to the lower ventromedial part of the contralateral optic tract. Sometimes a few fibres of this anterior loop from the most peripheral part of the lower nasal retina enter the terminal part of the optic nerve. It should be noted that the most peripheral nasal fibres, which lie on the superficial medial aspect of the optic nerve, maintain this superficial medial position in the optic tract, necessitating a single spiral twisting of all these fibres relative to one another during their passage through the central part of the chiasm.

The temporal macular fibres (Fig. 82c) from both eyes traverse the lateral parts of the optic chiasm as two distinct compact masses on the inner aspects of the temporal peripheral fibres and enter the ipsilateral optic tracts in that situation. The nasal macular fibres (Fig. 82c) from both eyes pass through the chiasm on the outer aspects of the nasal peripheral fibres and cross in the posterior part of the chiasm where the fibres from both eyes mingle with one another. In this situation they lie near the surface of the chiasm but, as they enter the contralateral optic tracts, they are covered on their inner aspects by the nasal peripheral fibres so that they become adjacent to the temporal macular fibres in the central part of the commencement of the optic tract.

The optic chiasm is supplied by a complex series of arteries including the internal carotid artery with its branch—the lateral or inferior chiasmal artery—which passes to the inferolateral aspect of the chiasm, the anterior cerebral artery with its branch—the superior chiasmal artery—which passes to the superoanterior aspect, the anterior communicating artery which sends branches to the superoanterior aspect, the anterior hypophyseal artery which sends a recurrent branch to the inferior aspect with ramifications which extend to the posterior aspect, the posterior communicating artery which sends branches to the inferoposterior aspect, and possible contributions from the middle cerebral artery, the anterior choroidal artery and the ophthalmic artery, which sometimes sends a prechiasmal branch to the anteroinferior aspect. These branches form a dense network of capillaries; in the lateral region the capillaries run in an anteroposterior direction, in the more central areas the capillaries pass across the midline, and in the median plane they form a free anastomosis so that the capillaries appear to follow the distribution of the groups of nerve fibres through the chiasm.

Lesions of the optic chiasm

Median pressure on the ventral surface of the optic chiasm from an expanding intrasellar lesion gives rise eventually to a *bitemporal hemianopia*, with an involvement of the upper temporal quadrants before the lower ones (Fig. 83). In both quadrants the visual field defects remain sharply limited by the vertical meridian although after an interval the lower nasal and the upper nasal quadrants may be ultimately affected. The involvement of the lower nasal quadrant before the upper nasal one is the result of the more medial position of the upper temporal fibres as compared with the lower temporal ones, so that the upper fibres are affected first by an expanding lesion despite their more dorsal situation. In contrast, median pressure on the dorsal surface of the optic chiasm from a purely suprasellar lesion, although it also causes a bitemporal hemianopia, changes the sequence of the involvement of these two quadrants so that the lower quadrant is affected before the upper one. In the event of the later development of a binasal hemianopia, however, the sequence of the involvement of the two quadrants, lower before upper, is retained.

It should be noted, however, that the visual field changes in chiasmal lesions are not confined to depression of the peripheral parts of the fields because central or paracentral changes may occur at any stage, even before the peripheral ones, in the progress of the lesion. Involvement of the anterior chiasmal angle (the junction of one of the optic nerves with the optic chiasm) is liable to produce an arcuate scotoma which curves in a paracentral position in the upper or lower temporal quadrant as far as the vertical meridian in addition to the peripheral field changes (Fig. 83). Similarly involvement of the posterior chiasmal angle (the junction of one of the optic tracts and the optic chiasm) is liable to produce changes in the central parts of the visual fields because of the presence of the macular fibres in the posterior part of the chiasm.

There are many lesions which produce chiasmal defects.

Injuries

Injury is rare except in a penetrating wound which is usually rapidly fatal because of the associated damage to the surrounding great vessels. Sometimes, however, the optic chiasm may be damaged by a violent frontal blow as the result of a disruption of the small chiasmal vessels which follows a sudden displacement of the brain relative to the skull.

Inflammatory conditions

Basal meningitis. This form of meningitis is often of an acute nature as the result of a primary infection or as the result of a secondary infection from some neighbouring source (nasal sinusitis, otitis media or cerebral

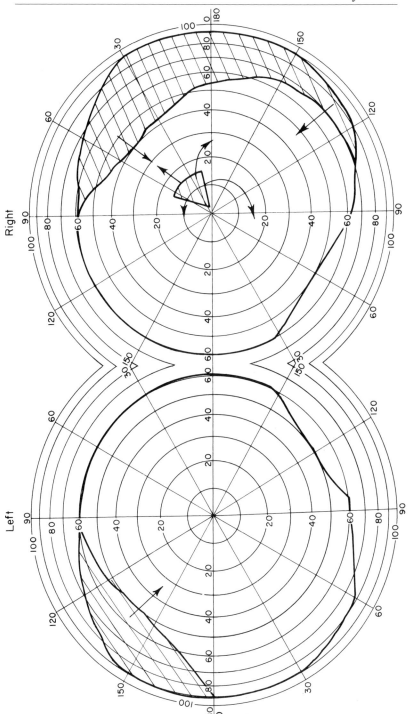

Fig. 83. The pattern of spread of peripheral and paracentral visual field defects in a chiasmal lesion.

abscess) so that the grave general manifestations predominate, but when it is of a chronic nature the ocular manifestations predominate.

Chiasmal arachnoiditis. This is a localized chronic inflammatory condition of the arachnoid membrane in the region of the optic chiasm, with the production of hyperplastic changes so that the visual fibres of the optic chiasm (initially their nutrient vessels) are compressed gradually. Many different types of infection have been postulated (e.g. tuberculosis, syphilis, actinomycosis) and sometimes previous trauma or subarachnoid haemorrhage may be the cause of the local adhesive inflammatory changes, but in most cases the exciting agent is unknown. Any type of chiasmal visual defect may occur, but there is a tendency for central or paracentral changes to be an early feature. Eventually some degree of optic atrophy occurs, but papilloedema is an unusual event. Headaches commonly occur. Rarely the neighbouring motor nerves to the extrinsic ocular muscles are involved.

Demyelinating conditions

Chiasmal neuritis. Rarely the optic chiasm may be involved in a process of demyelination in association with one of the demyelinating diseases (disseminated sclerosis, neuromyelitis optica, or encephalitis periaxialis diffusa); this is similar, therefore, to optic neuritis (p.153).

Vascular anomalies

Arteriosclerotic changes. Arteriosclerosis of the nutrient vessels may rarely account for a disturbance of the optic chiasm. Sometimes such changes in the arteries surrounding the optic chiasm produce direct pressure effects on the surface of the chiasm; for example, a hardening of the internal carotid artery may produce a nasal visual field defect (a rare form of chiasmal defect).

Aneurysm. An aneurysm of the supraclinoid part of the internal carotid artery or of the neighbouring arteries which are concerned in the formation of the circle of Willis is usually of congenital origin and may remain free from complications for many years (or even indefinitely), but sometimes it produces defects. First, its progressive enlargement may cause compression of the caudal part of the optic nerve or of the optic chiasm, with the production of typical visual field defects, or it may cause compression of the third cranial nerve with the production of an ophthalmoplegia (p.255). Second, it may permit a gradual or intermittent leakage of blood through its attenuated wall into the subarachnoid space, causing various form of ophthalmoplegia which may be transient but are often recurrent, usually associated with headache. Third, it may rupture suddenly with the formation of a massive subarachnoid haemorrhage; this is associated with severe headache, vomiting, ophthalmoplegia and coma. Death occurs rapidly in about 50% of such cases.

An aneurysm of the infraclinoid part of the internal carotid artery within the cavernous sinus may enlarge sufficiently to produce the pressure effects of a supraclinoid aneurysm, but more commonly it is associated with the formation of a caroticocavernous fistula (p.287).

Tumours

Craniopharyngioma. This is a congenitally determined tumour which arises in the epithelial remnants concerned in the formation of Rathke's pharyngeal pouch, the anterior lobe of the pituitary body or the hypophyseal duct. It may become evident at any age but occurs commonly in the early years of life. The general manifestations vary greatly but are often of a hypothalamic nature, including headaches, generalized weakness, progressive mental deterioration, drowsiness—sometimes with transient periods of unconsciousness, dystrophia adiposogenitalis and diabetes insipidus. Visual defects usually occur fairly early, but in the child are often ignored until they reach an advanced stage when there is obvious optic nerve atrophy, usually bilateral. The suprasellar situation of the tumour is demonstrated radiographically by ventriculography or CT scan, but a simple radiographic examination of the skull is also of great importance because, although an enlargement of the sella turcica is not common, other features such as decalcification of the clinoid processes, shortening of the dorsum sellae, or suprasellar calcification are frequently evident. Sometimes it is not possible for the neurosurgeon to remove the entire tumour without sacrificing the optic chiasm (or the caudal part of the involved optic nerve), although an aspiration of any cystic part of the tumour is of great value in relieving its immediate pressure effects; postoperative supervoltage X-irradiation may eradicate the tumour and prevent its recurrence.

Chromophobe adenoma. This pituitary tumour usually becomes evident in early adult life or in middle age. The general manifestations are varied and include headaches, generalized weakness, loss of libido, loss of body hair, amenorrhoea, mental sluggishness, fits of extreme temper and diabetes insipidus. Visual defects occur almost invariably with a suprasellar extension and are quite frequently early, although they tend to be ignored by the patient because of their trivial nature (a fluid appearance of the outlines of distant objects, transient attacks of misty vision, a slight impairment of reading vision), or disregarded by the examiner who considers them to be simply the result of some uncorrected error of refraction despite the fact that the provision of glasses fails to relieve the symptoms. The true nature of these visual defects is determined only by careful examination of the visual fields, particularly with red or small white targets, except in the later stages when optic nerve atrophy is apparent. Some form of ophthalmoplegia due to involvement of the third, fourth or sixth cranial nerves may rarely occur when the tumour spreads laterally. Simple radiographic examination of the skull reveals enlargement of the sella turcica which follows the intrasellar expansion of the tumour; it may also show thinning of the dorsum sellae or of the posterior clinoid processes, or undermining of the anterior clinoid processes, but the full extent of any suprasellar expansion is only demonstrated by more complicated methods (CT scan, ventriculography or carotid angiography). The treatment may be neurosurgical (craniotomy with a hypophysectomy, or trans-sphenoidal hypophysectomy), radiotherapeutic (supervoltage X-irradiation), or a combination of both procedures. Life-long hormonal supplements are required.

Chromophile adenoma. This pituitary tumour usually becomes evident in early adult life with gigantism or in middle age with acromegaly (in the acidophil type) or with Cushing's syndrome (in the basophil type). There is marked enlargement of the sella turcica (except in the basophil type), but a visual field defect is not an invariable feature because the tumour tends to remain intrasellar in situation.

Meningioma. This tumour affects the chiasm in different ways depending on whether it arises in a presellar, suprasellar or parasellar situation.
   Presellar meningioma—a meningioma of the olfactory groove— which causes anosmia due to pressure on the olfactory nerve, affects the caudal part of the optic nerve with the development of optic atrophy before causing a backwards and downwards displacement of the optic chiasm. This chiasmal involvement leads to various forms of visual field defect, but sometimes it produces bilateral central scotomata.
   Suprasellar meningioma—a meningioma arising from the region of the chiasmatic sulcus or tuberculum sellae—tends to affect the caudal part of the optic nerve (or sometimes both optic nerves) before causing a backwards and upwards displacement of the optic chiasm with the production of characteristic chiasmal defects involving the peripheral or central parts of the visual fields. In the later stages, signs of a pituitary defect (see p.329), of a hypothalamic disturbance, or of an internal hydrocephalus may become evident. *Internal hydrocephalus* is the result of a distortion of the third ventricle which leads to a blockage of the foramen of Monro by an extraventricular tumour, such as a suprasellar meningioma, or by an intraventricular tumour, such as a glioma or ependymoma, or as the result of a blockage of the aqueduct of Sylvius or the fourth ventricle by the extension of a tumour from the brainstem (midbrain and pons), pineal body, vermis of the cerebellum,

or eighth cranial nerve; it follows that a tumour of the posterior fossa, quite apart from causing papilloedema, is liable also sometimes to produce signs of chiasmal compression.

Parasellar meningioma—a meningioma from the region of the lesser wing of the sphenoid—causes involvement of the adjacent optic nerve (characteristically with the production of an upper altitudinal hemianopic defect of the ipsilateral visual field before leading to blindness of the eye) and subsequently involvement of the optic chiasm. A spread laterally produces the sphenoidal fissure syndrome (p.258).

Compression of the third cranial nerve over a long period may induce the picture of aberrant regeneration (p.255).

A characteristic radiological feature of meningiomas is the induction of hyperostosis of the adjacent bone.

Glioma. This tumour may occur as a primary event in the optic chiasm or as a glioma of the frontal lobe which spreads downwards to involve the optic nerves and optic chiasm (suprasellar involvement). Primary chiasmal gliomas are commonly associated with neurofibromatosis, tend to occur in adolescence and young adulthood, and may be associated with glioma of the optic nerve.

Tumours of the sphenoid bone. An osteoma, osteochondroma, haemangioma or sarcoma may cause pressure on the optic chiasm and sometimes also lead to proptosis, ophthalmoplegia and trigeminal neuralgia.

Tumours of the basal meninges. A primary tumour of the basal meninges is rare, but a metastatic carcinoma may spready rapidly with involvement of the optic nerves, optic chiasm, third, fourth, fifth and sixth cranial nerves, pituitary body and hypothalamus; death follows after a short interval.

Chordoma. This slow-growing tumour is derived from the notochord remnants in the dorsum sellae. It presents with multiple lower cranial nerve palsies (ninth to twelfth cranial nerves) but may produce inferior compression of the chiasm or optic tract.

The optic tract

In the most distal part of the optic tract the visual fibres maintain the same relative positions as in the posterior part of the chiasm: the temporal peripheral fibres lie dorsolaterally with the upper ones above the lower ones, the nasal peripheral fibres lie ventromedially with the upper ones above the lower ones and with the uniocular peripheral

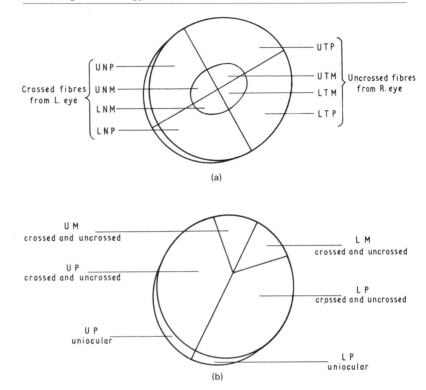

Fig. 84. The distribution of the visual fibres in the optic tract: (a) at the optic chiasm, and (b) midway between the optic chiasm and the lateral geniculate body (right optic tract, viewed in cross-section from behind). U = upper; L = lower; T = temporal; N = nasal; P = peripheral; M = macular.

fibres in a superficial position, and the macular fibres lie centrally with the temporal fibres lateral to the nasal ones and the upper fibres above the lower ones (Fig. 84a). There is, however, a rapid redistribution of the fibres in the tract so that the fibres from corresponding areas of each retina tend to be associated with one another; the upper peripheral binocular fibres (uncrossed and crossed) lie dorsomedially, the lower peripheral binocular fibres (uncrossed and crossed) lie ventrolaterally, the peripheral uniocular fibres (crossed only) lie on the superficial aspect of the ventromedial border, and the macular fibres (uncrossed and crossed) lie dorsolaterally with the upper fibres dorsal to the lower ones, although it is uncertain if the macular fibres extend as far as the surface of the optic tract (Fig. 84b). It is evident that there is some tilting of the main part of the optic tract whereby its upper border lies more laterally than its lower border.

In this way the horizontal meridian of the retina is represented by a line which passes from a dorsolateral position to a ventromedial one, the upper and lower halves of the vertical meridian of the retina are probably represented in the region of the junctions between the upper peripheral and upper macular fibres and the lower peripheral and lower macular fibres, the upper and lower halves of the circumferential meridian of the retina are represented by a line which passes round the dorsomedial and ventrolateral borders, and the fixation point in the retina is represented in the dorsolateral region.

The optic tract is supplied by the peripheral pial vascular network which is formed by branches from the anterior choroidal artery (usually a branch of the internal carotid artery), the middle cerebral artery, the posterior communicating artery and the posterior cerebral artery.

Lesions of the optic tract

The optic tract is the first part of the visual pathway in which lesions consistently produce *homonymous* field defects, as the result of the involvement of the visual fibres from corresponding areas of the retina of both eyes within a single lesion, although these are seldom congruous. In a complete hemianopia (loss of the nasal half-field of the ipsilateral eye and temporal half-field of the contralateral eye), the fovea is bisected vertically.

There are many lesions which produce optic tract defects—basal meningitis, demyelinating conditions, infraclinoid aneurysms (of the internal carotid artery, posterior communicating artery, middle cerebral artery or posterior cerebral artery), and rarely supraclinoid aneurysms which extend backwards—but the usual lesion is a tumour; the anterior part of the optic tract may be affected by a pituitary tumour which spreads backwards or by a parasellar meningioma, the posterior part of the optic tract by a tumour of the third ventricle or a tumour of the basal ganglia, and the lateral aspect of the optic tract by an expanding tumour of the temporal lobe. The associated involvement of neighbouring structures produces other features, including hemiplegia and hemianaesthesia in involvement of the internal capsule, dissociated gaze palsies in involvement of the medial longitudinal bundle or defective pupillary reactions when the region of the superior colliculus is involved.

The lateral geniculate body

The dorsal nucleus of the lateral geniculate body serves as a relay station in the projection of the visual fibres from the retina to the striate area of the visual cortex with the formation of synaptic junctions. The majority of the fibres from the optic tract enter the nucleus through its convex anterior surface, but some fibres enter through the hilum which lies in a concavity on the ventral surface of the medial part of the

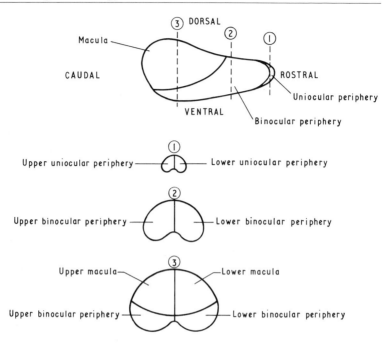

Fig. 85.   The distribution of the visual fibres in the dorsal nucleus of the right lateral geniculate body, viewed from the side and in cross-section through (1) the rostral part, (2) the central part, and (3) the caudal part of nucleus, viewed from behind.

nucleus. The visual fibres terminate in different parts of the nucleus according to their positions of origin in the retina (Fig 85): the crossed and uncrossed fibres from the hemimacula of each eye pass to a large median sector which lies in a dorsocentral position in the caudal two-thirds of the nucleus with a rounded caudal margin for the foveal fibres—the upper macular fibres terminating medially and the lower macular ones laterally. The crossed and uncrossed fibres from the peripheral binocular hemiretina of each eye pass ventrally on the medial and lateral aspects of the macular area—the upper retinal fibres terminating medially in the medial tubercle and in the rostral one-third of the nucleus and the lower fibres terminating laterally in the lateral horn. The crossed fibres from the peripheral uniocular retina pass to a narrow area on the ventral aspect of the rostral part of the nucleus—the upper fibres terminating medially and the lower fibres terminating laterally. The fibres terminate in the nucleus in different grey laminae (composed of nerve cells) which are separated from one another by white laminae (composed of medullated nerve fibres). In the macular and main binocular peripheral areas there are six grey laminae—laminae 1, 4, and 6 for crossed fibres and laminae 2, 3, and 5 for uncrossed fibres; in the rest of the binocular peripheral areas there are only four grey laminae—lamina 1 and a lamina composed of laminae 4 and 6 for crossed fibres and lamina 2 and a lamina composed of laminae 3 and 5 for uncrossed fibres; and in the uniocular peripheral area there are only two grey laminae, both for crossed fibres. There is evidence that corresponding retinal areas are represented in adjacent parts of all the laminae in a linear manner along a radius which passes through the nucleus in the direction of the centre of the hilum, so that there is a point-to-sector representation of the retina. The optic radiation emerges from the nucleus through its dorsocaudal surface.

In this way the horizontal meridian of the retina is represented by a plane which is more or less vertical through the lateral geniculate body in a rostrocaudal direction, the vertical meridian of the retina is represented by a plane which lies along the posterior border of the lateral geniculate body with the upper part of the vertical meridian extending medially and the lower part of the vertical meridian extending laterally, the circumferential meridian of the retina is represented by a plane which lies along the anterior border of the body with the upper part of the meridian extending medially and the lower part extending laterally, and the fixation point of the retina is represented in the central part of the most caudal region.

The function of the dorsal nucleus of the lateral geniculate body is not clearly understood, but it appears to serve largely as a relay station, with possibly an ability to exert integrating and modulating influences on the visual impulses. The suggestion that it is concerned with a distinction between the perceptions of light and colour with a trichromatic form of colour vision or with an appreciation of spatial relationships is not established with any certainty. It should be noted, however, that this is the first structure in the afferent visual pathway which emphasizes anatomically the functional importance of the macula by devoting such a large area to its fibres.

The lateral geniculate body is supplied mainly by the posterior cerebral artery or its posterior choroidal branch, but the anterior choroidal artery also plays some part.

There are no specific visual field changes in lesions of the lateral geniculate body and they tend to mimic those occurring in lesions of the optic tract or optic radiation.

The optic radiation (geniculo-calcarine pathway)

The optic radiation emerges from the lateral geniculate body as a compact band of fibres which, after passing through the posterior part of the internal capsule, spreads out as a broad band covering the outer surface of the lateral ventricle to its termination in the striate area of the visual cortex. The upper fibres of this broad band pass more or less directly backwards, but the lower fibres turn downwards before passing

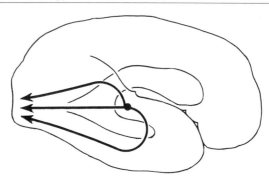

Fig. 86.   The optic radiation from the dorsal nucleus of the lateral geniculate body to the striate cortex (viewed from the lateral side). Note the relation of the lower fibres to the inferior horn of the lateral ventricle.

backwards, and some of these fibres pass forwards as well as downwards so that they form a loop in the region of the inferior horn of the lateral ventricle (the *loop of Meyer*) before turning back to join the main part of the radiation (Fig. 86).

There is evidence that the distribution of the visual fibres in the optic radiation has a uniform pattern throughout most of their course, with a fairly precise point-to-point arrangement according to their origins from corresponding areas of the retina of each eye, but it is likely that there are certain unusual features of the anterior part of the radiation, particularly within the loop of Meyer.

In the *anterior part of the optic radiation* it is likely that the visual fibres maintain to a large extent the arrangement which they have in the lateral geniculate body, with the exception that all the groups of fibres are rotated through 90°, so that the upper retinal fibres (macular and peripheral, crossed and uncrossed) lie dorsally, and the lower retinal fibres (macular and peripheral, crossed and uncrossed) lie ventrally. The macular fibres lie in the lateral part of the intermediate area, the binocular peripheral fibres lie in the medial part of the intermediate area and in the whole of the upper and lower areas, except for the most medial part of these areas in which lie the uniocular peripheral fibres (Fig. 87a). In this way the horizontal meridian of the retina is represented by the horizontal line which separates the radiation into its dorsal and ventral halves, the upper and lower halves of the vertical meridian of the retina are represented by the upper and lower halves of the lateral border of the radiation, the upper and lower halves of the circumferential meridian of the retina are represented by the upper and lower halves of the medial border of the radiation, and the fovea is represented by the central part of the lateral border (Fig. 87a).

In the *main part of the optic radiation* the upper retinal fibres (macular and peripheral, crossed and uncrossed) lie dorsally and the lower retinal fibres (macular and peripheral, crossed and uncrossed) lie

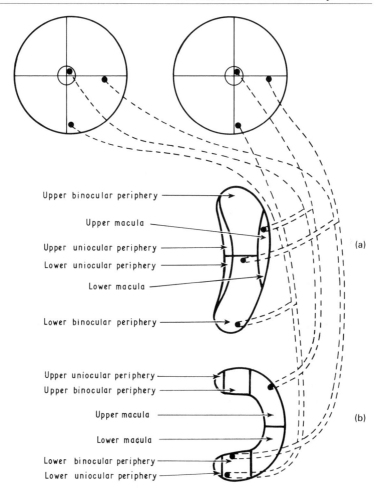

Upper binocular periphery
Upper macula
Upper uniocular periphery
Lower uniocular periphery
Lower macula
Lower binocular periphery

(a)

Upper uniocular periphery
Upper binocular periphery
Upper macula
Lower macula
Lower binocular periphery
Lower uniocular periphery

(b)

Fig. 87.   The distribution of the visual fibres in (a) the anterior part, and (b) the posterior part of the optic radiation (right optic radiation, viewed in cross-section from behind).

ventrally, as in the anterior part of the radiation, but within these areas the grouping of fibres is different. The macular fibres occupy the whole of a large intermediate area, the binocular peripheral fibres lie above and below this intermediate area with the upper and lower extremities occupied by the uniocular peripheral fibres (Fig. 87b). In this way the horizontal meridian of the retina is represented by the curved medial border, the upper and lower halves of the vertical meridian of the retina are represented by the upper and lower halves of the curved lateral border, the upper and lower halves of the circumferential meridian of the retina are represented by the upper and lower extremities of the radiation and by the upper and lower margins of the binocular peripheral areas, and the fovea is represented by the central part of the lateral border (Fig. 87b). It has been suggested, however, that the representations of the different retinal areas in the radiation may not be in a rigid series but rather in a system of layering, so that there is some overlap of the fibres from adjacent retinal areas, with the more peripheral area lying on the medial side of the more central one.

The *loop of Meyer* represents the lower fibres of the optic radiation which turn forwards in the region of the inferior horn of the lateral ventricle in the temporal lobe, although the exact relation of the fibres to the horn is in doubt; it is suggested that they sweep round the lateral side of the tip of the horn, that they cap the anterior surface of the horn, or that they turn backwards a short distance behind the horn—this last description is the most likely one because field defects are not common after opening the tip of the inferior horn by an anterior approach. It is suggested that the loop of Meyer, in contrast to the rest of the radiation, contains a greater proportion of uncrossed than crossed fibres, but it is more likely that there is an equal number of uncrossed and crossed fibres, although the uncrossed ones lie more superficially than the crossed ones.

The optic radiation is supplied anteriorly by the anterior choroidal artery and posteriorly by the posterior cerebral artery; the intermediate part is supplied also by the middle cerebral artery.

Lesions of the optic radiation

As a general rule, a lesion of the optic radiation produces a congruous type of homonymous visual field defect (Fig. 88a), but sometimes when the lesion involves the anterior part of the radiation the field defects are of an incongruous type with the larger defect in the ipsilateral field. This incongruity occurs when the lesion approaches the radiation from a lateral direction because in this position the ipsilateral fibres are more superficial than the contralateral ones, and it occurs also when there is an associated involvement of the nearby optic tract or lateral geniculate body, either directly or by interference with the blood supply. However, sometimes the incongruity may be more apparent than real because it may be the result simply of a sparing of the crossed uniocular peripheral fibres, suggesting a reduction of the field defect in the contralateral eye. The additional involvement of some other part of the optic pathway is the only likely explanation of the more rare cases of incongruity in which the contralateral defect is larger than the ipsilateral one.

Lesions of the upper or lower parts of the optic radiation usually cause a precise *quadrantanopia*, thereby suggesting that the upper and lower peripheral areas are separated by an anatomical interval. In

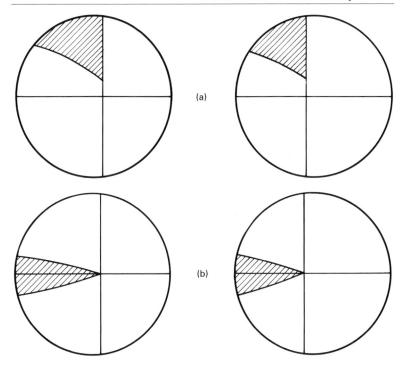

Fig. 88. Field defects due to lesions of the optic radiation: (a) upper homonymous congruous partial quadrantic defects; and (b) homonymous sector-shaped defects in the horizontal meridians.

lesions of the anterior part of the radiation, however, this precise quadrantanopia is often absent because of the contiguity of the upper and lower peripheral areas in that region, and when the lesion is limited to this area only the field defect consists of sector-shaped homonymous defects immediately above and below the horizontal meridian (Fig. 88b).

There are many lesions which affect the integrity of the optic radiation, including encephalitis, cerebral abscess, demyelinating conditions, vascular lesions (intracerebral haemorrhage caused by a rupture of an atheromatous artery, intracerebral thrombosis due to atheromatous occlusion or syphilitic endarteritis, or embolism), and tumours of the temporal, parietal or occipital lobes—primary (glioma, meningioma) or metastatic (carcinoma).

The visual cortex

The optic radiation fibres terminate in the medial aspect of the occipital cortex (*striate area*) in an orderly sequence with regard to their positions

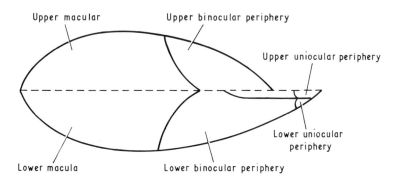

Fig. 89.   The distribution of the visual fibres in the striate area (left striate area, viewed medially). (Broken line = calcarine fissure.)

of origin in the corresponding areas of the retina of each eye, so that the point-to-point arrangement of the optic radiation is maintained in the visual cortex. The upper retinal fibres (macular and peripheral, crossed and uncrossed) lie dorsally and the lower retinal fibres (macular and peripheral, crossed and uncrossed) lie ventrally. To a large extent this separation of upper and lower fibres is fairly clear-cut because they are separated from each other by the deepest part of the cleft in the posterior part of the calcarine fissure, but in the anterior part of the calcarine fissure, beyond the level of the parieto-occipital fissure, both groups of fibres lie in the lower half of the fissure, although the dorsoventral arrangement of the two groups of fibres is maintained. The macular fibres terminate in a large portion of the more caudal part of the striate area, with the foveal fibres terminating in the extreme caudal region and extending usually on to a small part of the lateral surface of the occipital lobe. The binocular peripheral fibres terminate in the central part of the striate area with the most peripheral of these fibres extending beyond the level of the parieto-occipital fissure, and the uniocular peripheral fibres terminate in the most rostral part of the striate area below the calcarine fissure (Fig. 89). In this way the horizontal meridian of the retina is represented by the horizontal line which lies in the floor of the posterior part of the calcarine fissure, separating the striate area into its dorsal and ventral parts, and by the line which forms the junction between the dorsal and ventral parts of the striate area below the anterior part of the calcarine fissure; the upper and lower halves of the vertical meridian of the retina are represented by the upper and lower borders of the striate area; the upper and lower halves of the circumferential meridian are represented by the rostral extremity of the striate area and by the rostral border of the part for the binocular peripheral fibres; and the fovea is represented by the caudal extremity of the striate area (Fig. 90).

The main blood supply of the striate area is from the calcarine branch

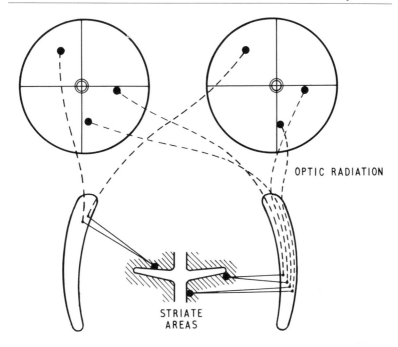

Fig. 90.   The distribution of the visual fibres in the striate areas (viewed in cross-section) with regard to their origin from the horizontal and vertical meridians of the retinae (right and left striate areas, viewed in cross-section from behind).

of the posterior cerebral artery, but the terminal branches of the middle cerebral artery also supply the caudal part of the area so that the macular region has a dual blood supply. Nutrient vessels arise from the vascular network which covers the striate area; short vessels pass to the grey matter of the cortex and longer vessels pass to the white matter, and there is evidence that these two types of vessels maintain some degree of independence.

Lesions of the visual cortex

Lesions of the striate area produce field defects which are characterized by their homonymous and congruous natures and also very often by the phenomenon of *macular sparing*, even in the presence of a hemianopic field defect. There is no conclusive evidence that macular sparing is the result of any bilateral representation of the macula in each striate area or of any link between the macular zones of the two striate areas through the corpus callosum; it is likely that it is largely the result of the failure of a lesion to involve the entire macular zone because of its large extent within the striate area. In some cases, however, macular sparing is present despite the known total destruction of one striate area, and it is suggested that this sparing is the result of a slight shift of fixation so that it is more apparent than real.

The lesions which affect the visual cortex are similar to those which affect the optic radiation, with the addition of trauma, which is liable to disrupt the visual cortex, particularly the part concerned with macular function, because of its position in the posterior part of the brain. The injury is usually a direct one in the occipital region (e.g. penetrating wound, fracture), but sometimes the effect may be of a contrecoup type as the result of a severe blow in the frontal region.

Encephalitis periaxialis diffusa (Schilder's disease). This is a widespread demyelinating disease which is mentioned here because its main effect is usually in the visual cortex, although it may involve the optic nerve, the optic chiasm, the optic tract or the optic radiation.

Cortical blindness

This term is applied to a severe defect of vision of both eyes, or even complete blindness, as the result of a lesion of the visual cortex. The suprageniculate situation of the lesion determines the absence of any ophthalmoscopic evidence of optic atrophy and the presence of normal pupillary responses to light (unless there is an accompanying infrageniculate lesion). It occurs in a variety of conditions, including encephalitis periaxialis diffusa (see p.155), vertebro-basilar insufficiency (p.127), uraemia (p.129) and hypertensive encephalopathy.

The higher visual mechanisms

The striate area of the visual cortex is the terminal sensory area for the fibres of the afferent visual pathway. However, there are other related areas—the *parastriate area* (which surrounds the striate area) and the *peristriate area* (which surrounds the parastriate area)—which are concerned with the higher visual (*visuopsychic*) functions, with an elaboration of the straightforward visual impressions into patterns which have meaning and which are interpreted in relation to past experience. Lesions in these visual association areas do not cause true blindness but rather a form of mind blindness (*visual object agnosia*) in which objects are observed but remain meaningless. The *supramarginal gyrus* (which is part of the parietal lobe) and the *angular gyrus* (which extends from the parietal lobe into the temporal lobe) also serve as important association areas which link the visual sensations with other sensory modalities (such as touch or hearing); lesions of these areas produce various forms of visual agnosia—*colour agnosia* (an inability to recognize colours) *visual spatial agnosia* (an inability to orientate different objects in space) and *corporeal agnosia* (an inability to identify the different parts of the body).

Visual hallucinations may represent real objects (formed), when they are usually due to lesions of the temporal lobe, or they may be unrecognizable bizarre shapes (unformed), which tend to occur in lesions of the occipital lobe. The fortification spectra of migraine may represent temporary ischaemia of the occipital cortex.

The determination of the visual field

This may be achieved by different methods which may be of a *kinetic* or *static* nature.

The confrontation test

This is a simple and rapid kinetic method and, although it is sometimes not capable of detecting subtle abnormalities, it is a most useful form of routine examination. The examiner stands opposite to and at arm's length from the patient so that the patient's right eye is fixing the examiner's left eye (and the patient's left eye is fixing the examiner's right eye); the patient closes each eye in turn and the examiner brings a moving object (his finger or preferably a white and then a red target) from the periphery inwards until the patient is just aware of the object. This determines the peripheral limit of the visual field and is compared with the examiner's (normal) visual field. It is possible also to detect defects (*scotomata*) within the visual field.

The perimeter

This instrument is placed on a table and contains an adjustable chin rest so that the patient is able to place his head in an upright position with each eye (in turn) directed towards a fixed target in the centre of a movable curved semicircular arc which is 33 cm from the eye. The arc is moved into six different positions for each quadrant of the visual field (with 15° between each position). With one eye fixing the central target (the other eye being occluded), a target is moved along the arc from a position beyond the extent of the visual field until it is just apparent; this point determines the extent of peripheral visual field in each position for the particular object. At this distance of 33 cm, a white object of 3 mm in diameter provides a measure of the full extent of the peripheral visual field; in the normal subject this is about 45° in the upper vertical meridian, 90° in the temporal horizontal meridian, 65° in the lower vertical meridian and 55° in the nasal horizontal meridian (the contours of the face, particularly the nose, determine the difference in these measurements in different meridians). The peripheral extents of

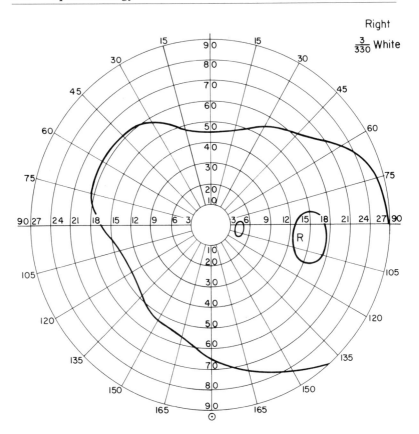

Fig. 91.   The normal peripheral visual field of the right eye.

the normal visual field in the right and left eye are shown in Figs. 91 and 92.

The visual field to colour targets is similar in outline to that with white targets, except that it is less in extent (green less than red and red less than blue) provided the point is recorded at which the colour (and not merely the movement) of the target is recognized by the observer.

The Bjerrum screen

This is another kinetic method. This flat screen provides detailed information of the state of the visual field within 30° of the fixation point. There are two sizes of Bjerrum screen—a smaller one with the patient seated 1m from the central fixation target and a larger one when the patient is 2m from the screen. Its main value is the determination of a scotoma in the central or paracentral part of the visual field which is

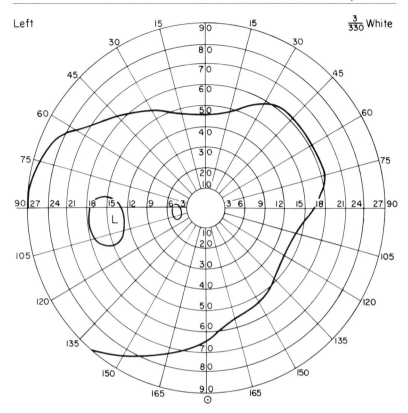

Fig. 92. The normal peripheral visual field of the left eye.

so small that it is difficult to determine on the perimeter. The patient (with one eye occluded) fixes a central target on the screen and indicates the disappearance of a target which is moved over the screen. The normal blind spot (which is produced by the optic nerve head) is plotted on the Bjerrum screen as an oval area (5.5° in the horizontal diameter and 7.5° in vertical diameter), the centre of which lies about 15° on the temporal side of the fixation point and mainly below the horizontal meridian (Figs. 91 and 92); this is determined first because its accurate appreciation confirms that the patient is co-operating in the test. The central visual field is then examined carefully for any central and paracentral defects; it is essential to employ targets of different sizes and different colours (the method of quantitative scotometry) in order to determine areas of the visual field in which there is a relative (as distinct from an absolute) loss of visual function—small white targets and coloured targets (red and green) may reveal scotomatous areas which are not determined by other means, particularly in such conditions as retrobulbar neuritis, chiasmal lesions and toxic amblyopia.

Modern bowl perimeters

To enhance comparability, modern bowl perimeters (such as the *Goldmann perimeter*) incorporate standard background illumination, and can project a spot of light of varying intensity or colour on to the inner surface of the bowl, thus enabling not only an accurate delineation of a scotoma and its density, but also an assessment of field by static, as opposed to kinetic, perimetry. This involves a gradual increase in the illumination of the immobile test object until the patient sees it (*threshold illumination*) and comparisons of thresholds throughout the field give a more sensitive assessment of field defects. An alternative approach to static perimetry involves the presentation of a number of light stimuli, the pattern and illumination of which can be simultaneously varied (*Friedman analyser*). It is important to correct any refractive error prior to field examination, particularly presbyopia, with the proviso that spectacle frames may sometimes induce artefactual field defects. Recently automated static perimetry techniques have been successfully used, particularly for monitoring changes in visual fields; for example, in the routine management of chronic simple glaucoma.

It is apparent that a careful assessment of the significance of any visual field defect which has been determined accurately is of great value in the localization of many forms of ocular and intracranial disease. The appearance of the optic disc is also of localizing importance because an infrageniculate lesion of the afferent visual pathway is usually followed within a period of about six weeks with some degree of optic atrophy, whereas a suprageniculate lesion is not accompanied by any alteration in the appearance of the optic disc.

17

Injuries

The limited scope of this book precludes any detailed account of ocular injuries, although in many chapters an account is given of the more common forms of injury. In this chapter brief mention is made of perforating injuries of the eyeball, and the sequelae of trauma.

Perforating injury of the eye

The cornea or sclera may be perforated in different ways: directly by a sharp pointed instrument (knife, scissors), directly by small particles (metal, glass), or indirectly by a severe contusion which leads to a rupture of the globe. There are several aspects in the management of such injuries.

Assessment of the injured eye

At presentation it is important to make a careful assessment of the injuries to enable the surgeon to give the patient a likely prognosis for vision, to choose the most appropriate surgical approach, and to provide a detailed account for any subsequent compensation claim. If the ocular media are opaque, then retinal and macular integrity can be assessed by establishing whether the patient can fix upon a light source, whether he is aware of a small movement of that source, and whether he can accurately locate the source when projected from different quadrants of the visual field. A relative afferent pupillary defect is often a helpful indicator of visual potential but may give false results in the presence of, for example, a dense vitreous haemorrhage. The anatomical integrity of intraocular structures is well assessed by ultrasonography, while their function may be assessed by electroretinography and by visual evoked responses.

Immediate treatment

Attention must first of all be directed to the general status of the patient, particularly following, for example, a road traffic accident. Tetanus immunoglobulin should be given in a perforating injury.

Primary surgical repair to restore the integrity of the eye is preceded by a careful examination of the globe, often requiring a general anaesthetic, to establish the extent of the injuries.

The lid. In suturing lid lacerations, especial care is taken to realign the lid margins. Torn canaliculi are sutured end-to-end following their identification by syringing with dye or by the insertion of polythene tubing into both the puncta.

The cornea and sclera. Lacerations are often irregular and shelving so that a restoration of normal contours involves careful suturing of the wounds after the removal of any devitalized tissue and after the abscission of any ocular structure (uvea, lens or vitreous) that has become incarcerated into the wound. The introduction of air or an inert stabilizing fluid such as Healonid into the anterior chamber greatly facilitates the correct apposition of the wound edges, thereby rendering a water-tight wound. This also enables reformation of the anterior chamber, thus preventing any subsequent adhesion of the underlying iris to the region of the wound or any development of adhesions between the iris and the cornea in the region of the filtration angle (peripheral anterior synechiae), thereby reducing the likelihood of a subsequent uveitis or secondary glaucoma.

The lens. Trauma may result in cataract formation or lens subluxation, or if the capsule is ruptured may lead to a lens-induced uveitis (p.95) and secondary glaucoma.

The iris. Perforating injuries of the iris are discussed on p.80.

The avoidance of infection

The use of antibiotics (by topical application, subconjunctival injection or systemically) reduces the risk of a septic type of inflammation of the eye (endophthalmitis, panophthalmitis), which is liable to lead to a rapid loss of the eye. A non-septic type of inflammation (uveitis) is not avoided by the use of antibiotics, but is less likely to occur when the integrity of the eye is restored rapidly after the injury, so that prolapsed uveal tissue is not present within the wound; it may be controlled by the use of topical or systemic steroids. The danger of a sympathetic ophthalmitis after an injury is discussed on p.94.

The removal of any retained foreign body

All forms of perforating injury of the eyeball should be subjected to careful radiographic examination in order to determine the presence of one or more intraocular foreign bodies. There are various specialised methods (e.g. *stereoscopic radiography*) which permit an accurate localization of the position of each foreign body; this is of particular value when a detailed view of the structures within the eye is prevented by disorganization of the cornea, by a traumatic cataract, or by haemorrhage within the anterior chamber of vitreous. Other specialized methods of detection (the *Roper-Hall foreign body detector* which works on the principle of the land-mine detector, or the use of ultrasonography or CT scan) are of value in certain cases.

There are many different substances which may enter the eye and their effects are variable:

Metallic particles. These commonly enter the eye at great speed and the heat which is generated at their liberation is retained until they enter the eye, so that they seldom lead to sepsis; the introduction of copper, however, may lead to the production of a sterile type of pus. The extent of the damage to the eye depends on the size of the foreign body, the tissues which are disrupted by its passage through the eye, and the site of its final termination. A retained particle of iron or steel gives rise, after an interval of several months (or even years), to widespread deposits of ferrous material on the lens capsule, in the uveal tract and in the retina with progressive degenerative changes and ultimately loss of vision; the affected tissues assume a characteristic rusty brown discoloration (*siderosis*). A retained particle of copper gives rise to similar deposits (*chalcosis*), which in the early stages are evident beneath the anterior lens capsule in a sunflower distribution, but eventually the deposits become more widespread, with the production of a panophthalmitis. A retained particle of brass causes similar changes to copper. Sometimes, however, these effects are avoided if the particle of iron, steel, copper or brass becomes encapsulated or if it becomes lodged in the lens where it is divorced from the circulation and biochemical degradation.

Other metallic particles—lead, aluminium, gold, silver and zinc—are less likely to cause reaction within the eye, so that they may remain relatively inert for an indefinite period.

Non-metallic particles. Stone and glass particles tend to remain relatively inert, but vegetable materials such as wood splinters are likely to lead to sepsis.

A magnetic metallic particle (iron and steel) may be removed by a magnet; when it lies in the anterior part of the eye it is removed readily by opening the anterior chamber at the limbus (the anterior approach), and when it lies in the posterior part of the eye it may be removed by a posterior scleral incision at a site determined by radiological localization. However, although this may satisfactorily remove the foreign body, it does not treat the vitreous disorganization from the entry point to the impaction site, which may later develop into a traction band and possibly lead to a retinal detachment. The introduction of closed intraocular microsurgery has provided the means for removal of intraocular foreign bodies under direct vision and the facility for a more extensive primary intraocular repair, such as removal of a cataractous lens (lensectomy), removal of vitreous haemorrhage, and prevention of transgel traction bands (vitrectomy). The instruments, all of 20 gauge calibre (vitreous cutter/aspirator, foreign body removal forceps, fibreoptic light source and infusion line) are introduced by way of the pars plana.

Long-term sequelae

The lids. Inaccurate closure of lid margins may lead to notching and inadequate tear film application. Cicatriceal fibrosis of lid lacerations may result in ectropion and epiphora, and exposure of the cornea requiring plastic surgical correction.

The cornea. Lacerations of the cornea resulting in axial scarring or irregular astigmatism may be corrected by suitable contact lenses, but dense axial scarring requires full-thickness corneal grafting after an appropriate interval.

The iris. Extensive loss of iris tissue may induce optical aberrations (spherical aberration).

Glaucoma. This may occur as a result of extensive peripheral anterior synechiae, chronic uveitis, or secondary to blunt injury where the iris root and ciliary body are avulsed from their scleral attachments giving rise to the appearance of a very wide angle to the anterior chamber (*angle recession*) which, if extensive enough, gives rise to late-onset glaucoma.

The lens. Post-traumatic cataract may develop at varying intervals of months or even years following injury.

The vitreous. Transgel traction may occur as described above.

The retina. Multiple retinal tears may occur at the time of injury or following vitreous traction, or may occur at the periphery presenting as a retinal dialysis, so that careful indentation indirect ophthalmoscopy is required once the eye has recovered from the original injury and surgery. As a result of contrecoup injuries, posterior pole oedema may be complicated by the development of a macular 'hole', with permanent impairment of vision.

Removal of an eye

It may be necessary to remove the eye after severe injury, particularly when there is a risk of the development of a sympathetic ophthalmitis, although the operation may be carried out simply because of a blind painful eye, or a blind eye which is cosmetically unsightly.

There are two main forms of the operation:

1. *Enucleation.* This involves the removal of the whole eye with a small portion of the optic nerve, but with retention of the conjunctiva, the bulbar fascia (to provide a lining for the socket) and the extrinsic ocular muscles, which are sutured to a buried implant to provide a fair degree of movement of the overlying prosthesis.

2. *Evisceration.* This involves the removal of the contents of the eye with a retention of the posterior part of the sclera so that there is no section of the optic nerve. Evisceration is the method of choice when the eye has been the site of a septic inflammation (panophthalmitis) because enucleation in such a case might cause a contamination of the cut end of the optic nerve, with the development of a spreading meningitis. However, the use of antibiotics in recent years has reduced the indications for an evisceration.

Artificial eyes. These are made of glass or of a plastic material; a plastic eye has certain advantages—it does not break, it is less likely to become rough and it is more durable. It is natural for an artificial eye to cause a certain amount of discharge from the socket because the conjunctival lining of the socket is a mucous surface; it follows that the artificial eye and the socket should be cleansed routinely each day, but in certain cases this has to be carried out much less frequently.

Contracted socket. Sometimes a socket may become contracted when the conjunctiva has been the site of some previous disease (e.g. trachoma, ocular pemphigoid) or more commonly when the artificial eye has not been worn for a prolonged period. An attempt may be made to enlarge the socket and then to line it with a skin graft which is retained by a mould of dental wax (although this lining of skin may produce a somewhat offensive discharge). Sometimes a satisfactory method is simply to enlarge the socket by dividing the adhesions and to maintain it by the insertion of a plastic mould at the time of the operation.

There is evidence that the growth of the orbit in early childhood is dependent to some extent on the presence of the eye, so that removal of an eye in early childhood or the absence of an eye (anophthalmos) from birth, or a gross degree of microphthalmos creates problems in later life in retaining a cosmetically satisfactory prosthesis. It is essential, therefore, to fit a sufficiently large prosthesis as soon as possible, and in the case of microphthalmos the prosthesis may be incorporated in a contact shell which fits over the eye, provided there is no useful visual function of the microphthalmic eye; in this context it should be remembered that peripheral visual function is of great practical value, even in the absence of central visual function.

18

Care of the Visually Handicapped

Definition of blindness

The statutory definition for the purposes of registration as a blind person is that the person is 'so blind as to be unable to perform any work for which eyesight is essential'; the test is not whether the person is unable to pursue his ordinary occupation or any particular occupation, but whether he is too blind to perform *any work* for which eyesight is essential , and only the visual conditions are taken into account—other bodily or mental infirmities are disregarded.

The principal factor to be considered is the corrected visual acuity of each eye separately or with both eyes together. The person examined may be classified in one of three groups:

Group 1—below 3/60 Snellen. In general, a person with visual acuity below 3/60 Snellen may be regarded as blind. In many cases, however, it is desirable to test the vision at 1m and not to regard a person having acuity of 1/18 Snellen as blind unless there is also considerable restriction of the visual field.

Group 2—3/60 but less than 6/60 Snellen. A person with visual acuity of 3/60 but less than 6/60 Snellen may be regarded as blind if the field of vision is considerably contracted, but should not be regarded as blind if the visual defect is of long-standing and is unaccompanied by any material contraction of the field of vision, for example, in cases of congenital nystagmus, albinism or myopia, particularly if there is a reasonable level of close reading vision.

Group 3—6/60 Snellen or more. A person with a visual acuity of 6/60 Snellen or better should ordinarily not be regarded as blind. He may, however, be regarded as blind if the field of vision is markedly contracted in the greater part of its extent, and particularly if the contraction is in the lower part of the field; a person suffering from homonymous or bitemporal hemianopia but retaining central visual acuity of 6/18 or better should not be regarded as blind.

The question of whether a defect of vision is recent or long standing has a special bearing on the certification of blindness. A person whose defect is recent is less able to adapt himself to his environment than a person with the same visual acuity whose defect has been of long standing. This is specially applicable in relation to Groups 2 and 3. Another factor of importance, particularly in relation to Group 2, is the age of the person at the onset of blindness. An old person with a recent failure of sight cannot adapt himself so readily as can a younger person with the same defect.

On rare occasions cases will arise which are not precisely covered by the foregoing observations, and such cases must be dealt with according to the judgement of the certifying ophthalmic surgeon.

In a person up to and including the age of 16 years, other factors may influence the local education authorities regarding the need for special educational facilities (p.359).

Partial sight

There is no statutory definition of partial sight, but the Department of Health and Social Security has advised that a person who is not blind within the meaning of the Act but who is, nevertheless, substantially and permanently handicapped by congenitally defective vision or in whom illness or injury had caused defective vision of a substantial and permanently handicapping character is within the scope of the welfare services which the local authority provides for handicapped persons, but is not entitled to supplementary benefit or a pension before the usual age or to income tax concessions.

The following criteria should be used as a general guide when determining whether a person falls within the scope of the welfare provisions for the partially sighted, as well as in recommending, where the person is under 16 years of age, the appropriate type of school for the particular child concerned:

1. For registration purposes and the provision of welfare services the following persons may be regarded as partially sighted:(a) 3/60 to 6/60 with full field; (b) up to 6/24 with moderate contraction of the field, opacities in media or aphakia; and (c) 6/18 or even better if there is a gross field defect (e.g. hemianopia) or there is marked contraction of the field as in tapetoretinal degeneration, glaucoma, etc.

2. For children whose visual acuity will have a bearing on the appropriate methods of education, disabilities may be classified as: (a) severe visual disabilities—to be educated in special schools by methods involving vision—3/60 to 6/24 with glasses; and (b) visual impairment—to be educated at ordinary schools with special consideration—better than 6/24 with glasses.

It should be emphasized that a determination of the level of close reading vision is essential in all children because in certain conditions (congenital nystagmus, Marfan's syndrome, etc.) this may be remarkably good, so that the child is able to cope with an ordinary school, provided he has a sufficient degree of intelligence, despite a marked restriction of the distant vision.

It is obvious that the classification of a child as partially sighted creates certain difficulties which can only be resolved when the child is sufficiently old to permit an accurate assessment of the visual acuity (uniocular and binocular, distant and near); indeed, it is recommended that any infant with a congenital anomaly causing a visual defect should be registered as partially sighted unless obviously blind. It follows that any infant or young child who is classified in this way should be re-examined every 12 months (or more frequently if necessary) in order to make an alteration in the category (to normally sighted or to blind) as early as possible. This also applies to the adult who is registered as partially sighted, because the category may change if sight is restored following successful medical or surgical treatment of the condition or if sight becomes worse following an inevitable deterioration of the condition.

The reading vision of a partially sighted adult may be sufficiently good to permit the use of books with a reasonable size of print; a selection of books with specially large print is available in most Public Libraries and the talking library is also available to the partially sighted on special certification.

The visually handicapped child

During the early development of the child, vision is of major importance for co-ordinating the responses to other sensory inputs, in learning skills and providing the incentive for exploration of the world around him, as well as contributing to mother/child bonding. The parents will therefore need instruction in developmental guidance to encourage aspects of development which are largely dependent upon vision.

The diagnosis of blindness in a child is a family crisis that necessarily requires family management. The parental response to the diagnosis is diverse and ranges from feelings of grief, disbelief, guilt and inadequacy to despair or even anger. It is important for the ophthalmologist to be aware of these emotions in subequent planning of supportive measures. The ophthalmologist must also try to understand the parents' perception of the diagnosis and carefully prepare them for the increased commitment which may severely encroach on their present lifestyle. Once the parents become reconciled to the permanence of the handicap, they can often face the problems of management more objectively and accept more readily the help that is available from the current excellent multidisciplinary visual and paediatric assessment centres. During these assessments they may encounter a bewildering number of personnel; parents should be given every opportunity to discuss their anxieties both together and separately, if desired, with the ophthalmologist.

Special consideration must be given to blindness in children. The definition of blindness in a child is related essentially to the educational methods which are going to prove to be necessary for his upbringing; in this way the blind child is one who is dependent on a form of education which does not involve the use of sight. It follows that children who are classified as blind by this definition have different degrees of blindness. Some may have true blindness—the total absence of light perception in both eyes—but others may have an awareness of light, an awareness of movement, or even an ability to discern to some extent large objects in the distance or near at hand. It is obvious that a blind child who has retained a certain amount of visual awareness has distinct advantages over a completely blind child, such as the ability to move more easily and more confidently in strange surroundings, but this ability in no way alters the necessity for him to be educated as a truly blind child.

The determination of blindness

This is a matter of great importance because it involves a decision that the child is going to be incapable of benefiting from a normal form of visual education or even from a modified form of education involving the use of special visual methods which is appropriate for the partially sighted, as distinct from the blind, child. It is also of great importance because it involves a decision that the blindness is incapable of being relieved to any significant extent by appropriate medical and surgical procedures. It is therefore essential for each case to be scrutinized with extreme care by an ophthalmic surgeon who is experienced in the diagnosis and treatment of the conditions which lead to blindness in childhood. The main difficulty occurs in the infant when it is not possible to determine the vision objectively. In such cases an indirect assessment may be made by observing the reaction of the child to a bright light; it is usual for a child, even when only a few days old, to be attracted to such a stimulus, although the gaze may be directed to the light only momentarily. The behaviour of the infant's eyes during feeding is also of significance because, despite the fact that the eyes generally remain closed, at certain times there is a tendency for the eyes to open and be directed to the mother's face and, provided the mother continues to gaze at the child, the child's eyes may move when she moves; a persistent absence of this phenomenon over a period of time is certainly suggestive of blindness. However, failure to be attracted to a light or to gaze at the mother may be due to mental retardation rather than the presence of any organic visual disturbance, so that a final decision is possible only after careful observation of all the relevant facts. Other aids in the diagnosis of impaired vision are the demonstration of optokinetic nystagmus, vestibulo-ocular reflexes, pupil responses, refraction and an estimation of the visual field.

With sensible organization, many special investigations may be carried out during an examination under anaesthetic, for example biomicroscopy of the anterior and posterior segments, measurement of corneal diameters, intraocular pressures, fundus fluorescein angiography, electrophysiological tests, and computerized tomography and ultrasound examination.

The most common causes of blindness in children are congenital or developmental anomalies which may be present at birth or may become apparent some time after birth. Sometimes these anomalies are confined to the eyes alone, but at other times they are associated with widespread changes in other parts of the body. A knowledge of the transmission of these inherited diseases may reduce their incidence by appropriate eugenic measures, but their elimination must await an elucidation of their basic mechanisms. Fortunately, many other forms of blindness following conditions such as ophthalmia neonatorum, infantile glaucoma, congenital cataract, etc., have been combated to varying extents by improved methods of prevention, diagnosis and treatment.

It is essential that the child be registered as blind whenever the determination of blindness has been made in order to allow him to benefit from the excellent facilities which are available. The management of the blind child varies according to his age.

The first five years of life

The baby and the infant up to the age of five years are the concern of the Social Services Department of the local authority, as an integral part of the National Health Service, which authorizes a qualified health visitor to supervise the child in his own home. This implies that unless there are exceptional circumstances, the blind child continues to live at home. It is generally recognized that during the early and formative years of the life of any child, there is nothing to replace an upbringing within the family because the love and affection which he receives there foster a sense of security which enables him to become established subsequently as an individual who is self-reliant and yet part of the community. This integration within the family is even more important for the blind infant, who is unduly dependent upon the influence of his parents because of his impaired means of communication which, of necessity, prolongs and makes more difficult the early period of training.

It is, of course, necessary for the parents to adapt themselves as quickly as possible to the vital part which they have to play in the early years of their blind child. Initially it is often difficult for them to overcome the emotional stress which quite naturally surrounds them after the final realization that the child is blind, but the happiness of the parents, of the blind child and of the whole family is dependent upon a rapid period of adjustment. An important factor in delaying this period is the failure of some parents to accept the verdict that the blindness is inevitable. In such circumstances it is the responsibility of the ophthalmic surgeon to show that his opinion is based on sound judgement which has been reached only after a careful and detailed examination of the patient. In many cases it is desirable for the surgeon to obtain confirmation of his diagnosis from a colleague, but every effort should be made to save the parents the needless anxiety which is produced by trailing the child unnecessarily from clinic to clinic, and sometimes even from country to country, in the forlorn hope of finding some miraculous cure.

It is the task of the parents, and particularly of the mother who is with him most of the time, to see that the blind child is allowed to progress as far as possible in a normal way; undue protection and excessive pampering are barriers to his progress and must be avoided. It is, of course, necessary to modify the approach to the child's development so that an effort is made to cultivate his other senses (the appreciation of touch, of changes in temperature, of hearing and of smell) which are usually unimpaired and which are indeed capable of much greater development than in the sighted child, in order to provide compensation for the loss of sight.

Normally, a child's visual awareness plays a large part in his increasing appreciation of his surroundings. It follows therefore that the blind baby should be handled much more than usual, although the initial contact with the child must always be very gentle so as not to startle him unduly. Also the blind baby should be spoken to frequently and be made conscious of the noises around him, otherwise there is a tendency for him to adopt a trance-like attitude. It is important at a very early stage to name the objects with which he is in contact and in this way he learns to recognize them readily by touch and by name. He therefore needs to be taught to explore and create a world around him. Speaking to the child also helps to develop his powers of speech; these are often late in development because the absence of sight prevents the young blind child from making the spontaneous comments which characterize the sighted child who is constantly aware of his surroundings. There are obviously special problems in teaching a blind child to feed himself, but these can be overcome by patience and by care in seeing that he is provided with food which can be manipulated fairly easily. Similarly there are problems in learning to walk because he requires more guidance and support than the sighted child.

Later, when the child is beginning to move around, he must be taught to become self-reliant so that he is able to move around a room by himself and then to move around the whole house, including the staircase. It is necessary, of course, to protect him from undue danger (but this applies also to a sighted child of that age), and it is a great help to him if his toys and the different articles of furniture are kept in constant positions so that he becomes adapted to his surroundings as quickly as possible with increasing assurance and self-confidence.

There is a tendency for the blind child to develop certain mannerisms, such as poking the eyes with the fingers or rocking to and fro when sitting down; these often occur because he is bored and feels isolated from his surroundings. It is desirable to prevent these mannerisms from becoming persistent and this is best achieved by diverting him to some form of useful activity—a further example of the necessity for constant care of the blind child. Unfortunately this poking of the eyes may be carried out in such a vigorous way in the older blind child (it is suggested that it is motivated because it induces pleasurable sensations), that it may lead to a rupture of fibres in the corneal stroma or even of Descemet's membrane, with the development of a bullous keratopathy (p.46), and the eye becomes painful as well as blind; this may necessitate removal of the eye.

After the age of five years

When the blind child reaches the age of five years it is necessary for the parents to arrange for his education. The decision about placement for education is made between parents and local authorities, with advice from the paediatric and visual assessment centres. In recent years, there has been emphasis upon the need to keep the visually handicapped child within his home environment and to defer residential schooling for as long as is practicable. Thus day schooling is advised, at least until the age of eight and thereafter if possible, depending on parental and local authority commitment. The alternative is for placement in a weekly boarding school. It is of course possible for the parents to make their own arrangements for his education, but these must have the approval of the educational authorities. Naturally, particular stress is laid on the learning of Braille, which is the blind person's medium for reading and writing. Sometimes the blind child has an additional handicap, such as deafness or mental deficiency, and there are special schools which cater for the blind and deaf child and for the blind and educationally subnormal (ESN) child. Even so, development of such children is often better within the home environment if the parents and social services can arrange the appropriate support, though periods of a residential placement may be necessary.

Thereafter the blind child's education may continue at a secondary school and every opportunity is given for the child subsequently to enter a university. The less gifted child may proceed to a secondary technical college, which provides a further education designed to prepare him for a career in such activities as typing, piano-tuning or music. The blind child remains the responsibility of the local education officer during the school and university period, but thereafter the blind

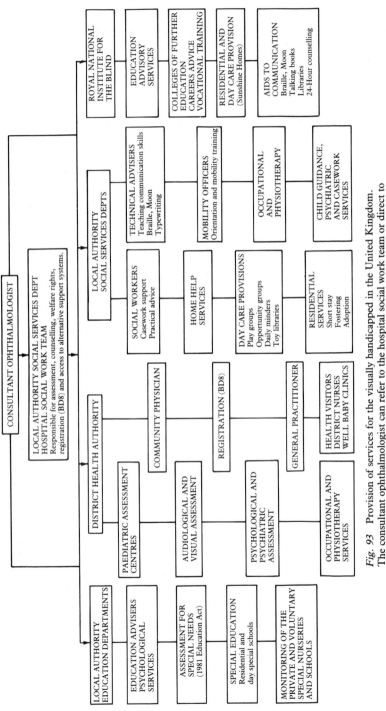

Fig. 93 Provision of services for the visually handicapped in the United Kingdom.
The consultant ophthalmologist can refer to the hospital social work team or direct to
the relevant agency.

person enters the care of the Department of Employment which is concerned with maintaining him in suitable employment. In all the different stages of the education of the child, an important person is the home teacher of the blind who is an officer of the welfare department. She maintains contact with the blind child throughout the period of training, and her experience is valuable in fostering progress and in helping the parents to appreciate the ways in which they are able to contribute to the child's well-being. A scheme for the provision of services for the visually handicapped is shown in Fig. 93.

The visually handicapped adult

The blind adult who has been blinded in childhood will pass automatically into a sphere of employment which is suitable for his capabilities. The person will be referred to the Careers Adviser of the local authority or the RNIB with a view to employment training. The normally-sighted adult who becomes blind as the result of some injury or disease faces entirely different problems. There are, however, facilities which are available through the Manpower Services in co-operation with the Blind Persons' Resettlement Officer at certain Job Centres. This officer covers a specified group of Job Centres and he assists the registered blind adult to re-enter employment with confidence and courage. Recently efforts have been made to keep the newly blind person in his present employment by providing low-vision aids if appropriate and by enlisting the help of the employer. In England, a third of the blind of working age are employed and more than half of these are in normal competitive occupations. As a general rule a course at a residential rehabilitation centre which provides instruction in the basic requirements of the blind person (Braille, typewriting and mobility training) is followed by some form of specialized training in light engineering at a government training centre, or in shorthand typewriting, telephone switchboard operating or physiotherapy at the Royal National Institute for the Blind. Special facilities are available for the ex-Service blind at St Dunstan's Hospital and recently these services have been expanded to include 'uniformed professions' blinded whilst on duty.

The National Library for the Blind provides a comprehensive selection of books of all kinds (technical, classics, novels, etc.) in Braille which are sold or loaned. Local authorities provide the British Talking Book Service for the Blind and may also act as an agent for local talking newspaper services. The talking library provides books on records or tapes for those who are too old to learn Braille because of intellectual difficulties or frequently because their fingers are not sufficiently sensitive to achieve any degree of fluency; in such cases the simpler MOON books are more readily mastered and have proved a great comfort to the lonely and elderly, although the method is less versatile than Braille because it can only be read, not typed.

The blind person receives certain benefits including social services provided by the Local Authority, supplementary benefits when applicable through the Department of Health and Social Security, certain income tax concessions, a postal vote and travel permits.

Index